An introduction to the

Symptoms and Signs of Clinical Medicine

An Introduction to the Symptoms and Signs of Clinical Medicine

Edited by

David Gray DM, MPH, FRCP
Reader in Medicine and Honorary Consultant Physician,
Department of Medicine, Queen's Medical Centre, Nottingham, UK

Peter Toghill MD, FRCP
Emeritus Consultant Physician, Queen's Medical Centre, Nottingham, UK and
Previously Director of CME, Royal College of Physicians, London, UK

ARNOLD

A member of the Hodder Headline Group
LONDON
Co-published in the USA by
Oxford University Press Inc., New York

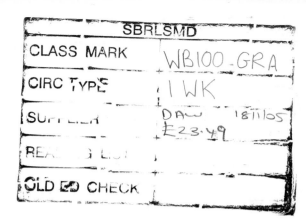

First published in Great Britain in 2001 by
Arnold, a member of the Hodder Headline Group,
338 Euston Road, London NW1 3BH

http://www.arnoldpublishers.com

Arnold International Students' Edition published 2001
Arnold International Students' Editions are low-priced un-abridged editions of imported textbooks. They are only for sale in developing countries.

Co-published in the USA by
Oxford University Press Inc.,
198 Madison Avenue, New York, NY10016
Oxford is a registered trademark of Oxford University Press

British Library Cataloguing in Publication Data
A catalogue record for this book is available from the British Library

Library of Congress Cataloging-in-Publication Data
A catalog record for this book is available from the Library of Congress

ISBN 0 340 73207 5
ISBN 0 340 76045 1 (International Students' Edition)
1 2 3 4 5 6 7 8 9 10

Commissioning Editor: Georgina Bentliff
Project Editor: Paula O'Connell
Project Manager: Jane Duncan
Production Editor: Wendy Rooke
Production Controller: Iain McWilliams

Typeset in 10/11 pt Palatino by Scribe Design, Gillingham, Kent, UK
Printed by Gutenberg Press Ltd, Malta

Contents

Contributors

Allen BR, MB, FRCP Consultant Dermatologist, Department of Dermatology, University Hospital, Queen's Medical Centre, Nottingham, UK

Arie THD, CBE, FRCP, FRCPsych, FFPHM Professor Emeritus of Health Care of the Elderly, Ageing and Disability Research Unit, The Medical School, University of Nottingham, Nottingham, UK

Bendall MJ, DM, FRCP Consultant Physician, Department of Health Care of the Elderly, Queen's Medical Centre, Nottingham, UK

Bignell CJ, MB, FRCP Consultant Physician, Department of Genitourinary Medicine, Nottingham City Hospital, Nottingham, UK

Brown GV, MB, BS, FRACP, FAFPHM, PhD, MPH James Stewart Professor of Medicine, Department of Medicine The University of Melbourne, Royal Melbourne Hospital, Victoria, Australia

Galloway NR, MD, FRCS Consultant Ophthalmic Surgeon, Department of Ophthalmology, Queen's Medical Centre, Nottingham, UK

Gibbin KP, MB, FRCS Consultant Otolaryngologist, Directorate of Otorhinolaryngology and Head and Neck Surgery, Department of Medicine, Queen's Medical Centre, Nottingham, UK

Gray D, MPH, FRCP Reader in Medicine and Honorary Consultant Physician, Division of Cardiovascular Medicine, Queen's Medical Centre, Nottingham, UK

Hampton JR, MD, FRCP Professor of Cardiology and Honorary Consultant Physician, Division of Cardiovascular Medicine, Queen's Medical Centre, Nottingham, UK

Johnston IDA, MD, FRCP Consultant Physician, Department of Respiratory Medicine, Queen's Medical Centre, Nottingham, UK

Page SR, MD, FRCP Consultant Physician, Department of Diabetes, Endocrinology and Nutrition, Queen's Medical Centre, Nottingham, UK

Puri BK, MB, BChir, MRCPsych Consultant Psychiatrist and Senior Lecturer, MRC Clinical Sciences Centre and MRI Unit, Imperial College School of Medicine, Hammersmith Hospital, London, UK

Rubin PC, DM, FRCP Dean of the Medical School, Professor of Therapeutics, and Honorary Consultant Physician, Queen's Medical Centre, Nottingham, UK

Toghill PJ, MD, FRCP Consultant Physician Emeritus, Queen's Medical Centre, Nottingham, UK; Previously Director, Continuing Medical Education, Royal College of Physicians, Regent's Park, London, UK

Preface

Our primary object in editing this book is to produce a simple, hands-on guide for clinical students during their early days on the wards. To be good doctors we need to listen to our patients to understand their symptoms and we need to examine them using our critical senses. The acquisition of these two skills is undoubtedly the most important task in one's medical education and it is the basis of all doctor/patient relationships.

We believe that the best way of learning medicine is as medical apprentices. Watch and listen to your teachers as they deal with their patients. Then, as you gain experience, practise the techniques, first under supervision, and later on your own. There is no substitute for seeing real patients in the setting of the hospital or the consulting room. We are not enthusiasts for the box-ticking method of taking histories or indeed for using surrogate patients. We are fortunate in the UK that most patients, when they are ill, willingly accept the presence and training activities of medical students on the wards and in their homes. Indeed patients often subsequently recall with affection the 'student doctors' who helped to look after them. The privilege of learning from patients must never be abused.

In the majority of illnesses a working diagnosis can be reached following a careful history and examination, even before investigations are undertaken. To enable students to reach this working diagnosis we have indicated the methods of presentation of the commoner illnesses and the circumstances in which they might occur. We have also emphasized which symptoms are potentially serious and which may be relatively trivial. It is a waste of time constructing a wide differential diagnosis if one does not know what is common and what is rare. As patients usually arrive with symptoms rather than diagnoses we have included a problem-based section.

Our book is intended to complement the excellent textbook by Sir Norman Browse, *An Introduction to the Symptoms and Signs of Surgical Disease*, which is also published by Arnold. It deliberately reverses the trend for ever-enlarging encyclopaedic texts and has evolved from PT's earlier book *Examining Patients*. We have been concerned that modern students are now faced with the impossible task of trying to keep up with the explosion of knowledge. Fortunately, virtually unlimited access to information is now available to medical practitioners (and patients) on the Internet. As a consequence the assembly of factual knowledge has become much less important than the acquisition of skills and experience.

David Gray
Peter Toghill

Nottingham, 2000

Acknowledgements

We are most grateful to our colleagues here in Nottingham and elsewhere who have given their valuable time and expertise to contribute to this book. Many others have given us illustrations from their personal collections. Our sincere thanks also go to those patients who have allowed themselves to be photographed for educational purposes. Most of these photographs have been taken, over a period of several years by the Audio-Visual Department of the Queen's Medical Centre Nottingham. We are also grateful to those students who have allowed us to show, as examples, their early attempts to write up clinical notes.

The editorial staff of Arnold encouraged us to produce this textbook to complement the excellent surgical textbook by Sir Norman Browse, which is also published by Arnold. Fiona Goodgame was most supportive in getting the project under way and Jane Duncan has been helpful and patient in co-ordinating everyone's efforts and putting the book together.

David Gray
Peter Toghill
Nottingham 2000

Glossary

A glossary of terms which have not necessarily been defined in the text

Abduction Movement away from the midline of body or limb.
Adduction Movement towards the midline of body or limb.
– algia A suffix meaning 'pain arising in or from'.
Amnesia Loss of memory.
Anastomosis (pl. es) Junction, cross-connection
Aneurysm Dilatation of an artery.
Anorexia Loss of appetite.
Anosmia Loss of sense of smell.
Anosognosia Lack of awareness or acceptance of severe disability, usually a left hemiplegia.
Anuria Failure of secretion of urine.
Aplasia Lack of development or growth.
Ascites Fluid in the peritoneal cavity.
Blepharitis Inflammation or redness of the eyelid margins.
Brady – A prefix meaning slow.
Bruit A noise due to turbulent flow in a blood vessel.
Bulla (pl. ae) Large blisters in the skin.
Cachexia Wasting.
Chemosis Oedema of the conjunctiva.
Cholestasis Stagnation of bile.
Circadian A description of a rhythm recurring on a daily basis.
Coarctation A narrowing of a blood vessel.
Crepitus Grating or creaking with joint or bone movement.
Cyanosis Blue colour of the skin due to deoxygenation of the blood.
– cytopenia A suffix meaning a reduced number of cells
Diascopy Looking through a glass slide pressed on the skin.
Diverticulum (pl. a) A blind sac.
Drusen Colloid bodies on retina.
Dys – A prefix meaning pain or difficulty with certain activities.
Dysarthria Difficulty in articulation.
Dysphagia Difficulty or pain on swallowing.
Dysphasia A language defect in putting thoughts into words (expressive) or understanding the spoken word (receptive).
Dysphonia Difficulty in phonation.
Dysplasia Abnormal development of growth.
Dyspnoea Breathlessness or difficulty in breathing.
Dyspraxia Difficulty in formulating and synthesizing movement patterns.
Dysuria Scalding or pain on micturition.
Ecchymosis (pl. es) Bruise.
Effusion A collection of fluid in a potential space.
Embolus (pl. i) Substance carried in the blood stream and large enough to occlude a vessel.
Epigastrium Upper abdomen.
Erythema Redness or flushing of the skin due to dilatation of superficial blood vessels.
Erythrodermia Red skin.
Expophthalmos Protrusion of the globe of the eye in thyroid disease.
Fistula (pl. ae) An abnormal track between two hollow organs or between an organ and the skin surface.
Fossa (pl. ae) A hollow.
Frequency Frequent passage of small volumes of urine.
Gangrene Death and infective necrosis of tissue.
Gingivitis Inflammation of the gums.
Haematemesis (pl. es) Vomiting of blood.
Haematuria Blood in the urine.
Haemolysis Breakdown or destruction of erythrocytes.

Haemoptysis (pl. es) Coughing up blood.
Hallucinations Abnormal perceptions of objects.
Hemianopia Half of the visual field on one side.
Homonymous On the same side, as in vision.
Hyper– A prefix meaning overactivity or more than normal.
Hyperacusis Sounds seeming to be unduly loud.
Hyperaemia Increased blood flow.
Hyperhidrosis Excess sweating.
Hyperphagia Increased eating.
Hypo– A prefix implying underactivity or less than normal.
Iatrogenic Caused by doctors or as a result of treatment.
Ichthyosis Scaly, fish-like skin.
Idiopathic Cause unknown.
–itis A suffix implying 'inflammation of'.
Illusions Misinterpretations of stimuli.
Intertrigo Eczema at skin flexures.
Koilonychia Spoon shaped nails.
Kyphos An increase in the forward flexion of the thoracic spine by sharp angulation at one point.
Kyphosis An increase in the anteroposterior curvature of the spine.
Lanugo Soft fine hair as in the newborn.
Macro– Large.
Macule A small, visible but non-palpable skin lesion.
Mydriasis Dilatation of the pupil.
Naevus (pl. i) A skin blemish, not necessarily vascular in origin.
Nocturia Passing urine at night.
–nychia A suffix meaning 'of the nail'.
Oedema Fluid in tissues.
Oligo– Prefix meaning reduced or little.
Oligomenorrhoea Scanty periods.
Oliguria Secretion of small volumes of urine.
Onycholysis Separation of the distal nail from the nail bed.
-orrhoea A suffix meaning 'discharge from'.
Orthopnoea Breathlessness on lying flat.
Osteomalacia Failure of calcification of new osteoid.
Osteoporosis Reduction in bone mass.
Paper money sign Confluent spider naevi, like the background of an American dollar note.
Phlebitis Inflammation of a vein.
–plasty A suffix denoting repair or correction by surgery.
Pleurisy Pain arising from the pleura.
Pneumo– Prefix meaning air in an organ or cavity.
–pnoea A suffix meaning 'related to breathing'.
Polycythaemia Excess of erythrocytes in the blood.
Polyphagia Increased appetite.
Polyuria Passing large volumes of urine.
Prognathos Protrusion of the lower jaw.
Proptosis Protrusion of the globe.
Pruritus Skin itching.
Ptosis Drooping of the eyelid.
Rhinophyma A bluish, red discolouration and swelling of the nose.
Scoliosis A lateral curvature of the spine.
Stenosis (pl. es) A narrowing.
Stigma (pl. ata) A characteristic sign.
Sulcus (pl. i) A groove or furrow.
Tachy– A prefix meaning fast.
Telangiectasia Enduring dilatation of blood vessels in skin.
–uria A suffix used relating to the urine.
Vesicles Small blisters in the skin.
Viscus (pl. era) Hollow internal organ.
Xanthoma (pl. s) Deposits of lipids in the skin.
Xanthelasma (pl. s) Plaques of lipids in the skin of the eyelids.

History taking and clinical examination: the basics

A

History taking

1

TAKING A HISTORY

Each disease tends to present in a fairly characteristic way. Doctors try to tie together the symptoms a patient reports, the signs of bodily change seen on clinical examination and the physiological and pathological changes found in various blood and other tests into a recognizable pattern typical of a specific disease. Having thus made a *diagnosis*, the doctor, drawing on experience and knowledge, can discuss with the patient the expected *prognosis* and the range of options for treatment. The process of talking with and examining a patient (and writing in the notes) is generally referred to as 'clerking a patient'. The most important part of the whole process is 'taking a history'.

What is a history?

A history is a detailed account of the patient's current illness; significant factors which might predispose to illness; details of any previous medical history; current and previous drug treatment; any relevant history of familial illnesses; and personal and social history and habits.

A patient's symptoms are important because they provide most of the clues to diagnosis and so help direct a thorough physical examination appropriately and indicate the sorts of tests that are most likely to confirm the clinical suspicion and make the diagnosis. For some diseases like migraine, there are no helpful investigations, so the diagnosis rests solely on a well-taken history. In angina, the description of effort-related chest pain or angina may be sufficient to make a confident diagnosis without tests.

While taking a history, you learn about patients' attitudes to their illness and about their fears, either from non-verbal clues or from 'throw away' comments' such as 'I told my daughter it isn't cancer because I haven't coughed up any blood'.

Some basic advice on talking with patients

You may feel intimidated and insecure when you first talk with patients. Generally however, you will find patients to be very supportive and helpful, especially if you tell them that you are 'a student doctor working in Dr X's team'.

You may find that some patients provide a detailed blow by blow account of seemingly disconnected events which you soon gather to be completely irrelevant. To the patient, these may appear to be the reasons why they became ill. Politely interrupt and ask a slightly different question to put them back on track.

Don't be misled by a patient's own diagnosis, or that offered by a relative or even the family doctor – you will need to make up your own mind after speaking with, then examining, the patient. Also, don't be put off if the patient starts mentioning things in a different sequence to that listed in Revision Panel 1.1 at the end of this section. Simply make a mental note of what is said and if necessary clarify any detail you may have forgotten.

Maintain eye contact as much as possible as this helps establish a working relationship with your patient and reinforces the impression of your being interested. Try to avoid interrupting your patient. Politely say 'I'm sorry, can you just clarify for me...'. Make rough notes (in as few words as possible) as the patient talks – this running record will form the framework of your fuller notes later.

Some DOs and DON'Ts

When you talk with patients, DO:

- Introduce yourself and explain why you have come to see the patient.
- Ask if you may talk with and examine the patient.
- Talk with, and not to, your patient.
- Learn to be a good listener.
- Be polite and respectful at all times.
- Act courteously and avoid using a patient's first name unless asked to.
- Avoid using patronizing terms such as 'gran' or 'dear'.
- Allow more time for the very young or very old and those with impaired hearing.
- Ask specific questions to make up for any lapses of the patient's memory.
- Pass on to medical colleagues any concerns the patient may have.
- Respect the information given as confidential.
- Summarize what the patient said and confirm that this is what the patient really means.
- Record information legibly.
- Get a professional interpreter if necessary who will be trained to translate the questions you ask – speaking through a family member is not a good substitute.
- Guide the conversation but do not put words in the patient's mouth.
- Note any obvious body language.
- Seek information from the patient first and then obtain supplementary information from a relative, partner or friend if necesssary.
- Put the patient's complaint into social context – details of the family background, work, type of house or bungalow and hobbies may be relevant.
- Ask what the patient thinks is going on.
- Try to get the timing and sequence of events clearly established.
- Take short-cuts if your patient appears very ill.
- Speak with a patient's family, friends and family doctor if your patient has difficulty communicating such as after a stroke (Fig. 1.1).

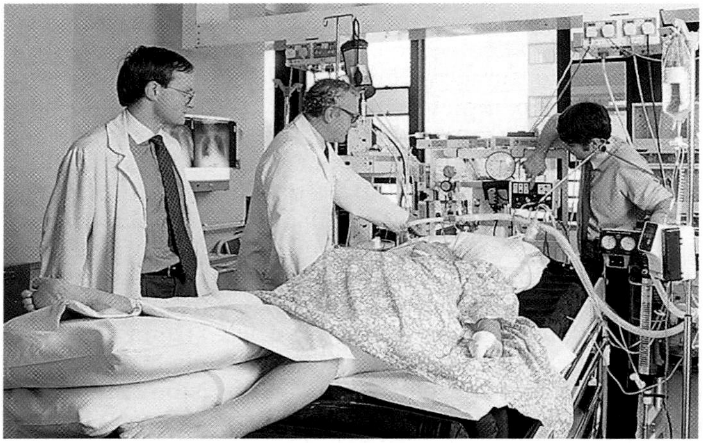

FIG. 1.1 Sometimes with very ill patients it will be impossible to establish personal contact. Make sure that you talk to anyone who can offer useful information. This includes friends, relatives, carers and ambulance men.

Revision Panel 1.1

Learning what to present and what to leave out

A detailed Family and Social History is crucial to the management of a 25-year-old patient disabled by multiple sclerosis but is not immediately helpful to a previously fit teenager with acute appendicitis.

- Remember that examination and tests together contribute far less to diagnosis than does a well-taken history.

And remember DON'T:

- Worry if there is a 'pregnant pause' every now and again.
- Interrupt the patient unless it is obvious that a question has been misunderstood.
- Write while the patient is talking.
- Ask leading questions – try to keep them as general as possible.
- Use scientific words and jargon that the patient will not understand.
- Give an opinion on diagnosis or treatment.
- Use complex language – particularly when talking with patients for whom English is a second language.
- Harass a vague patient – this only makes things worse.
- Criticize doctors' views or treatment.

DEVELOPING THE ART OF TAKING A GOOD HISTORY

It is usually much easier to practise on patients in clinic than on patients who have just arrived in hospital acutely unwell – there is less pressure on members of the medical team to get to the bottom of things quickly. So accept any opportunity to visit clinic and talk with patients. Another useful source of practice are patients recovering from an acute illness who are often only too glad to have someone to talk to, not least to help pass the long hours of the hospital day. Try not to look at the patient's notes until you have seen the patient.

It really is unimportant what clinical specialty you are attached to. You simply need exposure to patients of all kinds. You will probably find it difficult to remember all the questions you are supposed to ask and will rely heavily on your 'pocket guide to taking a history'. This does not matter. Practice, aided by a rapidly expanding knowledge of disease, puts this right very quickly.

Remember to start by asking a simple 'open' question and then seeking to refine the detail, for example 'When did you notice things went wrong?' and then 'What happened after that?'

Common mistakes

As a novice, you will spend much time recording seemingly endless detail about a patient's complaint and appear to be getting nowhere. Don't be afraid to politely interrupt if it seems that the patient has got hold of the wrong end of the stick. Rephrasing a question (perhaps using more familiar language) will redirect your patient and shorten an otherwise rambling response.

It is tempting to jump to conclusions too soon about the cause of an illness. Always ask yourself if it all makes sense. If not, check over the entire history, to make sure that you have a clear description of the time sequence of symptoms. Check if you have omitted anything.

How to direct the course of an interview

Patients are very different. Some will have written down a list of their complaints in immense detail and in chronological order; others will present you with a fluent array of apparently disconnected minor symptoms; still others will answer questions in a monosyllabic way so that you will be hard pressed to get them talking.

As a first strategy, just ask an open-ended question and sit back and await an answer. Many patients will have rehearsed what they wish to say to 'get it off their chest.' You may find some of the information will be relevant so try not to interrupt. Once they have finished their speech, you can probably go back to the beginning with 'It sounds like your main problems are chest pain and getting out of breath. What seemed to bring these on?'

Some patients are very loquacious and keen to inform you of every nuance in their illness. Keeping a rambling patient on track may seem impossible at first but avoid appearing bored and disinterested. Most patients will not be offended if you *politely* interrupt them (to curtail clearly unnecessary detail) as you will come across as someone who is interested in the problems.

The most difficult patient is inarticulate almost to the point of being monosyllabic. Some patients may need encouragement with very simple, often direct, questions until their confidence builds up.

And finally, remember that it takes time, patience and practice to develop expertise in any skill. Interviewing patients is no exception.

Getting down to details – the presenting complaint

Background information of the patient's age, sex, ethnic group, present (and sometimes previous) occupation and particularly social circumstances helps to put the impact of any disease into context.

Document the presenting complaint, whenever possible using the patient's own words as symptoms can mean different things to different people. 'Blackouts' are commonly described by patients and may be due to a wide variety of diseases. A carefully taken history and a clear description will help point at least to the appropriate system of the body and sometimes to a specific diagnosis.

It is important to map out critical events of an illness, as a specific sequence of events may indicate a particular diagnosis. In meningitis, flu-like symptoms may be followed by sweating, sensitivity to bright lights, nausea and a stiff neck.

Sometimes the timing of these critical events can be tied to a particular TV programme (for symptoms which progress rapidly) to holidays and birthdays for illnesses which progress slowly. Using familiar times like these help patients recall details they might otherwise have not mentioned.

Practical Point

Some causes of blackouts

Stokes–Adams attacks.
Epilepsy.
Simple faints.
Postural hypotension.

Patients may remember some events more readily than others so you may need to ask direct questions to obtain more detail. Asking 'Dizziness is very common. What sort of dizziness do you have?' may elicit more detail, but occasionally you may need to ask direct questions such as 'Do you feel faint when you get out of bed in the morning?'

The timing and sequence of events often helps differentiate one disease process from another so the history should provide a concise, clear and chronological record of the patient's symptoms. Try to avoid expressions such as 'Last Thursday'. While undoubtedly accurate, this is less helpful than 'Three days ago' which gives a better guide to anyone reading the notes a few days (months or even years) later. Even better is 'Chest pain on exertion three days ago, getting progressively worse one day ago and severe chest pain which woke from sleep six hours ago.'

You should first enquire about the *current problem*, when things first started going wrong and how things changed after that. Ask a very general question such as 'What is your main problem at present?' followed by 'When was the first time you realised you weren't well?' At this stage, always record the patient's own words – you can convert them into medical jargon later.

Beware putting words into the patient's mouth. If a patient comments that the stools changed colour, ask 'what colour do you mean?' rather than saying 'Black?' if you suspect melaena from a bleeding peptic ulcer.

Systematic enquiry

Patients never recall and volunteer all the information you will need to assess the impact of disease on every bodily system. The systematic enquiry helps jog the patient's memory using direct questions. Often in young people, the responses will be negative, but with increasing age and accumulating medical problems, responses are more likely to be positive; here, you may need to delve a little more deeply to enquire for example 'What exactly do you mean when you say that you get palpitations?'

You will quickly learn that you can assess an entire body system by asking just a few questions, listed in Revision Panel 1.2.

> Revision Panel 1.2
> **Symptomatic enquiry**
>
> *General well-being*
> Weight, appetite, fever, sleep, mood.
>
> *Cardiovascular/respiratory*
> Exercise tolerance, breathlessness, chest pain, cough, ankle swelling, nocturnal dyspnoea, wheeze.
>
> *Alimentary*
> Abdominal pain, nausea, vomiting, bowel habit routine.
>
> *Genitourinary*
> Micturition frequency, dysuria, incontinence, menstruation.
>
> *Nervous*
> Headaches, limb weakness, altered sensation, speech and hearing problems.
>
> *Locomotor*
> Joint pains, stiffness, backache.

Previous medical history

Many patients will keenly describe previous illnesses, especially if the doctor got the diagnosis wrong or underestimated the patient's powers of recovery. Otherwise you will need to enquire about illnesses which have caused loss of work or absence from school. How long it took to get back to normal is a useful guide to severity. Hospitalization for a week and full recovery in three months is the norm after a heart attack, any longer suggests a major complication such as heart failure or ongoing exertional chest pain. Hospital records and the family doctor's referral letter help too.

Elderly patients have survived an era when serious illnesses like tuberculosis and rheumatic fever were common; advancing age increases the risk of diabetes, hypertension and myocardial infarction, so it is helpful to ask about these.

Family and social history

Patients may report that cancer or heart disease 'runs in the family'. When you enquire about a family history, you are asking about the likelihood of inherited disease and an adverse genetic profile. Discovering that a patient's relatives all died in their 80s from heart disease may be interesting but is not diagnostic of an inherited problem. A family with thalassaemia presents very different problems.

Anniversaries of a relative's death often trigger unreasonable fears among surviving family and this may precipitate unnecessary visits to the doctor with minor complaints; this is particularly true of heart attack and cancer.

If you do suspect a familial disease, you need to construct a family tree as shown in Fig. 1.2(a), using the symbols detailed in Fig. 1.2(b).

With elderly patients, find out if they are independent or who is the main carer. House design also becomes important in the elderly because of limited mobility and difficulty with stairs. Social Service input and access to caring neighbours should also be recorded.

If you suspect that there may be money problems, tactful enquiries may reveal financial difficulties and warrant urgent action to sort out social benefits and free prescriptions.

Generally, doctors take a very poor social history, mainly because of time constraints. Any suggestion of work-related illness should trigger enquiry about the type of work, expo-

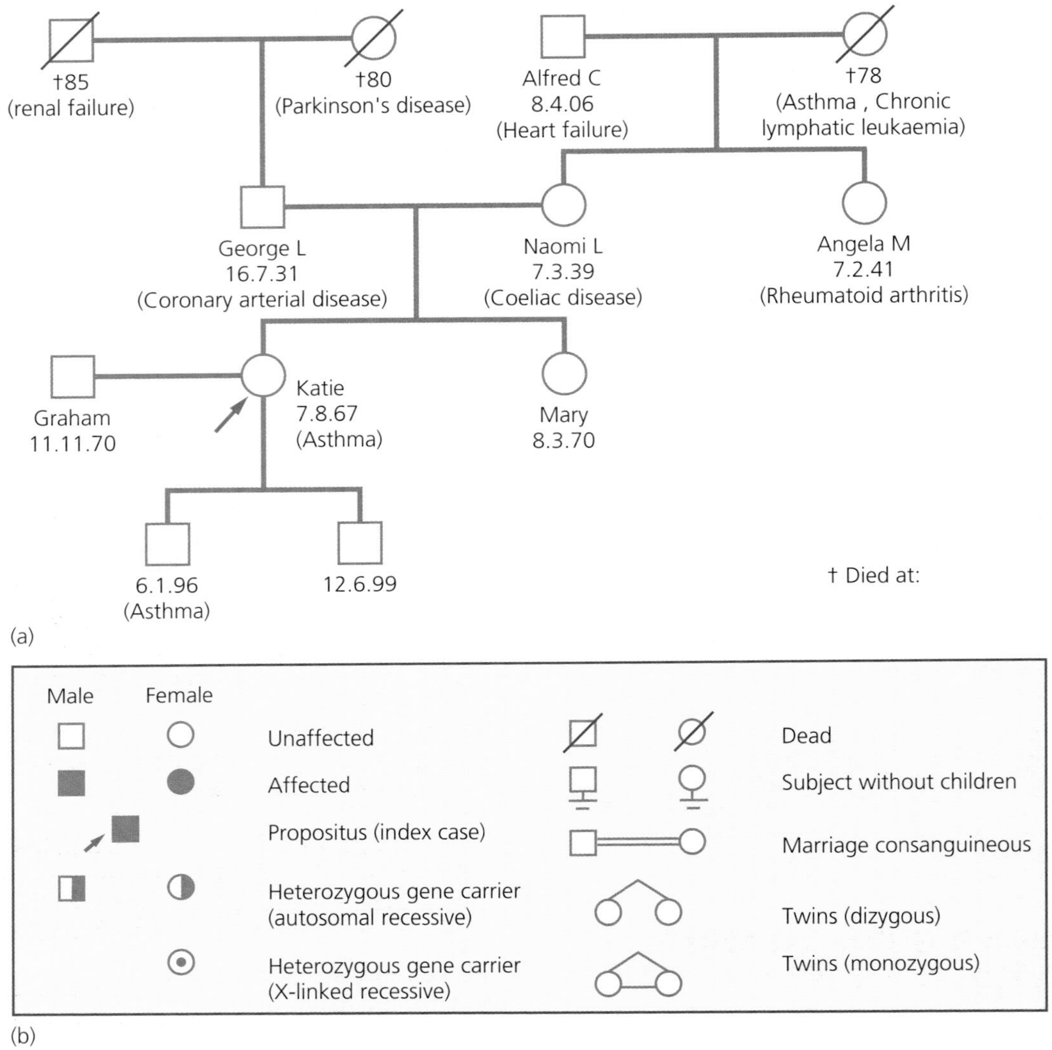

FIG. 1.2 (a) How a family history might be recorded in the hospital notes for Katie L who has been admitted to hospital with asthma. (b) Symbols used in constructing a pedigree for a family with a genetic disease.

sure to noxious chemicals and hazards like asbestos, and the overall working environment. If necessary, the work history from leaving school may prove essential. Try to avoid general terms like 'engineer' – this may mean anything from the man who mends the washing machine to someone who designs jet engines.

Doctors are particularly bad at taking an alcohol history. 'Big' drinkers include Merchant Navy and Servicemen, publicans, businessmen and doctors themselves. Most people underestimate the amount they drink. With these professions start negotiations on the true level of alcohol consumption along the lines of 'Many people in your line of work drink a lot, usually around five or six pints a night. Does that apply to you?'

In contrast, most patients who smoke tell the truth about their consumption. The number of cigarettes smoked is probably easier for a patient to monitor than it is for alcohol.

Leisure activities rarely cause health problems in older patients but sports-minded youngsters may seek help to resume their activities.

It is not usual to ask about sexual activities unless there are specific reasons (see Chapter 19).

Drug history

With advancing age, a patient may accumulate several medical problems, requiring an array of medication to control or suppress symptoms. Always make a point of inspecting any medication a patient brings. Some medicines may be current and others 'old' or even expired which can cause confusion in an elderly patient.

Try to make a habit of recording what each drug is for. You will soon learn to recognize the commonly prescribed ones, such as non-steroidal anti-inflammatory agents, anti-depressants, and a range of drugs for cardiac and respiratory problems.

A SIMPLE GUIDE TO WRITING UP A GOOD HISTORY

Patient's notes are valuable sources of information. They provide:

- A detailed record of a patient's original presenting complaint; subsequent management plan and response to treatment.
- The results of investigations performed to establish or reject a diagnosis.
- A record of major illnesses in an individual's medical history.

Practical Point

Test results should be recorded and filed.
Your patient's notes should be:
Accurate.
Legible.
Tidy.
Up-to-date.

- A legal record.
- Audit and research data.
- Additional information from relatives and the patient's GP.

Remember these points when writing in a patient's notes. Above all, ensure that the record is accurate and legible, kept tidy and up-to-date with all test results recorded and filed. Use bullet points to draw attention to important information. Where information is lacking, speak with the General Practitioner or a member of the family.

While on the subject of writing up notes, it is important that, for patients in hospital, you should record in the notes:

- A progress report every day.
- Any significant test result which helps with diagnosis (this may be a 'positive' or a 'negative' result) – red ink or block capitals will help these stand out when you present on ward rounds.
- Whenever you discuss with the patient (or relative) any medical, family or social problems relevant to medical care.
- Whenever you discuss the results of important tests.
- Whenever there is any clinical deterioration.
- Concise summaries of discussions during ward rounds.
- Any change in management decisions, especially with regard to any policy on resuscitation from cardiac arrest or sudden decline in health.

Revision Panel 1.3

Synopsis of a history

1 *Essential information*
Name. Age and date of birth. Sex. Marital status. Occupation. Ethnic group.

2 *Presenting complaint (PC)*
Record the patient's own words.

3 *History of presenting complaint (HPC)* Chronological order of all symptoms. Change in character especially severity. Treatment given (including self-prescribed) and response. Record important positive and negative answers to direct questions that assist with diagnosis.

4 *Systematic direct enquiry (SE)*

(a) *Alimentary system and abdomen (AS)*
Appetite. Weight. Nausea, vomiting and regurgitation. Swallowing difficulty. 'Indigestion and heartburn'. Signs of blood loss in vomit or stools. Abdominal pain and distension. Regular bowel habit and any change. Stool character. Jaundice.

(b) *Respiratory system (RS)*
Cough and any blood loss. Sputum. Breathlessness at rest or on exertion. Hoarseness. Wheezing. Chest pain or discomfort.

(c) *Cardiovascular system (CVS)*
Breathlessness at rest, on exertion, on lying flat in bed or waking from sleep. Chest pain. Cough. Ankle swelling. Exercise tolerance. Leg pains on walking. Palpitations. Syncope.

(d) *Urogenital system (UGS)*
Loin pain. Swelling of ankles, hands or face. Micturition frequency, urgency, hesitancy, pain or bleeding. Thirst. Problems with sexual intercourse. Menstrual history including menarche and menopause. Pregnancies and complications.

(e) *Nervous system (NS)*
Faints and loss of consciousness. Fits. Muscle weakness, paralysis, stiffness and tremor. Sensory symptoms. Change of smell, vision, hearing, balance, personality or behaviour. Headaches. Speech.

(f) *Musculoskeletal system (MSK)*
Muscle or joint pain, swelling or stiffness. Weakness. Difficulty with walking.

5 *Previous medical history (PMH)*
Previous illness, operations or accidents. History of major illness such as diabetes, rheumatic fever, diphtheria, tuberculosis, myocardial infarction. Allergies including drugs.

6 *Drug history*
Detailed record including dose and frequency.

7 *Family, personal and social history (FH/SH)*
Cause of death of close relatives and any familial diseases and premature death. Marital status. Type of accommodation. Present (and any relevant previous) occupation. Exposure to industrial hazards. Any relevant overseas travel. Smoking and alcohol habits.

Putting it all together

When you think you have established clearly what has led the patient to seek medical help, briefly summarize what you have gleaned. This provides an opportunity to make sure you have got the story straight. You will find this difficult at first, but with practice, experience, general reading and observing the medical team on ward rounds, you will soon learn how to put together a sensible list of potential diagnoses. Now you can concentrate on looking for specific signs associated with each of these possible diagnoses when you examine the patient.

The clinical examination

2

WHY DO A CLINICAL EXAMINATION?

There is no doubt the patient–doctor relationship is crucial for the proper and successful conduct of clinical medicine. This is established by taking a history and examining the patient yourself. Many might argue, quite reasonably, that in a modern, technological age there is no need to perform a clinical examination. After all:

- Echocardiography will tell us about the heart valves.
- Computerized tomography (CT) scanning will show solid tumours in the chest.
- Magnetic resonance imaging (MRI) will reveal abnormalities in the brain.

Why, therefore, should you as a medical student still need to know how to perform a clinical examination that is accurate, comprehensive and compassionate?

Practical Point

Why is clinical examination necessary?

It is a personal skill which can be taken with you to any part of the world.

Certain physical signs depend on your special senses and cannot be reproduced by machines.

It establishes a special rapport between you and the patient.

The most compelling reason is that much of the world's population still does not have access to relatively simple X-rays, let alone more sophisticated investigations such as MRI scanning. Assessment, diagnosis and treatment are determined by clinical findings alone.

You must remember too that the discovery and interpretation of a large number of physical signs cannot be matched by investigations or advanced imaging technology. So far we have yet to produce a machine that tells us that 'the patient looks ill', a subtle skill which remains entirely within the province of the experienced clinician. More specifically the hearing of triple rhythm, the sight of spider naevi and the smell of hepatic fetor are physical signs that cannot easily be replaced by investigations.

This is not to decry the desirability of selected investigations. A thorough physical examination will suggest which investigations are most appropriate to clinch a diagnosis and avoid 'routine' screening procedures which may be time-consuming, unnecessary, immensely expensive and not without risk to the patient.

Practical Point

Learn a standard examination routine.
Practise on as many patients as possible.
Establish the range of 'normality'.
Don't cut corners until you have mastered basic skills.
Learn to use the simple 'tools of the trade'.

FIRST IMPRESSIONS

In everyday life, first impressions convey a lot and medicine is no exception. You shouldn't forget that the process of 'first impressions' is two-way, and at the same time your patient (and their relatives) will be forming an opinion of you. Remember that your patient may be as anxious as you are. Open the conversation by introducing yourself and explaining why you are there. Most will be sympathetic and some will be overhelpful, providing you with too much material to digest. Occasionally you may come across a patient who is a bit brusque and grumpy and in short not at their best. Arranging to visit another time might seem a good idea. You will not have this luxury as a doctor, so persevere and try to make the most of the experience.

It is important to remember that the clinical assessment of a patient doesn't divide itself conveniently into history, examination and investigations. Whilst taking the history, inevitably and perhaps almost unconsciously, you will have been taking note of features that may influence the way in which you deal with a particular patient.

Before you start the clinical examination

Having taken the history from your patient, you should have in mind what diagnoses are the most likely to account for the patient's symptoms. If you cannot devise a differential diagnosis at this stage, you should at least have a good idea of the nature of the problem and the system that is primarily involved. If not, you should take a minute to review the history again as you may have missed something important.

Once you are satisfied that you have a differential diagnosis in mind, you are ready to start the formal clinical examination. The differential diagnosis provides key pointers to guide you through your clinical examination. In particular:

- It focusses your attention on looking for diagnostic clues in specific areas – e.g. looking for spider naevi, hepatomegaly, gynaecomastia and ascites in suspected chronic liver disease or neck stiffness, fever and rash in suspected acute meningitis.

With more experience you will develop clinical instinct, become adept at devising a differential diagnosis, and putting in place, from a quick glance, a useful framework on which you can build your more detailed assessments.

An overall view of your patient

First impressions are important whether your patient is at home, in the surgery, in hospital or at his place of work.

Whilst talking to your patient you should try to:

- Assess social background and lifestyle.
- Establish your patient's perception of the clinical problem.
- Estimate how severe is any pain.
- Decide whether your patient is seriously ill.
- Identify unusual and/or significant facial appearances.
- Assess body physique.
- Observe abnormalities of posture or gait.
- Make any obvious 'spot diagnoses'.

You need to be aware of how we form some of these first impressions.

Social background and life style

We are all accustomed to assessing people socially in terms of ethnicity, social class and status, friendliness or hostility, attitudes and other factors. All of these will influence how we deal with medical problems. The management of a newly arrived, articulate, co-operative student from West Africa with a high fever will, of necessity, be quite different from that of a drunk, aggressive football fan with a severe head injury.

The face betrays lifestyles. The alcoholic advertises himself with a beaming rhinophymic nose, rheumy eyes and florid skin, signposting the diagnosis which will be con-

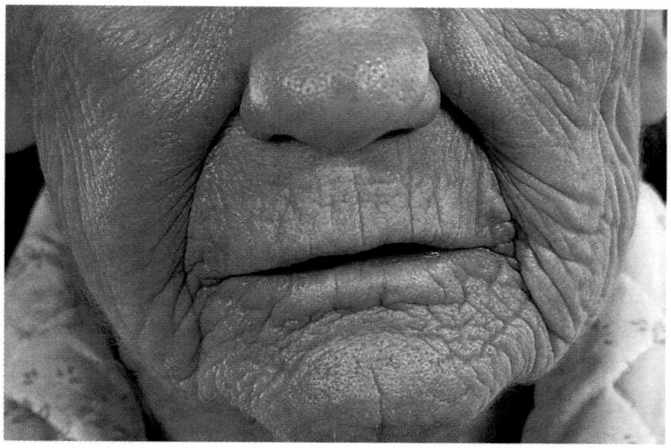

FIG. 2.1 Severe skin wrinkling in a heavy-smoking 62-year-old.

firmed later by noting sweaty palms, tremor and the whiff of alcohol in the breath. Smokers generally reek of tobacco but bear gross and premature skin wrinkling as a sign of heavy smoking that is unfortunately still poorly recognized (Fig. 2.1).

How the patient perceives the problem

There may be some truth in the comment that there are three sorts of symptoms:

- Those that worry patients but don't worry doctors.
- Those that don't worry patients but do worry doctors.
- Those that worry both patients and their doctors.

Patients cannot be expected to know all those symptoms that are serious and those that are not so serious. What concerns the patient most may not be obvious during the first few minutes but will certainly emerge during the history taking. Is the patient taking a realistic view of his or her illness? Many are clearly unaware of its seriousness and others seem relatively unconcerned. Some have to be dragged to consult their doctors by a worried partner. At the other extreme some are terrified of the possible implications of their symptoms, often magnified by inappropriate comments in the press or on TV.

Doctors are well aware that the patient's last 'throw away line' on finally moving towards the surgery door is frequently the most important of the whole interview, that is the real reason for the patient seeking the doctor's advice: 'By the way doctor, I've felt a lump in my neck. Is that alright?'

Is the patient seriously ill?

With acute and serious illness requiring urgent admission to hospital, diagnosis can be easy. The pallor and sweating of massive gastrointestinal bleeding, the stertorous breathing of the collapsed, elderly man with a stroke, and the laboured wheezy breathing of the asthmatic housewife will all indicate even to the layman that something is seriously amiss.

It is the more subtle changes of chronic ill-health which tax the diagnostic skills of the most experienced doctor. What confronts the doctor or medical student at that initial interview is a

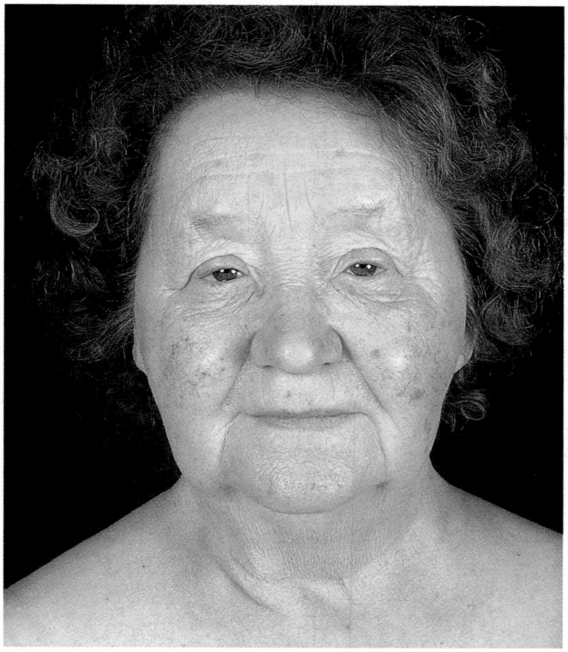

FIG. 2.2 Myxoedema. The changes were not noticed by the patient's doctor who had been seeing her regularly for generalized aches and pains.

single snapshot of a patient in a continuing and possibly progressive illness. Close relatives and friends have an advantage in having witnessed changes that occurred in recent days, weeks or months. By contrast, in some chronic diseases such as myxoedema (Fig. 2.2), the changes may be so slow as to be virtually imperceptible to those near and dear, but immediately obvious to a new and unfamiliar observer.

A frequent feature of serious disease, in particular malignancy, is loss of weight. Fat and muscle bulk is lost and the skin becomes too big for the body. This results in loose redundant folds of skin on the limbs and trunk. Your patient does not need to tell you of the weight loss – the gaping collar, loose trousers and tightened belt present abundant evidence.

Illness is often accompanied by anaemia but the diagnosis of anaemia on clinical grounds is not simple because:

- Elderly, indoor workers and town dwellers often look pale but are not anaemic.
- Weather-beaten, outdoor workers often have ruddy complexions which can at times conceal real anaemia.
- Chronically ill people usually look pale and sallow as a result of a combination of anaemia and increased melanin deposition in the skin.
- Uraemia causes a muddy complexion due in part to increased deposition of urochromes.
- The palpebral conjunctiva and the mucous membranes of the mouth may look pale in healthy individuals.

The only reliable method is to measure the haemoglobin level.

Spot diagnoses

A 'spot diagnosis' of a medical problem that can be recognized at first glance is not that common. Some fairly obvious ones you may come across are shown in Revision Panel 2.1.

A word of warning. If you do make a spot diagnosis do not close your mind to the possibility that the patient may well have other quite unrelated problems.

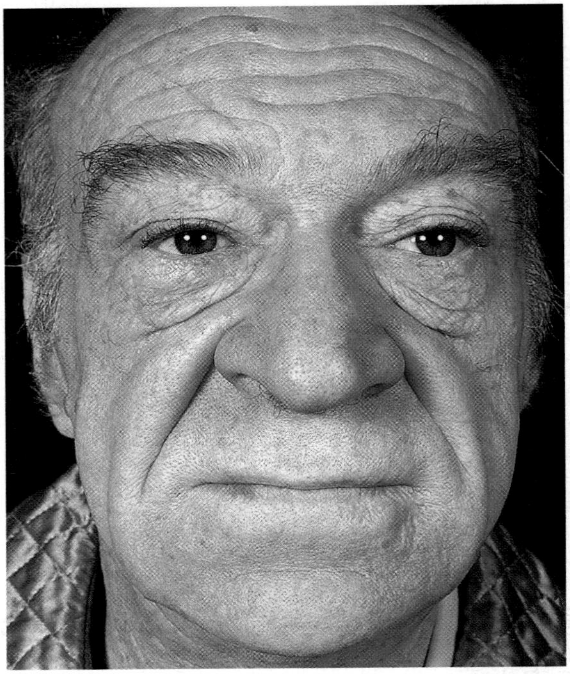

FIG. 2.3 Acromegaly. Diagnosis that can be made at a glance! This man's friends told him his appearance was changing.

Revision Panel 2.1

A selection of spot diagnoses

Coarse features, prominent nasolabial folds, heavy jaw (Fig. 2.3).	Acromegaly.
Prominent eyes (Fig. 2.4).	Thyrotoxicosis.
Tremor, shuffling gait and impassive facies.	Parkinson's disease.
Deafness, big head (Fig. 2.5).	Paget's disease.
Poker back and stiff neck.	Ankylosing spondylitis.
White patches on face and hands (Fig. 2.6).	Vitiligo.
Extreme suntan in a white-skinned person (Fig. 2.7).	Addison's disease.

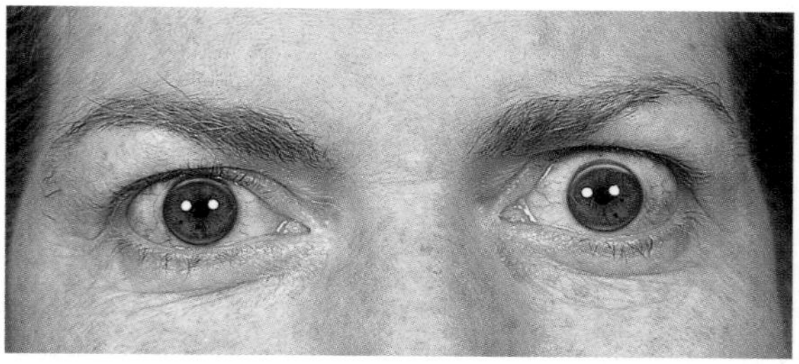

FIG. 2.4 Prominent staring eyes in thyrotoxicosis.

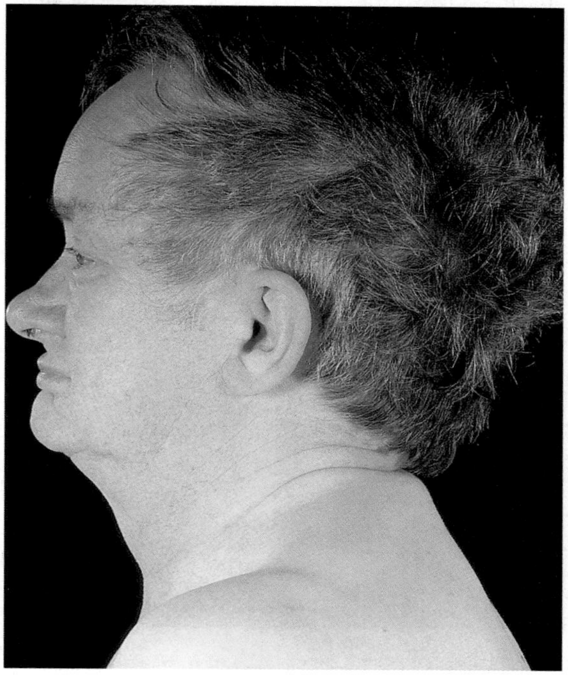

FIG. 2.5 The large head in Paget's disease. The vault of the skull bulges over the eyes and ears.

Facial appearance

While you have been taking the history you will have had the opportunity of examining the face of your patient and of assessing responses to your questions. You will have learned a good deal about your patient's perception of the problem and you will have picked up a few clinical pointers.

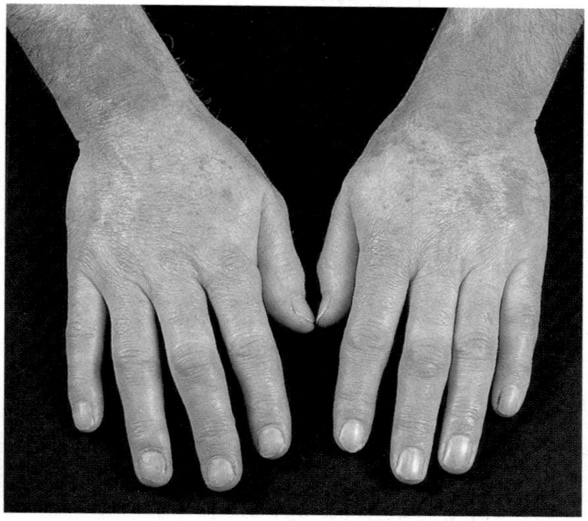

FIG. 2.6 Vitiligo of the hands. Note the geographical outline.

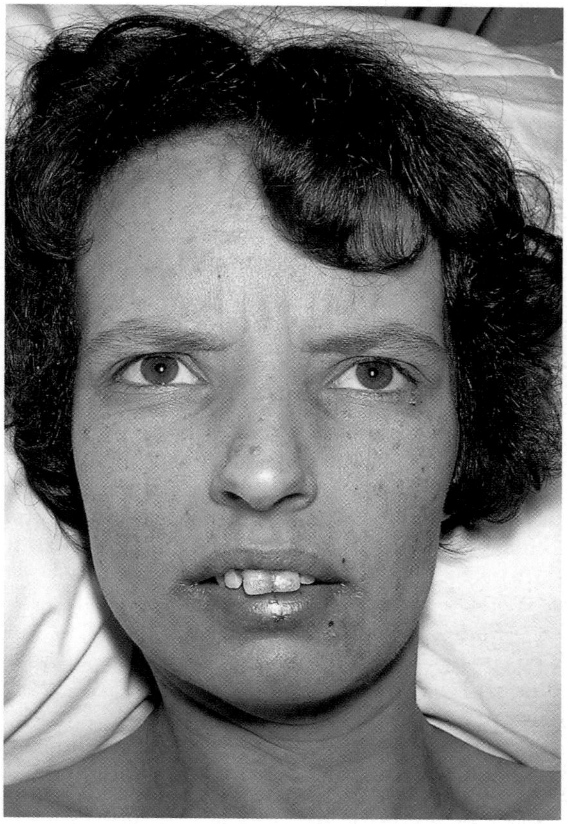

FIG. 2.7 Deep pigmentation of the skin in Addison's disease.

Observing a red face may suggest abuse of alcohol but you should also consider the red flush of embarrassment, especially (but not exclusively) in adolescents, menopausal flushing in a middle-aged woman, excessive red blood cells (polycythaemia rubra vera) accompanied by a grossly plethoric face and cyanotic ear lobes and nose, or a localized flush over the cheekbones, the malar flush, due to a stenosed mitral valve.

Whilst by no means diagnostic of hyperlipidaemia, an arcus senilis and xanthelasmata are commonly associated with atheromatous disease.

Ear lobe clefts (see Fig. 17.2) are now also well recognized as being linked with coronary artery disease. A facial rash may be a clue to a more extensive or 'systemic' disease. The telangiectasia, pinched nose and puckered mouth in a middle-aged women indicates scleroderma, whereas the bulbous red nose of lupus pernio is local evidence of sacoidosis.

Most importantly the face offers clues as to psychiatric disease, for example the lugubrious, impassive and unresponsive face of the severely depressed patient – although the differentiation between true depression and unhappiness may be difficult. At the other end of the scale the hypomanic patient may exhibit a spectrum of facial expressions during a conversation ranging from unusual frankness to rudeness.

Body physique

People come in all shapes and sizes and part of the physician's expertise and experience is to attempt to identify those who fall outside the normal range. As a broad generalization people relate to the shape of their parents. Confucius says that 'geese are not bred from flamingos'!

Thinness and loss of weight

Loss of weight is a feature of serious chronic illness. Seeing the patient for the first time the doctor has to decide whether the patient is just thin or has indeed lost weight. This may not be easy as few people weigh themselves regularly.

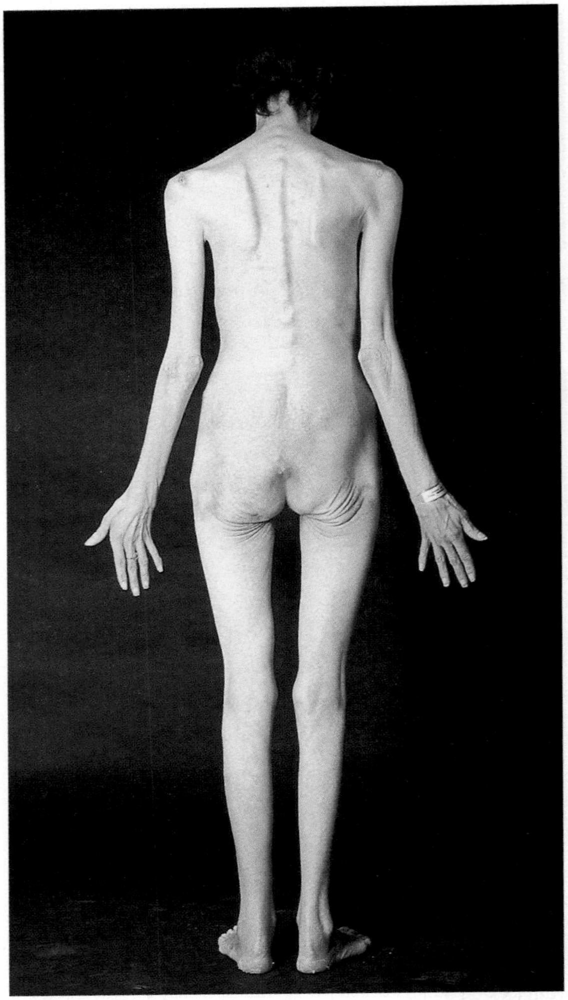

FIG. 2.8 Gross loss of weight in adult coeliac disease. This patient had been admitted to a psychiatric hospital with disturbed behaviour which improved as the coeliac disease came under control.

Some common causes of loss of weight are seen in Revision Panel 2.2. These can be broadly classified according to age. In the underdeveloped world, malnutrition is sadly still a common cause of weight loss in children while in the Western world weight loss in teenage girls is frequently due to anorexia nervosa. In middle-age diabetes, thyrotoxicosis and malignancy figure high on the list. Less well recognized causes are chronic anoxia sec-

Revision Panel 2.2

Loss of weight in the young, middle-aged and elderly

Age group	*Loss of weight*
Young.	Malnutrition.[a] Diabetes. Malabsorption. Tuberculosis.[a] Anorexia nervosa. AIDS. Chronic infections.[a]
Middle age.	Malignancy. Diabetes. Thyrotoxicosis. Malabsorption (Fig. 2.8). Cardiac cachexia. Chronic hypoxia.
Old age	As in middle age. Senile cachexia. Malnutrition and neglect.

[a]Mainly in the tropics
AIDS: Acquired immunodeficiency syndrome.

ondary to lung disease and cachexia related to chronic heart failure. The elderly tend to lose weight in the last year or two of life.

Patterns of disease throughout the world vary and continue to change. The continuing menace of the human immunodeficiency virus (HIV) infection in Central Africa and parts of North America brings it to the fore as a common cause of weight loss in young adults. In China and in the Indian subcontinent tuberculosis is still common. Whereas chronic infections (apart from HIV) are now unusual causes of loss of weight in the Western World, they remain serious health hazards for all ages in the tropics.

Obesity

Everyone can recognize a fat person though the distribution of the obesity varies from one person to another. In general men have more generalized obesity whereas women may have, in addition to truncal obesity, fat breasts, buttocks and thighs. The distribution of the obesity is usually genetically determined though environmental influences and lifestyles may override this. Various forms of lipodystrophies exist, one of the most common being obesity distributed in a 'below the belt' pattern. Some of the causes of obesity are shown in Revision Panel 2.3.

Attempts have been made to define obesity scientifically in terms of a Body Mass Index (BMI) derived from Quetelet's formula (W/H^2) where W is the weight in kg and H is the height in metres. Using this method the obese are divided into three grades:

I: BMI 25–29.9
II: BMI 30–39.9
III: BMI > 40.

By this definition one-third of the population of the United Kingdom is obese.

Revision Panel 2.3

Causes of obesity

General
Genetic influences.
Gluttony.
Inactivity (often an effect as well as a cause).

Endocrine
Cushing's syndrome.
Hypothyroidism.
Hypothalamic disorders.

Drugs
Steroids and anabolic agents.

Too short or too tall?

Most people are short because of genetic and racial influences but you should always consider other causes in an unusually short person or in the child of normally sized parents. Some of the causes of short stature are listed in Revision Panel 2.4 and will also be dealt with elsewhere, but particularly worthy of note is the syndrome of achondroplasia which produces a characteristic appearance and an instantly identifiable syndrome. The legs and arms are very short, the head appears large and the bridge of the nose is depressed.

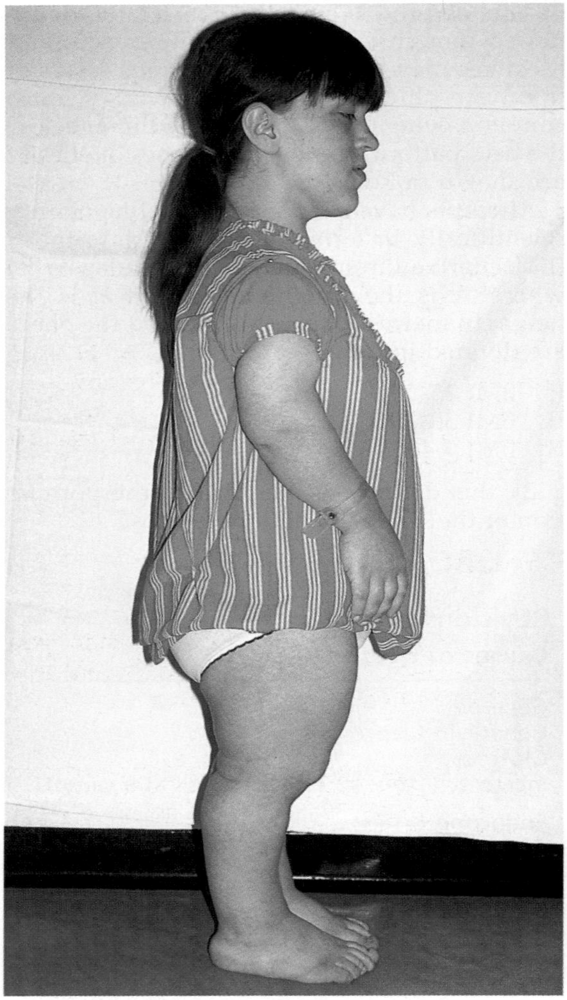

FIG. 2.9 Achondroplasia.

Revision Panel 2.4
Causes of shortness

Genetic
Simple hereditary shortness.
Achondroplasia (Fig. 2.9).

Nutritional
Malnutrition.
Rickets (dietary).
Coeliac disease.

Endocrine
Cretinism.
Pituitary syndromes.

Chromosomal
Down's syndrome (Fig. 2.10).
Turner's syndrome.

Psychiatric
Emotional deprivation.

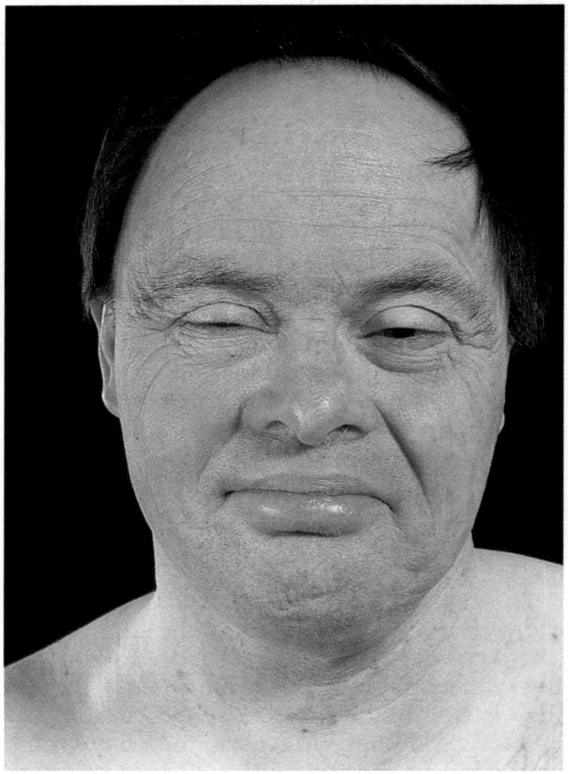

FIG. 2.10 Down's syndrome. This 40-year-old man was 4ft 10 in (147 cm in height).

With improved diet and life style many populations are getting taller and physically stronger; this is seen particularly in South East Asia, China and Japan. As with the other variations in body size, tallness is otherwise usually genetically determined. Nevertheless on seeing unusually tall patients one should just bear in mind such rarities as the gigantism/acromegaly syndrome and Klinefelter's and Marfan syndromes.

Gait and posture

Watch how your patient moves. As your patient approaches you it may be possible to define involuntary movements, a hemiplegia, a fixed hip and many other neurological and orthopaedic conditions. Of course watching your patient move is an essential part of the subsequent formal examination. Those patients with severe musculoskeletal pains will move cautiously and guardedly. View with suspicion the patient complaining of excruciating back pain who leaps easily onto the examination couch. Likewise bedfast patients with severe abdominal pain are unlikely to move unnecessarily though colicky pain may cause the patient to writhe in agony.

Having formed your first impressions, you can now proceed to examine your patient.

THE FORMAL CLINICAL EXAMINATION

Now that you have taken the history and formed a series of impressions about your patient you can press on with the formal part of the clinical examination. Here you must use all your senses to detect physical signs. Strictly speaking you are looking for *abnormal* physical signs. Everyone will have physical signs but traditionally when we ask, 'Are there any physical signs?' we are referring to *abnormal* ones.

Establishing what might reasonably be called *normal* is one of the first lessons you will have to learn when examining patients. There is a wide range of normality that you will soon come to recognize with practice and experience. Take the opportunity to examine as many patients as you can.

You will also need to handle simple 'tools of the trade'. In subsequent chapters you will learn how to supplement your examination by using instruments such as the sphygmomanometer and the ophthalmoscope.

The quickest way to master clinical examination is to have a standard routine that you carry out on every patient. This may seem tedious but you will be less likely to miss out essential parts of the examination. Only after having mastered the basic skills can you then learn how, and when, you can safely cut corners.

After taking a history, the experienced clinician will have made a mental list of potential diagnoses and will often go straight to the system or site most likely to yield signs that confirm or refute these tentative diagnoses. If the initial findings on examination are at odds with the clinical suspicions, the rest of the examination can never be ignored.

Later in this book you will learn how to examine each system in detail. For now you simply need to get to grips with the basic principles and a standard scheme which can be adopted for all medical patients.

BEFORE YOU START

Don't make things more difficult than you need. It is best to get things right before you start the examination (Fig. 2.11).

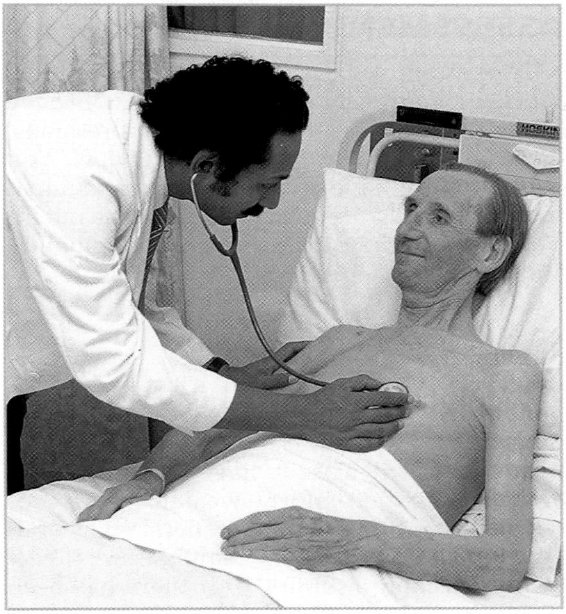

FIG. 2.11 Make sure that your patient is comfortable and prepared. Ensure that the bed is at the right height and that all instruments are at hand.

Try to make sure that your patient is comfortable by:

- Ensuring privacy with curtains or screens.
- Maintaining their dignity at all times; covering up exposed areas when you have finished examining those parts.
- Explaining what you are going to do.

For your own comfort:

- Stand on the patient's right-hand side.
- Set the couch or bed at the right height for you.
- Make sure that any instrument you may need is at hand.

All this may seem obvious but is often neglected. Occasionally of course, conditions may be less than perfect. In a patient's home you may be forced to examine from the wrong side of a low bed, in a gloomy room while competing with a crying baby and a loud television in the background. At least the latter can be switched off.

START WITH THE GENERAL ASSESSMENT

Much of your general assessment will have been taken care of in those 'first impressions' during the earlier parts of the interview. You will certainly have to modify your examination to take into account your patient's intelligence, comprehension, co-operation, mobility and modesty.

TAKING AN OVERALL VIEW

By now you will already have noted evidence of distress, discomfort, weakness, loss of weight, breathlessness and general signs of ill health. Make a note of the temperature, if necessary checking it yourself. If there has been exposure to cold and you suspect hypothermia, record the aural or rectal temperature using a low-reading thermometer. As part of this initial survey think of and look for:

- Anaemia – but remember that pallor does not equate with anaemia.
- Cyanosis – central or peripheral.
- Jaundice.

You may develop your own sequence as you gain more experience, but the advice here will ensure you miss nothing important. Follow the same pattern each time and eventually it will become routine.

The traditional method of examining patients is to work through each system in the same order each time. Many physicians go straight to the system they think is implicated in the history, especially in acutely ill patients. This does take experience and as a beginner you are advised to follow a standard approach until you have developed the necessary confidence and skill. Sometimes you may find yourself modifying your initial diagnosis as the examination proceeds.

Start with a general overview, then progress through the major systems – cardiovascular, respiratory, gastrointestinal and central nervous systems, followed by musculoskeletal, lymphatic and renal/genitourinary systems as appropriate and in as much detail as required.

Practical Point

Initial leads from the history are not always correct

An elderly woman consulted her doctor because of a six-month history of breathlessness on exertion and persistently swollen legs. The cardiovascular system was examined first as the doctor suspected mild heart failure. Heart sounds were normal, there were no murmurs, the jugular venous pressure was not raised and the lungs were clear. The only abnormality noted was pitting oedema of the lower legs. While completing the remainder of the examination, a mass was felt in the lower abdomen. Investigations revealed an ovarian carcinoma as the cause of her problems.

What follows is a scheme for routine examination of the systems but this routine may have to be modified when dealing with an acutely ill patient in hospital or a patient being examined at home.

In each section there is a suggested sequence for performing the examination, followed by a list of points that have to be noted. Use the latter as a checklist. At the end of each section there will be a note of the instruments that may be required to complete the examination.

The hand

Start by picking up your patient's hand and checking the pulse. This gives you the first opportunity of establishing physical contact, which is one of the ways in which further confidence can be established. Whilst checking the pulse look at the nails and skin. Some abnormalities are associated with specific systemic disorders (Fig. 2.12) (See Revision Panel 2.5).

The hand may also tell you about the patient's background, occupation and personal hygiene. Note any tattoos. Exotic designs have often been acquired during military service, especially in the Far East; simpler designs after a drunken night out with a group of pals; and crude ones may have been self-inflicted, sometimes while serving a prison sentence.

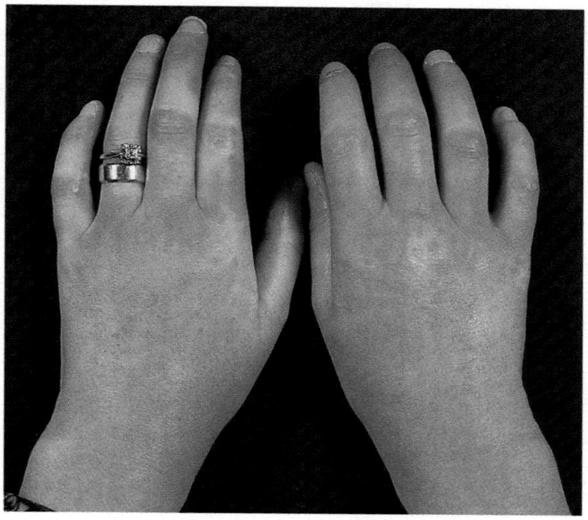

FIG. 2.12 The hands in scleroderma showing tight skin, ischaemia and loss of tissue at the ends of the digits.

Those doing manual jobs such as carpenters or gardeners usually have big, hefty hands. Note any Heberden's nodes, osteoarthritis or rheumatoid arthritis (Fig. 2.13).

In the elderly, particularly women, there may be dark red bruises on the backs of the hands and forearms, apparently spontaneous, which are termed senile purpura. Also note the skin thickness which may be like tissue paper in the very old, those on long-term

Revision Panel 2.5

What can be learned from examining the nails?

Abnormality	*Common causes*
Clubbing.	Suppurative lung disease. Carcinoma of bronchus. Fibrosing alveolitis. Cirrhosis of liver. Infective endocarditis. Chronic diarrhoea.
Koilonychia and ridging.	Chronic iron deficiency.
Pitting.	Psoriatic arthropathy.
Nail infarcts (splinters).	Trauma. Infective endocarditis. Vasculitis.
Transverse ridging (Beau's lines).	Severe illness, courses of chemotherapy.

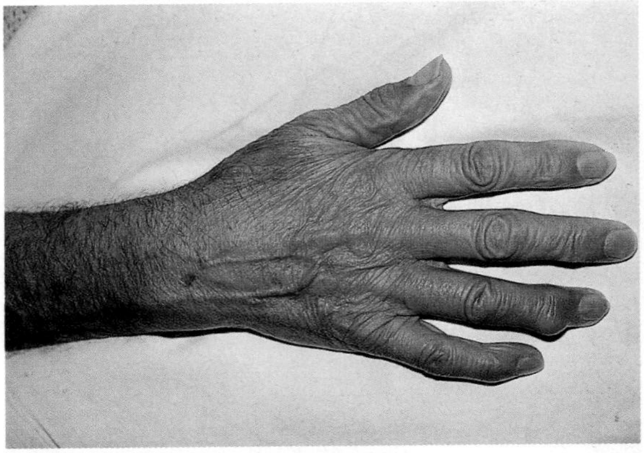

FIG. 2.13 Heberden's nodes.

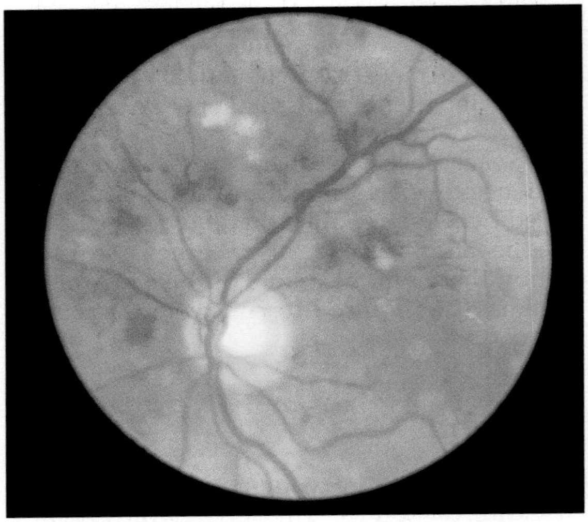

FIG. 2.14 The fundus in accelerated hypertension.

steroid therapy and in women with osteoporosis. In the hand, note:

- Pulse.
- Nails.
- Skin.
- Joints.
- Vascular changes.

Cardiovascular system

You will already have checked the pulse whilst looking at the hand but the following is a useful sequence:

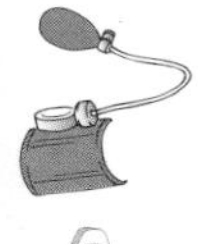

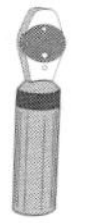

- Pulse – rate, rhythm, character and volume.
- Blood pressure.
- Evidence of heart failure. Right-raised jugular venous pressure, sacral and leg oedema, hepatomegaly, ascites. Left-crackles at the lung bases.
- Palpate precordium for abnormal pulsation.
- Note position and character of the apex beat and parasternal heave of right ventricular hypertrophy.
- Heart sounds, murmurs and exocardial sounds.
- Palpate peripheral pulses and note veins.
- Fundoscopy for hypertensive changes (Fig. 2.14).
- **Required:** sphygmomanometer and ophthalmoscope.

Respiratory system

You will already have inspected the hand for possible clubbing and cyanosis. Look for tremor that might be present with carbon dioxide retention. Note any respiratory distress or stridor. Then move to the neck to feel the position of the trachea. After this, examine the chest, front and back, by inspection, palpation, percussion and auscultation.

- Hands – clubbing, cyanosis, tremor.
- Respiration – character, rate, depth, evidence of stridor.
- Face – cyanosis, plethora, oedema associated with superior vena caval obstruction.
- Chest features – barrel shape, depressed sternum, asymmetry, scars, dilated vessels, skin lumps (Fig. 2.15).
- Palpate position of trachea.
- Inspect and palpate for chest movement and symmetry.
- Check for either tactile vocal fremitus or vocal resonance.
- Percuss the lungs.
- Auscultate the breath sounds; note added sounds.
- **Required:** peak flow meter.

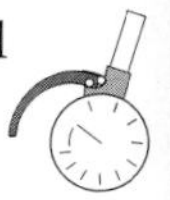

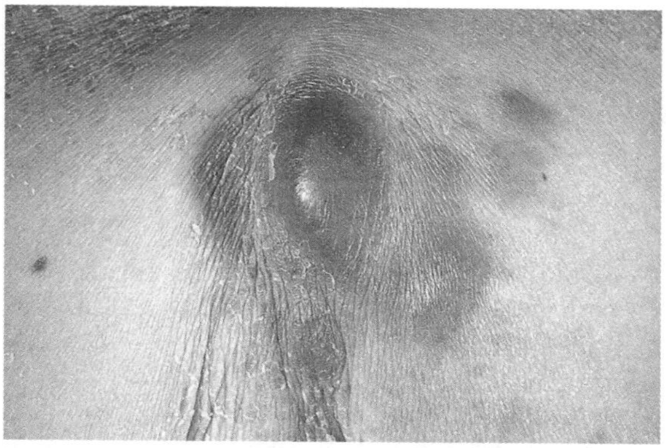

FIG. 2.15 Malignant deposits on the chest wall. In this woman the skin lumps were deposits of myeloma, a relatively rare physical sign.

Gastrointestinal system (including genitourinary)

The gastrointestinal tract includes the mouth, pharynx, rectum and anus, all of which are accessible for simple clinical examination. In patients with liver disease always look for evidence of systemic manifestations. Start the examination with the mouth and pharynx, then move on to the abdomen and complete your examination with inspection of the anus and rectal examination. Note that you will cover the examination of more general aspects of the genitourinary system at the same time.

- Jaundice.
- Stigmata of chronic liver disease – spider naevi, liver palms, white clubbed nails.
- Mouth and pharynx:
  - oral fetor,
  - lips,
  - tongue: appearance and degree of hydration,
  - teeth, gums and dentures,
  - oral mucosa,
  - tonsils.
- Abdomen:
  - abdominal wall – scars, distended veins, hernial orifices, umbilicus,
  - distension, visible peristalsis or pulsation,
  - palpation – tenderness, rigidity, release pain, enlarged liver, spleen, kidneys, distended bladder, abnormal masses, aortic pulsation,
  - percussion of liver, spleen, kidneys, bladder, shifting dullness,
  - auscultation: bowel sounds, bruits,
  - genitalia,
  - inspection of anus,
  - rectal examination,
  - vaginal examination if necessary.
- **Required:** tongue depressor, torch, glove for rectal examination.

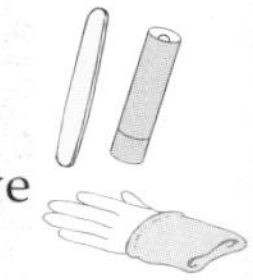

Central nervous system

There is less 'routine' in neurological examination than in any other system and in many patients assessment of general intelligence, memory, mood and level of consciousness is of crucial importance. Simple observation of the patient walking into and moving around the clinic room can be very informative. Abnormal movements may be immediately obvious, or may only appear at rest.

Begin with an overall assessment of intellect, memory and speech. Then go on to examine the patient from the head down starting with the cranial nerves moving to the neck, upper limbs, trunk and lower limbs.

- General:
  - cognitive functions, mood, emotional state,
  - conscious level,
  - speech,
  - involuntary movements.
- Cranial nerves in sequence, paying particular attention to:
  - pupillary reactions,
  - fundi,
  - eye movements,
  - hearing.
- Neck:
  - deformities,
  - stiffness.
- Abdomen:
  - abdominal reflexes,
  - state of bladder.

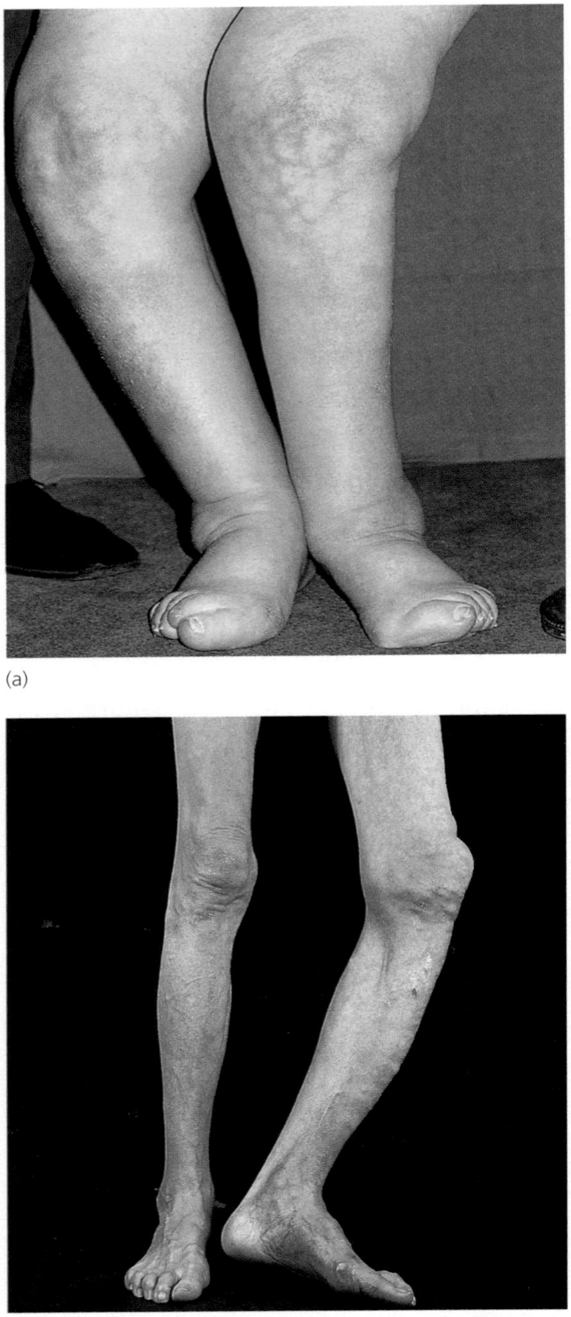

(a)

(b)

FIG. 2.16 Two conditions causing acquired deformity of the legs. (a) Bilateral osteoarthritis of the knees showing windswept legs. (b) Paget's disease of the left tibia. Note the swelling, and forward and lateral bowing of the bone.

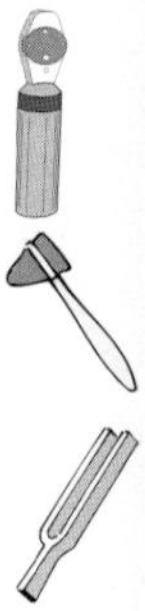

- Upper and lower limbs:
  - tone,
  - power,
  - co-ordination,
  - wasting,
  - reflexes,
  - sensation.
- **Required:** ophthalmoscope, tendon hammer, materials for testing the sensory modalities including tuning fork.

Musculoskeletal system

You will already have formed an overall impression of your patient's mobility. Examine the spinal movements first, then deal with the upper limb and lower limb in a systematic way, starting proximally at the shoulder and hip.

- Build and posture.
- Axial skeleton:
  - kyphosis, lordosis, scoliosis,
  - shortening,
  - rigid spine.
- Joints (Fig. 2.16a,b):
  - pain, swelling, limited movement,
  - record abnormal joints.

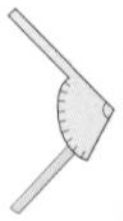

- **Required:** goniometer to measure joint movement.

Anaemia and the lymphatic system

You will already have covered most of this with your general assessment. Deal with the lymphatic system by palpating the nodes in order starting with the epitrochlear nodes, then progressing to axillae, the neck and finally the groins. Don't forget that the spleen, which will have been examined earlier, is part of the lymphatic system.

- Buccal and conjunctival mucosa for anaemia.
- Skin for purpura and ecchymoses.
- Epitrochlear, occipital, cervical, axillary and inguinal nodes.
- Spleen.

Putting it all together

Going through a physical examination in a systematic way takes time and may seem tedious or even unnecessary. Nevertheless, it is the only way to ensure that nothing is missed. With experience you will learn that, according to circumstances, parts of the examination may be omitted. For example, you are unlikely to perform a routine examination of the joints in an elderly man with a severe pneumonia; however, if his mobilization is slow, you will need to know if musculoskeletal problems are contributing to his delayed recovery.

Finally

It is sensible to finish off with a brief summary of the main points of the history and examination, taking no more than three lines. This will lead you nicely into a differential diagnosis, which will help you to decide what investigations are necessary to reach a definite diagnosis.

Revision Panel 2.6
Physical examination

Don't rush.

Make sure your patient is comfortable and understands what is going on.

Work systematically.

Don't be afraid to use a check list.

Utilize simple instruments to supplement your findings.

3 In practice

COMMON MISTAKES AND HOW TO AVOID THEM

Striking the right balance

So far we have emphasized the importance of performing a comprehensive, routine physical examination. The reason for this is to familiarize yourself with a workable sequence and to ensure that nothing is missed out. Once you have learned this it is essential to strike the right balance in emphasis. Clearly it is a waste of time examining sensation in the legs in great detail when your patient has developed jaundice after what sounds like an attack of biliary colic.

Nevertheless it would be highly relevant to assess carefully the cognitive state of a patient with worsening jaundice due to infective hepatitis. Experience alone will tell you how to strike the right balance.

Don't make things difficult for yourself

Most mistakes arise by hurrying through the examination:

- Do make sure that all the apparatus you need is to hand.
- Do allocate sufficient time to carry out a thorough examination.
- Don't rush.
- Don't cut corners by trying to examine a patient who is lying uncomfortably in bed and who is not suitably undressed.

Record only what you examine and what you find

There are many circumstances when there is insufficient time to complete a full examination. If for some reason you do not examine a particular system, say so. In the notes you might record this as:

- Central nervous system – Not examined.

Records must be accurate if they are to be meaningful so you should never record a minimum statement such as:

- Central nervous system – No abnormality detected.

This implies that you have carried out a full examination and found no significant abnormality. In other words, the nervous system is normal. It is better to describe what you actually examined:

- Fundi normal.
- Cranial nerves examined and normal.
- Upper and lower limbs: normal tone, power, co-ordination, reflexes and sensation.

If a patient later develops say a spastic paraparesis, it may help with a differential diagnosis to know that at a particular point in time both central and peripheral nervous systems had been comprehensively checked and were intact.

Avoid hedging your bets

Students often say that 'borderline clubbing is present' or that 'the optic disc edge is possibly blurred'. You cannot have it both ways. Try to come to a firm conclusion as to whether or not an abnormal physical sign is present. This does get easier with practice.

Don't invent physical signs that you think should be there

Very often the history points strongly towards a specific condition and some of the findings on examination confirm clinical suspicions. This does not mean that all the signs must fit. For example, consider an elderly man with angina who is found to have a loud systolic murmur over the precordium, radiating to the neck. Quite reasonably this raises the diagnostic possibility of aortic stenosis. Not infrequently students then invent a slow rising pulse (one of several features of severe aortic stenosis) when the pulse is normal. Not every supporting physical sign is required (or is present) to make a clinical diagnosis. It is diagnostic greed to expect every physical sign to be present in every patient.

Common errors in eliciting physical signs

These are dealt with in subsequent chapters but Revision Panel 3.1 lists a few examples.

Revision Panel 3.1

Some common errors made when assessing patients

System	*Error*	*Comment*
Cardiovascular	Assessing height of jugular venous pressure (JVP) using external jugular vein.	Use internal jugular vein.
	Assuming that the valves lie beneath those areas traditionally described as aortic, mitral, pulmonary and tricuspid areas.	See text (p. 57).
	Checking for oedema at ankles in a bedfast patient.	Look in sacral area.
Respiratory	Diagnosing longitudinally curved nails as clubbing.	See text (p. 74).
	Equating the term 'diminished air entry' with all causes of reduced breath signs.	Describe what you hear, not what you think the underlying cause is.
	Ascribing dullness and absent breath signs at the base to a pleural effusion when the liver is enlarged.	Check the other physical signs.
	Placing too much emphasis on tactile fremitus.	Never makes any difference to interpretation of physical signs.
Gastrointestinal	Overdiagnosing jaundice in Black people.	Sclerae often yellow in health.
	Regarding visible peristalsis as abnormal in the elderly.	Seen normally in thin old people.
	Feeling mass in right iliac fossa.	Caecum palpable in slim women.
Central nervous	Assessing pupillary reaction to light with torch directly in front of eye.	Patients look at light and accommodate. Shine light source from side.
	Looking for fasciculation of tongue with tongue protruded.	View tongue whilst still in mouth.
	Claiming reflexes to be absent without using reinforcement.	See text (p. 132).

Avoid introducing your own bias

Always record what you have found, not what you think you should find. This avoids introducing your own prejudices into the clinical arena.

Blood pressure (BP) is one measurement which is open to observer bias. Many students have a 'digit preference', especially for 'round' numbers. For example, they record blood pressures and pulse (P) rates in units of five or ten:

- BP: 120/85
- P: 90 per minute

If you take the trouble to measure these carefully, what you may find is that:

- BP: 124/86
- P: 94 per minute.

Perhaps the only clinical sign that does not require precise recording is respiratory rate. Here, it is usually sufficient to state that the rate is visibly faster than the observer's.

Only use well-accepted abbreviations

Unfortunately many doctors lapse into 'abbreviation speak'. Some of this passes off as medical 'shorthand' such as:

- The HP phoned to say that the SHO in A+E has admitted an MI with an SVT and a BP of 90/70 who has been having frequent attacks of PND and who is now in LVF.*

Using a language and shorthand known to members of a particular specialty but not necessarily to others is another form of shorthand. Unfortunately, it is not particularly elegant, may be confusing to the non-specialist and more important, it may be downright dangerous.

*The House Physician phoned to say that the Senior House Officer in Accident and Emergency has admitted a patient with myocardial infarction, plus supraventricular tachycardia and a blood pressure of 90/70, who has been having frequent attacks of paroxysmal nocturnal dyspnoea and who is now in left ventricular failure.

> Revision Panel 3.2
> **Emphasize relevant points**
>
> Don't waste time on superfluous detail.
>
> Avoid using abbreviations like NAD (instead of 'no abnormality detected').
>
> If you have not fully examined a system, record only what you did examine.
>
> Don't make up signs because you think they should be there.

A SIMPLE GUIDE TO WRITING UP EXAMINATION FINDINGS

The routine examination

There is no standard or perfect way of writing up findings from your clinical examination. Much depends on circumstances and individual preferences. Many doctors prefer to start with the system the history suggests may be at fault. This is essential when rapid assessment may be life-saving.

This section however provides a simple standard format with suggestions that will suffice for most non-urgent situations.

General appearance – the 'thumbnail sketch'

It is always useful to start with a short 'thumbnail sketch' to convey to anyone reading your notes what your overall impression of the patient was at that particular time. 'A lively, spirited 85-year-old widow who has clearly lost much weight' will immediately convey the sense that, though ill, this old lady is clearly going to make a fight of it. Contrast this with the bland comment 'Obvious loss of weight' which so often appears at the beginning of the notes.

Be careful about using what you may think are slick and coded comments such as 'Lacks cerebral neurons' – never assume that your patient (or their relatives) won't understand. You will also avoid embarrassment if an aggrieved patient and his solicitor request to see the medical records at some future date.

How to do it

Below are a few helpful ideas (Example 1). The left column shows how the physical findings might be recorded for an elderly retired steel worker who has been admitted to hospital as an emergency with severe breathlessness due to collapse of the right lung as a result of bronchial carcinoma. Set against this description, on the right, are comments with suggestions for alternative methods of recording findings which may be helpful in different circumstances.

EXAMPLE 1

Patient Mr PCL
11am, 2 May 1999

Whenever you examine a patient, make it a rule always to start your clerking with the date and time you saw the patient

On examination
General appearance
A somewhat emaciated, depressed but alert, grizzled, old man who is breathless at rest.
Cyanosed ++.
Gross loss of weight.
Not clinically anaemic.
T 37.5°C.

This thumbnail sketch helps personalize the record. It also makes the patient more memorable.

Whenever possible, record the current weight.

Record the temperature (T) This may well be recorded in the nursing observations but forms an important part of the medical record too. It is not enough to note 'T – normal'. Write down the actual result. If it is low, check with a low-reading thermometer and record that you have done so.

Alternative
You may record temperature, pulse, respiration and blood pressure at the beginning and cyanosis in the Respiratory section if you prefer.

Cardiovascular system
P: regular 90 per min, occasional extra beats.
BP: 124/78 right arm, sitting, Phase V.
JVP: not elevated.
No hepatomegaly, sacral or ankle oedema.
Apex beat 5th left intercostal space 10 cm from midline.
No abnormal praecordial pulsation.
Heart sounds 1 and 2 normal. No added sounds or murmurs.

Always record the position the patient is in, the limb in which blood pressure was measured.

You may abbreviate heart sounds as

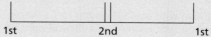

Respiratory system
Breathless at rest, respiratory rate 28/min.
No stridor or obvious wheeze.
Central cyanosis.
Gross 'drumstick' clubbing of fingers and toes.
No swelling of wrists or ankles.
Trachea deviated to right.
Chest movements reduced on right.
Generally dull percussion note over whole of right chest anteriorly and posteriorly.
Breath sounds reduced over right chest, especially at base.
Generalized inspiratory wheeze bilaterally.
Crackles at right base.

The chest signs may be recorded in a simple diagram.

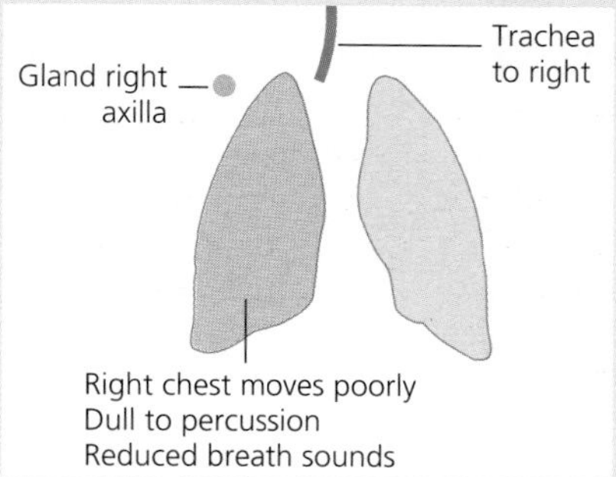

continued

Gastrointestinal system

Tongue dirty.
Edentulous.
Thin walled abdomen with visible peristalsis.
Liver (L), spleen (S) and kidneys (K) not palpable.
Rectal examination – large firm regular prostate.

Again, abdominal findings can be recorded in a diagram like this.

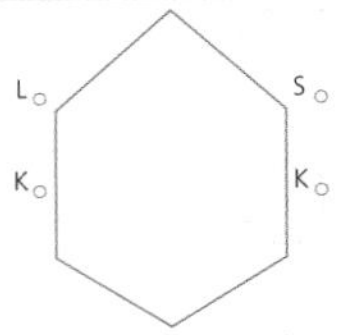

Central nervous system

Appears fully alert but intellectual function not tested due to general condition.
Speech normal.
Pupils react equally to light and accomodation.
Optic discs normal.
Nerve deafness on left.

Under other circumstances mental functions may well have to be examined in some detail – see Mini Mental Test (Chapter 13).

Musculoskeletal system

Limbs generally weak but no significant wasting.
Biceps, pronator, triceps, knee and ankle jerks all normal.
Flexor plantar response.
Sensation not tested. Patient fatigued.

Reflexes can be recorded as.

Reflexes	Right		Left
Biceps	+		+
Pronator	+		+
Triceps	+		+
Abdominal	+		+
		+	
Knee	+		+
Ankle	+		+
Plantar	+		+
	↓		↓

Lymphatic system

Enlarged gland in right axilla 2.5 cm diameter.

It is better to record size in cm rather than refer to fruit and vegetables for comparison.

In summary

An ill-looking man with obvious weight loss, a heavy smoker presenting with haemoptysis. Clinical signs of clubbing, node in axilla and collapse of right lung.

Try to sum up all the salient points in a few lines

Diagnosis

Carcinoma of bronchus causing collapse of right lung and metastatic lymph node in right axilla.

In other circumstances, where the signs are less obvious, a differential diagnosis may be more appropriate, listing the most likely cause first.

Revision Panel 3.3
Recording the physical examination

Record the date and time of examination.

Start with a 'thumbnail sketch'.

Set out your findings in a systematic way.

Add in diagrams where appropriate.

Try to devise a differential diagnosis at the end.

If you don't know what is wrong, say so.

'Good' and 'not-so-good' practice

As in most aspects of medical practice, there is no substitute for experience. Having taken a good history and having carried out a thorough examination, your efforts will have been wasted if you do not record your findings properly. As a general rule, 'if it is not written down, it wasn't done'.

The account doesn't have to be immensely detailed but it must include:

- All the significant positive physical signs.
- Any physical signs you looked for but did not find, bearing in mind your differential diagnosis.

The degree of detail recorded is a matter for experience. It is not necessary, for example, to list all the individual features of clubbing if it is obvious to all that the patient *does* have gross clubbing. However, if you note that both wrists are somewhat painful, hot and swollen as well, then it is essential to record this in view of the possible association with hypertrophic pulmonary osteoarthropathy.

Some general rules

Even if you are a most untidy person, always ensure that:

- You record the details immediately whenever you examine a patient.
- Whatever you write in the patient's notes is legible.
- Notes are kept tidy. Check and then file all test results correctly and promptly.
- Important results are recorded in a prominent place so they stand out. Red ink helps.
- If serial tests are requested (such as cardiac enzymes), write all the results together so that any rise diagnostic of heart attack is obvious.

Example of simple table to show serial 'cardiac' test results 'at a glance'

	Day 1	*Day 2*	*Day 3*
CK			
Troponin			

CK: creatine kinase.

- You leave some space in case you forget to record something.
- You never alter records retrospectively unless you also record the date of the alteration or addition clearly.

Practising writing up is as important as practising any other clinical skill – the more you do it, the easier it becomes. You will find it helpful to look at the way the doctors on your team write up their findings. You will quickly learn how important good medical records can be when you are called to review a patient you have never seen before who has suddenly deteriorated. Concise, well-laid out notes will let you get to grips with medical problems with a minimum of delay.

Practical Point

Remember

If it is not written down, it wasn't done.

How *not* to do it

Now we might look at how not to write up the physical findings. The following case is taken from an early attempt at clerking a patient.

In this case (Example 2) a middle-aged woman presented with a six-month history of loss of appetite, easy bruising and swelling of the abdomen. She consumed large quantities of alcohol but told the junior medical student that she only drank 'socially'. Though the signs are recorded correctly, the reader has no impression of her background or lifestyle from what is actually recorded.

Diagnosis

Ascites

The problem with this is that it might be describing anyone with ascites. In fact the comment 'Woman with ascites and jaundice' would convey as much as is in the notes. The writer is just not thinking 'on his feet'.

An opening statement of 'a dishevelled and unkept jaundiced middle-aged woman, smelling strongly of alcohol' not only presents a very clear image of the patient but also immediately directs attention to the possibility of alcoholic cirrhosis as the likely cause of her problems.

Next should follow a comment on any stigmata of chronic liver disease. Although 'spiders' have been mentioned, it would be helpful to know that there were 'numerous spider naevi, some confluent, distributed over the face, arms and trunk' and then a description of other stigmata of liver disease such as liver palms, white nails and clubbing.

In the abdomen, there is no mention of how much ascites, or the size, smoothness and regularity of the liver. The comment about the spleen, '? palpable', is worthless.

Practical Points

DO

Give a succinct overall description of your patient at the onset.
Concentrate on the abnormal signs.
Record other essential features such as blood pressure, temperature and pulse.
Emphasize negative signs if these have a bearing on the diagnosis.

DON'T

Waste time listing unrelated negative findings.

EXAMPLE 2

On examination

General appearance

Satisfactory.
Jaundiced. A few spiders.

Cardiovascular system

NAD
P: 72
BP: 120/80
Heart sounds: normal.

Respiratory system

NAD except clubbing.

Alimentary system

Distended abdomen due to ascites +. Liver enlarged.
? Spleen palpable. No masses.
PR negative.

Central nervous system

Grossly normal.
PERLA.
KJs and AJs Negative.

Diagnosis

Ascites

In the examination of the central nervous system one suspects that the examiner here has done no more than confirm that the patient is conscious by testing pupillary reaction and tapping the knee and ankle joints. Probably most students know that PERLA means 'pupils equal and react to light and accomodation' and KJ/AJ represent knee jerks and ankle jerks but a slavish addiction to abbreviations can often be frustrating and irritating to the reader.

Finally

On pages 33–37 some examples are given of notes taken by medical students, which have been annotated to identify good points and bad.

K M C

Consultant:......................................
Ward:..

Unit No:..........................
Surname:.........................
Forename(s).....................

Date & Time	IN-PATIENT CLINICAL NOTES
PC **date? time?**	66yr former publican with history of MI $3\frac{1}{2}$ years previously and 4 subsequent admissions for ↑SOB and palpitations presented with ↑SOB this evening **What was the diagnosis then?**
HPC	Sudden onset of ↑SOB at rest this evening similar to previous episodes Worse lying flat Not relieved by GTN; not worse on deep inspiration °CP °sweating °nausea °palpitations °Cough °sputum °wheeze °haemoptysis **What does this abbreviation mean?** Son brought her to A & E ↳ Given iv frusemide 50 mg + salbutamol/Atrovent via a nebulizer which improved SOB considerably **Could you devise a differential diagnosis from this history?**
good	Risk factors **for cardiac disease** MI Feb 1999 AF 2° to LVF April 1999 ↑BP ↑cholesterol Strong FHx of MI: father + 2 brothers died of MI in their fifties + mother died of a stroke Ex-smoker–4/12 ago (15/day for 50 years) °dm °rh. fever **Better not to use dm as an abbreviation for diabetes mellitus – not generally accepted**
SR	NAD
PMH	MI Feb 1999 (anticoagulated for mural thrombus) ↑bp 1994 TB–3 episodes (last one aged 32 years, treated with streptomycin + PAS) Arthritis in both legs Basal cell Ca on tip of nose, treated c̄ RT °dm °TIA °Rh fever °COPD °asthma **repetition**
FH	As above **not needed again**
DH	amiodarone perindopril 4mg od warfarin 4.5mg od **usually variable dosing** frusemide 40mg od simvastatin 20mg od GTN as required **What do these drugs do?** NB previously on sotalol for AF but this worsened her LVF on an earlier admission In May 1999 discontinued + started on amiodarone instead **good**

Kings Medical Clinic, University Hospital NHS Trust, Borchester

KMC

Consultant:......................................
Ward:...

Unit No:..........................
Surname:.........................
Forename(s)......................

Date & Time	IN-PATIENT CLINICAL NOTES
SH	Retired publican — **repetition** Widower 4 children, one c̄ Down's syndrome, lives locally Lives alone in a bungalow Independent + active — **repetition** Ex-smoker - quit 4/12 ago (15/day for 50 years) ° Alcohol — **unusual for a retired publican? worth a comment?** Anxious +++
O/E	Looked well, able to complete sentences ✓ GCS 15, alert orientated 36)C° (° J ° A ° Cy ° Cl ° O ° L) — **These are unacceptable abbreviations which aren't generally known**
CVS	Pulse 80 AF, Apex N, Parasternal heave JVP → ° carotid bruits BP 130/70 — **arm? position? phase?** HS I, II+0 All pulses present 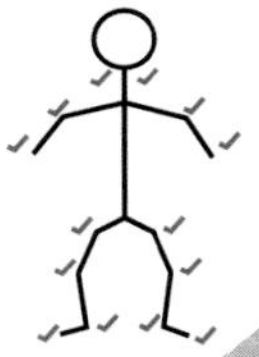
RS	RR 16 Trachea central CE R = L AE R = L Mild expt wheeze Bibasal creps to midzones PN-resonant TVF/TVR N 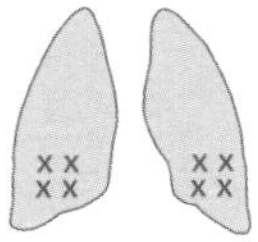
GI	° Distension ° Discolouration (° AA) ° Herniae ° Masses ° Organomegaly ° AB soft, nontender ° BS 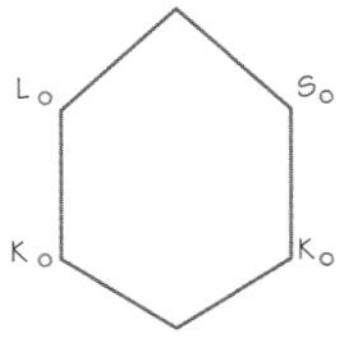
CNS	CGS = 15, alert, orientated, All 4 limbs moving **A lot of abbreviations!** **Summary?** **Differential diagnosis?** **Tests required?**

Kings Medical Clinic, University Hospital NHS Trust, Borchester

K
M
C

Consultant:......................................

Ward:...

Unit No:..........................

Surname:.........................

Forename(s)......................

Date & Time	IN-PATIENT CLINICAL NOTES
4/6/99	ECG: AF Q-wave in a VL ? ST in V_4 - V_6
	CXR: bilat. widespread patchy shadowing R>L Pulmonary oedema
	This is your "clinical impression" and what you are treating as cause of symptoms, based on results of tests
	Bloods: Acute LVF +/– superimposed infection? Repeat ECG Urea 10 ↑ Ck 70 WCC 16.3 ↑ LDH 549 INR 158 ALP 99 Cr 119 ↑ AST 23 Na 140 GT 34 U 3.9 ALB 33 Bilirubin 7
5/6/99	Acute LVF resolved Chest clear Pulse 60 reg JVP → HS I, II + 0
	good *you might add 1) whether treatment has been changed 2) precipitating factors:* *myocardial infarction?* *rhythm abnormality?* *myocardial pump failure?* *all triggered by infection?*

Kings Medical Clinic, University Hospital NHS Trust, Borchester

K M C

Consultant:......................................

Ward:...

Unit No:..........................

Surname:.........................

Forename(s).....................

Date & Time		IN-PATIENT CLINICAL NOTES
6.6.99.		72y ♀
		Severe CP
	HPC	Woke up on Friday night with chest pain spreading through to her back + L arm
		This settled down and eventually she returned to bed
		Saturday am the pain started again
		Central crushing chest pain
		↳ Back + L arm as before
		Made worse by lying flat
		Not relieved by Gaviscon
		Assoc w mild SOB (° palpn ° nausea ° sweating)
		On Sunday morning the pain ↑ severe
		10/10 pain score assoc w nausea + cold sweats
	SR	NAD
		(except occ palpn + ankle swelling (in hot weather)
	AMH	OA 1991
		↑ bp 1991
		° Dm ° asthma ° TB ° TIA ° MI ° COPD
		° Operations
		Otherwise relatively fit and well
	FH	Nil of note
	DH	NKA
		On admission:
		Inderal 160 mg od
		co-proxamol
		co-amilofruse
	SH	Lives with husband and son, daughter lives locally.
		Cares for husband who is wheelchair bound.
		Ex-smoker (50 yrs ago; can't recall amount)
		Alcohol.
		Self-caring + independent

Annotations:

- **abbreviations!** (on "72y ♀ / Severe CP")
- **When was this? 2 days ago? 1 week ago? Be specific** (on "Woke up on Friday night")
- **good** (on "Central crushing chest pain")
- **Aggravating and alleviating factors can be helpful with diagnosis** (on "Made worse by lying flat / Not relieved by Gaviscon")
- **good** (on "10/10 pain score assoc w nausea + cold sweats")
- **Was this the first problem? Or was this one of many previous episodes? Always record any previous events. If you are not sure if "cardiac" ask about alternative causes of chest pain-e.g. peptic ulcer, reflux, musculoskeletal.**
- **Make a new section on "cardiac risk factors" if you suspect coronary disease**
- **Include: Smoking, diabetes mellitus, hypertension, cholesterol, family history, previous angina/ heart attack, other vascular disease**
- **You have not recorded dose frequency for most of these**
- **Good social history**
- **How much alcohol?**

Kings Medical Clinic, University Hospital NHS Trust, Borchester

K
M
C

Consultant:......................................
Ward:..

Unit No:............................
Surname:..........................
Forename(s).......................

Date & Time	IN-PATIENT CLINICAL NOTES

O/E

Well
Pain ↓ c̄ GTN — **Not required here**
Pulse 70 regular
Sats 95% O/A — **Does this mean "saturation 95% on air"? or does it mean 95% saturation on admission? Beware abbreviations!**
° J ° A ° Cy ° Cl ° O ° L
Apyrexial
Poor dentition

CVS

Pulse 70 reg; BP 170/90 — **Record which arm, position of patient + phase**
Apex N parasternal heave — **Do you mean normal?**
JVP →
HS I, II+O — **"+ No murmurs"**
Peripheral pulses present

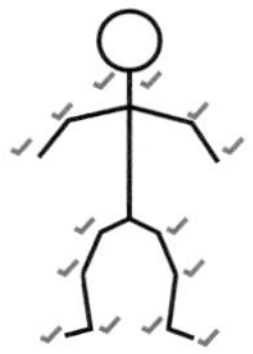

In view of history of hypertension + pain radiating to back, did you consider aortic dissection? Important to record blood pressure in each arm.

RS

RR 18/min
Trachea central — **Abbreviations! What does CE/AE mean?**
CE R = L
AE R = L, vesicular BS
Few creps bibasally
° Wheeze

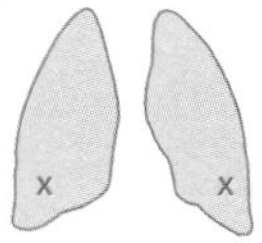

GI

Obese
° Masses
° Organomegaly
Ab soft, nontender
BS ✓

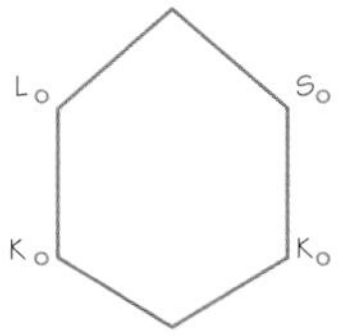

CNS

Not formally assessed

You have omitted Summary; Differential diagnosis; List of investigations requested. What did you think was the cause of her symptoms? Your differential diagnosis was probably myocardial infarction; unstable angina, aortic dissection.

CXR

Cardiomegaly AP film

ECG

NSR, 94 per min
Imm ST ↑ V_2–V_4
Early T inversion in ant leads
↳ Anterior MI

Plan

Admit for 5/7
Reg nitrate, aspirin, diuretics
Start ACE tomorrow
Check cholesterol, fasting gluc
Serial CE and ECGs

Kings Medical Clinic, University Hospital NHS Trust, Borchester

Practical Point

Personalize your description of the patient.

Make up your mind about physical signs – are they present or not?

Think about and revise your differential diagnosis as you carry out your examination.

Try to avoid abbreviations.

Practical Point

It is much easier to recall the important features of an illness when you have seen a patient than if you try to remember information from a textbook.

HOW TO PRESENT A CONCISE HISTORY ON A WARD ROUND

Many students become very anxious when asked to present a patient's history and examination findings to the entire medical team on a ward round. Most doctors will be sympathetic, providing that you have done your homework and suitably prepared your notes.

The idea is to give other members of the medical team (who may not have seen the patient before) a synopsis of the patient's history, important examination findings, working diagnosis, test results and progress. It is also an opportunity to show how your skills are developing. This is not the time to find that your notes are chaotic, illegible or incomplete.

- Practise your presentation skills in front of your fellow students. This will make 'the real thing' less stressful.
- Speak in a clear and (hopefully) confident voice. Everyone in the team needs to hear.
- Nervousness may make you speak a little faster than normal. This will get better with practice.
- Don't be concerned that the version of the story you have obtained differs slightly from others. Patients do recall more information when the same question has been asked several times.
- Report the patient's presenting complaint using the patient's own words.
- Aim to describe more precisely in what order and when symptoms developed. Making sense of apparently disjointed 'facts' is part of the skill you will need to develop.
- Do include recognized precipitating or risk factors, anything which may provoke symptoms. This affords an opportunity to assess the risk of recurrent disease after discharge.
- Do mention any features of the family and social history* which may affect present or future care.
- Do not report *every* operation or hospital admission the patient has had unless these have a direct bearing on the current illness. For example, sudden onset of breathlessness with chest pain worse on inspiration is suggestive of a pulmonary embolus; a history of hip replacement surgery two weeks previously is highly relevant, but gallbladder removal ten years previously is not.
- Do bear in mind that the situation may have changed since you first interviewed the patient.
- Try to avoid reading everything word for word. Present salient features but be prepared to expand should the boss want more detail. Don't be afraid of making eye contact with your supervisor, so remember to look up every now and then. As you gain confidence, you will reach a stage where your notes are used less and less and you will be able to present the major features from memory.

---

*Some consultants like a potted social history first – this puts the disease and patient in some sort of context.

Revision Panel 3.4
Common mistakes

Your first presentations will:

Be too long (because you don't know what to leave out).

Be too vague (because you don't know what to put in).

Not help with diagnosis (because your knowledge of disease is 'thin').

Be disjointed (because taking a history requires practice).

If you know that you may be asked to present, try to read your notes before attending the ward round. It will impress if you can simply use your notes as a 'back-up' because you described most of the history from memory.

Although you may have recorded the responses to every question you asked, many of these will bear little on the major problem, so, in a patient with a heart problem, whenever possible dismiss these with a statement such as 'there were no symptoms suggestive of significant respiratory, gastroenterological or neurological disease'. Cutting corners like this saves time.

Mistakes are inevitable. You may not have got to the bottom of the main problem; the patient's answers may make little sense and you can't put all the bits together. Regular practice in history taking and in presentation soon leads to a skill which once learned is never forgotten.

Talking with the acutely ill patient

Having built up a battery of experience with patients in clinic or on a ward, at some time you will need to learn to talk to patients who are acutely ill. This is discussed fully in Section B of this book, but the important points are:

- There is often insufficient time to take a comprehensive history.
- There may not be any history available.
- There may not be time to examine the patient fully.
- Your course of action is dictated by the likely diagnosis, the circumstances, the age of the patient and the speed of onset of the illness.

Taking a history from an acutely ill patient is difficult. There are several reasons for this:

- The patient may be in pain or confused.
- The patient may be very ill.
- The patient may have no patience for a student.
- You may feel embarrassed at being 'slow'.
- Relatives may be anxious.

It is very important that you learn how to cope with all of these problems. As a house officer you will be expected to see any patient who warrants it.

The best strategy is the simplest – learning by watching. You will gain much by accompanying a junior house officer on 'medical take' who will look for visual clues to disease while asking the patient questions and perhaps taking blood for tests at the same time. Senior house officers are often particularly adept because they are refining their skills in readiness for their higher postgraduate exams.

It may appear a haphazard process, but with time, experience and confidence you will soon appreciate how to save time taking a history and examining a sick patient and when you can (safely) cut corners.

It is also helpful to listen to doctors presenting to a registrar or consultant on ward rounds. You may be surprised that much detail is omitted. You shouldn't assume that many questions have been forgotten during the clerking. It is simply that much of the information is not relevant to the immediate problem.

Understanding body systems

B

Making sense of cardiovascular disease

4

The relationship between anatomy, physiology, symptoms and clinical examination is seen more clearly in the cardiovascular system than in any other system, often enabling a firm diagnosis to be made at an early stage.

The anatomy of the cardiovascular system is fairly accessible, which means that much can be learned from physical examination, and the investigations of cardiovascular disease produce images that are easy to understand in anatomical and physiological terms.

SYMPTOMS OF CARDIOVASCULAR DISEASE

Cardiovascular problems cause four main symptoms:

- Pain.
- Breathlessness.
- Ankle swelling.
- Palpitations and syncope.

None of these is limited to cardiovascular disease and a 'differential' diagnosis always has to be considered.

Pain

This can be experienced in any muscle that becomes ischaemic. If the coronary arteries are narrow there may be sufficient blood flow to oxygenate the heart muscle at rest, but insufficient to supply the extra oxygen demand of exercise. Heart muscle then becomes painful and exercise-induced ischaemic pain is called angina. Complete blockage of a coronary artery causes a similar pain, but this is more severe and persists longer.

Practical Point

Features of angina are:

Central chest pain which may also radiate to the arms, back, throat and jaw.

The pain comes on with exertion and is relieved with rest.

It is worse after heavy meals and in cold weather.

If the blood supply to the leg muscles is adequate at rest but provides inadequate oxygen for exercise, because of blockage of peripheral vessels, a cramp-like pain develops called 'intermittent claudication'. Increasing ischaemia can cause pain at rest, and eventually gangrene (Fig. 4.1).

Chest pain can come from any structure within the chest but its characteristics differ depending on its origin (see Revision Panel 4.1).

Breathlessness

When breathlessness is due to cardiac disease it is usually first noticed only on exertion, but with increasing disease it occurs more and

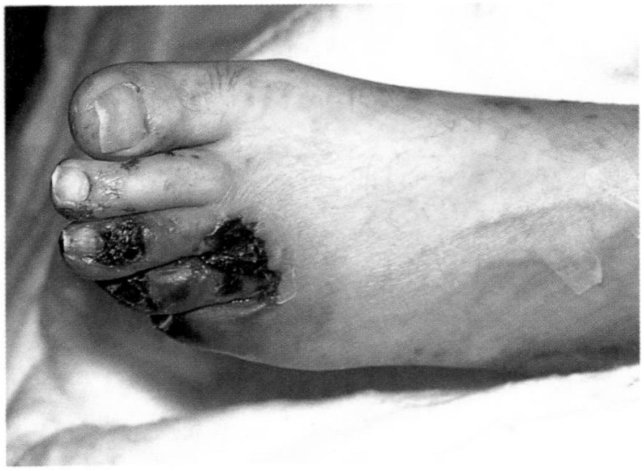

FIG. 4.1 Gangrene of the foot.

more easily until eventually it is present at rest. Severity of breathlessness may be easily classified on a four-point scale (New York Heart Association), in which NYHA grade I describes mild breathlessness and NYHA IV severe breathlessness with symptoms at rest.

Cardiac breathlessness is sometimes associated with wheezing; the old-fashioned (and confusing) term for this was 'cardiac asthma'. Breathlessness is due to congestion of the lung capillaries with blood, the result of high left-ventricular end-diastolic pressure, which in turn raises left atrial, pulmonary vein, and pulmonary capillary pressure. This causes the lungs to become stiff. In severe circumstances the haemodynamic capillary pressure exceeds the plasma oncotic pressure so fluid leaks into the alveoli causing pulmonary oedema. The patient may then cough up thin, frothy, blood-tinged fluid.

Orthopnoea

The inability to lie flat because of breathlessness is characteristic of heart disease. A high left atrial pressure (usually the result of high left ventricular pressure at the end of diastole, but sometimes due to mitral stenosis) makes it difficult for blood to enter the left atrium. If the patient sits up a hydrostatic 'head' of pressure will be available to help blood flow from the upper parts of the lung to the left atrium, aided by reflex redistribution of flow to the

Revision Panel 4.1

The origins of chest pain

Cause of pain	*Characteristics of pain*
Cardiac ischaemia	Central, tight, radiates to arms, back, neck, jaw.
▪ Chronic stable angina	Predictable on exercise and relieved by rest. Worse in cold or windy weather, induced by emotional stress, rapid relief by glyceryl trinitrate.
▪ Unstable angina	Similar to chronic stable angina but occurs at rest.
▪ Myocardial infarction	Similar distribution of pain but persistent, much more severe and often associated with nausea and vomiting.
Pericarditis	Localized anterior central pain, worse on breathing and lying flat.
Aortic dissection	Usually sudden onset, severe with radiation to the back.
Pleural pain	Lateralized, worse on breathing and associated with cough.
Oesophageal pain	Central, may radiate to back, worse on eating and associated with vomiting.
Spinal pain	Mainly in the back but may radiate round to front in a nerve root distribution.
Skin pain	Usually due to 'shingles' (herpes zoster), a blistering, scabbing, and scarring rash in nerve root distribution.
'Musculo-skeletal'	Usually localized to left side of chest, with chest wall and joints between sternum and costal cartilages particularly tender to palpation.
'Non-specific' chest pain	Often a similar distribution to chronic stable angina but seldom severe, not predictable, and not affected by cold, wind or emotional stress and may persist for hours.

upper zones. Conversely, of course, venous return from the lower lobe is worse, and it is here that oedema fluid collects.

Breathlessness has many causes other than cardiac disease, including:

- Obesity.
- Lack of physical fitness.
- Anxiety – a 'need to take a deep breath'.
- Lung disease – infective, obstructive (such as tumours) or intrinsic (alveolitis, pulmonary embolus).
- Severe anaemia.

These are discussed in Section C.

Ankle swelling

This occurs when the venous pressure (the haemodynamic pressure within veins and capillaries) exceeds the oncotic (osmotic) pressure of the blood. This is common in old people who spend much time seated but it is important to remember that ankle swelling can develop in normal people who have been sitting still for a long time as in long journeys.

Cardiovascular disease causes ankle swelling in two ways: from venous disease and from heart failure. The history may not be helpful in separating these except that ankle swelling due to heart failure is symmetrical and painless, while in venous disease it is asymmetrical and often painful.

Ankle swelling is also a feature of a low plasma albumin, which causes a low plasma oncotic pressure and is made worse by varicose veins.

Palpitations and syncope

Different people use the words 'palpitations' and 'syncope' in different ways. Normally an individual is unaware of his or her heart, so 'an awareness of the heart beat' is the best definition of palpitations. Syncope means collapse, usually with loss of consciousness, but without any features suggesting an epileptic fit.

Palpitations and syncope can only be understood with reference to the electrocardiogram (ECG) and a final diagnosis can only be made if an ECG is recorded at the time a patient actually has the symptoms of which he complains. However, a clear description of a patient's symptoms is essential.

When a patient complains of palpitations he may be describing one of three things, each with its own characteristics:

- An undue awareness of the normal rhythm – sinus rhythm.
- Extra beats – extrasystoles or 'ectopics' as they arise from an ectopic, or abnormal, focus in the heart.
- Sustained tachycardia – or paroxysmal tachycardia that comes and goes.

Since most people will be asymptomatic at the time they are actually seen, the patient's description of the original symptoms becomes very important (Revision Panel 4.2).

Revision Panel 4.2
Patient description of palpitations

Heart rhythm	*Patient description*
Sinus rhythm	Heavy regular beats that speed up and die down as when running upstairs; noticed at times of stress.
Extrasystoles	Heart beat irregular and unable to count the rate, sensation of 'missed beat' or 'jumping into the throat'; often at rest or lying down at night; made worse by smoking, alcohol, coffee or tea.
Paroxysmal tachycardia	Sudden onset of rapid heart beat 'too fast to count' or, if counted, more than 140 per minute; may be regular, or irregular if atrial fibrillation; associated with chest pain, breathlessness or dizziness. Characteristically stops suddenly, but often described as dying away.

Syncopal attacks may be associated with complete heart block, when they are called 'Stokes–Adams' attacks. In complete block the

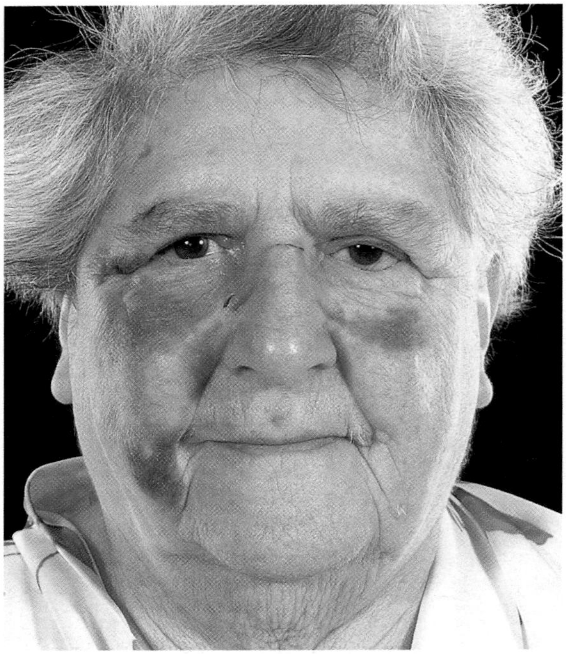

(a)

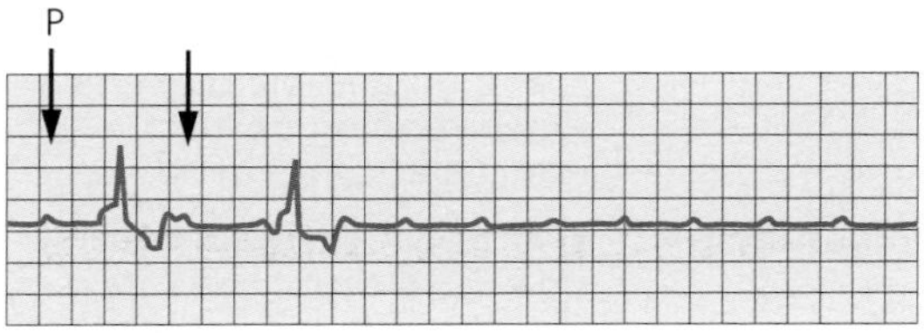

(b)

FIG. 4.2(a) This woman collapsed without warning, falling forwards and injuring her face. (b) The cause is shown on her ECG tracing – complete heart block followed by ventricular standstill.

ventricular rate is always slow and an inadequate output may cause breathlessness at rest. However, if the rate slows further the patient may collapse to the ground (Fig. 4.2) and subsequently even have a fit due to inadequate oxygen supply to the brain. During the attack the patient is characteristically pale, but flushes red on recovery.

Most people with syncopal attacks do not have complete heart block. The differential diagnosis includes:

- Simple faints – these can be recognized from the circumstances in which they occur (unusually hot or crowded places). They always occur while standing.
- Micturition syncope – occurs after getting up in the night to urinate.
- Postural hypotension – this causes dizziness on standing up, due to blood volume loss or drugs given for hypertension.

THE REST OF THE HISTORY

There may be clues to the diagnosis of cardiovascular disease in the systems review, the family history, the social history, and above all in the past history, so you should have a pretty good idea of the diagnosis before you begin to examine the patient. When the present problem seems to follow an episode in the past this should, of course, be included under 'History of the presenting complaint'.

Practical Point

Most people with syncopal attacks do not have complete heart block but heart block is a diagnosis that must not be missed.

Past history

Things to enquire about include:

- Rheumatic fever in childhood – usually described as a long illness with painful joints and much time off school. 'St Vitus Dance' – abnormal involuntary movements – can be part of this.
- Heart murmurs heard while undergoing a routine medical examination.
- Previous heart attacks and angina.
- Previous palpitations.

Systems review

Direct questions relating to symptoms and systems other than the cardiovascular system may reveal symptoms that are actually due to,

Revision Panel 4.3

A check list for the 'systems review' for a patient with cardiovascular disease

System	*What the patient may complain of*	*Possible cardiovascular interpretation or association*
Respiratory	Breathlessness. 'Asthma'. Wheezing at night. Coughing up sputum or blood.	Left ventricular failure. Pulmonary emboli. Mitral stenosis.
Gastrointestinal	'Heartburn'. Vomiting. Anorexia or weight loss. Jaundice.	Angina. Digoxin toxicity. Infective endocarditis. Hepatic congestion due to cardiac failure.
Nervous	Headache. Visual problems. Dizzy turns and blackouts.	Severe hypertension. Cranial arteritis. Cerebral emboli. Tachy- and brady-arrhythmias.
Renal and urinary	Urinary infections. Blood in urine.	Chronic pyelonephritis → hypertension. Renal emboli, endocarditis.
Musculoskeletal	'Growing-pains' in childhood.	Rheumatic fever leading to chronic rheumatic disease.
	'Arthritis'.	Aortic incompetence and/or pericarditis due to systemic lupus erythematosus.
	Painful back.	Aortic incompetence due to ankylosing spondylitis.

or are associated with, cardiovascular disease (Revision Panel 4.3).

Family history

Ischaemic (coronary) heart disease does run in families, but a family history is only significant when close relatives have had a heart attack before the age of 50.

Social history

Smoking is the main cause of arterial (both peripheral and coronary) disease and it takes ten years for the excess risk to disappear on stopping smoking.

While a small regular amount of alcohol protects against heart attacks, heavy drinking is a cause of hypertension, atrial fibrillation, and heart muscle disease (cardiomyopathy).

THE PHYSICAL EXAMINATION

Examination of the cardiovascular system should be performed in four stages:

- General appearance.
- Physical signs associated with the arterial circulation.
- Physical signs associated with the venous circulation.
- Physical signs associated with the heart itself.

In each stage it is important to think logically and to relate the findings to the anatomy and physiology of the circulation. Although the usual sequence of 'inspection, palpation, percussion and auscultation' should be remembered, these four methods of examination have variable importance in each stage.

General appearance

From the end of the bed check for:

- Signs of pain – is the patient uncomfortable, pale, sweating?
- Breathlessness – is there any audible wheeze or visible distress?
- Position in bed – is the patient lying comfortably or does he or she feel the need to sit up?
- Cough – look in the sputum container to see what the patient has coughed up, looking especially for blood (haemoptysis).
- Cyanosis – this gives the patient a blue or purplish colour. Central cyanosis affects the mouth, lips and tongue and indicates a predominance of deoxygenated haemoglobin in the circulation due to heart failure, a right-to-left intracardiac shunt (see below), chronic lung disease, or polycythaemia. Peripheral cyanosis, affecting only the hands or feet, indicates sluggish blood flow through the skin with high oxygen extraction.
- Amputation of a limb – although this may be due to previous trauma, it may indicate peripheral arterial disease or embolization.
- Fever – this is seen for a day or two after a myocardial infarction, but is persistent in infective endocarditis.
- Finger clubbing – in its extreme, finger clubbing includes curvature of the finger nails both laterally and longitudinally, filling in of the nail fold angle, sponginess of the nail bed, and sideways widening of the distal phalanges. Clubbing is present when any two or three of these features are present. Clubbing associated with central cyanosis indicates cyanotic congenital heart disease with shunting of blood from the right side of the heart to the left; without cyanosis it may result from infective endocarditis. It is a non-specific sign that occurs in many cancers, longstanding infections like bronchiectasis and many other chronic lung and gastrointestinal conditions (see Revision Panel 5.6).
- Splinter haemorrhages – these are linear red or black streaks under the finger or toenails (Fig. 4.3). These are usually due to trauma but may be a sign of infective endocarditis.

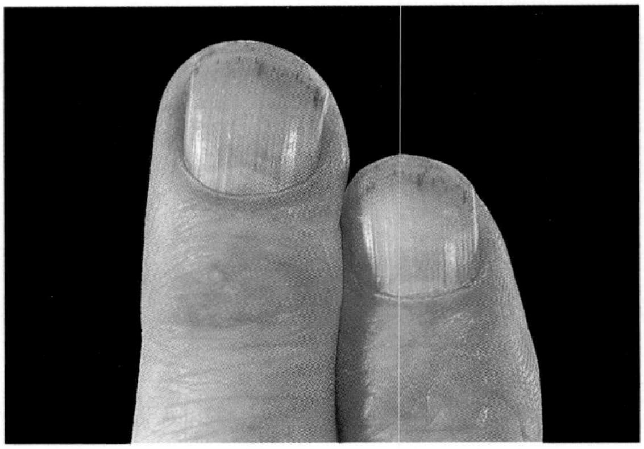

FIG. 4.3 Splinter haemorrhages.

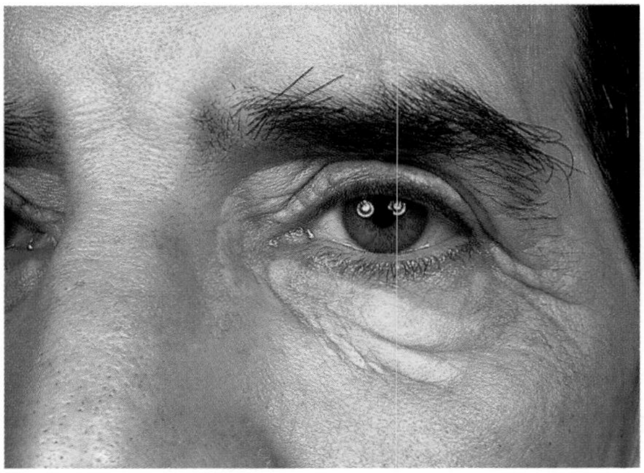

FIG. 4.4 Xanthelasma.

- Anaemia – check the mucous membranes (conjunctivae and nail beds for pallor). Anaemia may explain breathlessness and can contribute to angina.
- Lipid deposits – patients with high plasma cholesterol levels may develop deposits around the eyes (xanthelasma – Fig. 4.4). High cholesterol levels are a risk factor for coronary disease, so the presence of lipid deposits provides indirect evidence of ischaemia.
- Signs of specific diseases – some diseases or syndromes that may be associated with cardiovascular problems can be recognized from the end of the bed. Some are listed in Revision Panel 4.4.

Revision Panel 4.4

'Spot diagnosis' – syndromes associated with cardiovascular disease

Syndrome	*Cardiovascular problems*
Chromosomal	
Down's.	Septal defects.
Endocrine	
Thyrotoxicosis.	Atrial fibrillation, heart failure.
Myxoedema.	Angina, pericardial effusion.
Acromegaly.	Enlarged heart, heart failure.
Addison's disease.	Hypotension.
Musculoskeletal	
Marfan's syndrome.	Dissection of aorta.
Ankylosing spondylitis.	Aortic regurgitation.
Rheumatoid arthritis.	Pericarditis.
Scleroderma.	Cardiomyopathy.
Paget's.	High output heart failure.
Miscellaneous	
(such as alcoholism)	Cardiomyopathy.

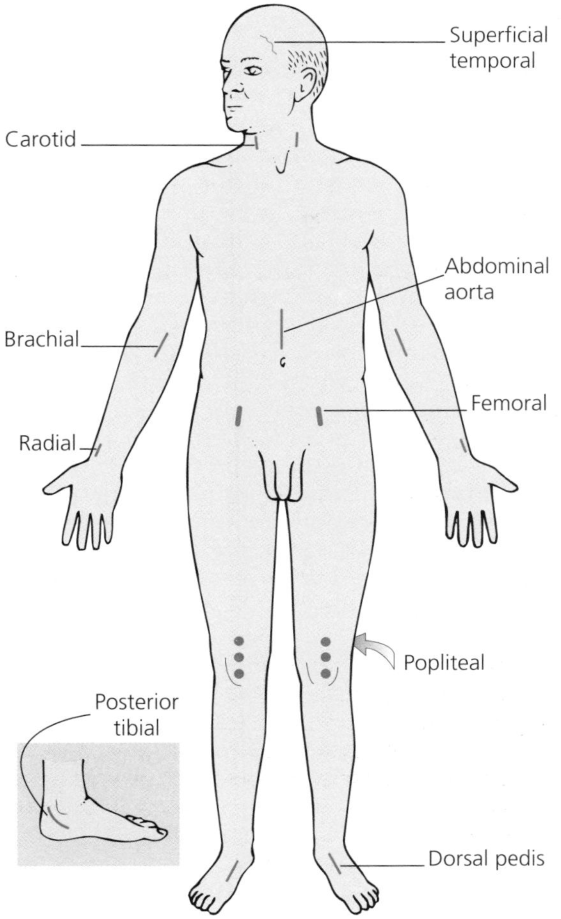

FIG. 4.5 The site of the main arterial pulses. Palpation of the leg pulses is of critical importance in patients with peripheral vascular disease. The dorsalis pedis artery can be felt along a line from midway between the malleoli to the proximal part of the first metatarsal space. The posterior tibial artery can be palpated midway between the medial malleolus and the prominence of the heel.

Examination of the arterial circulation

When an artery is close to the surface of the skin it can be felt as a 'pulse'. Characteristics of pulses that should be recorded are:

- Presence or absence.
- Rate.
- Rhythm.
- Character.
- Presence of bruits.
- Blood pressure.

The pulses that should be identified are the superficial temporals, carotids, brachials, radials, abdominal aorta, femorals, popliteals, dorsalis pedis and posterior tibials (Fig. 4.5).

First note and record whether all the pulses can be felt. Absence suggests the artery may be blocked by atheroma and thrombosis or by an embolus. The superficial temporal arteries have a special significance in that they can be affected by an inflammatory disease called temporal arteritis (see also Fig. 26.3). This makes the arteries painful and tender, and often causes them to thrombose so that pulsation is lost.

The pulse character, best felt in the carotid arteries, describes the arterial pressure waveform. With practice and by comparison with your own pulse you can appreciate that in some patients the rise in pressure is unusually slow (a sign of aortic valve stenosis) and that in others the pressure falls away rapidly (as in aortic regurgitation).

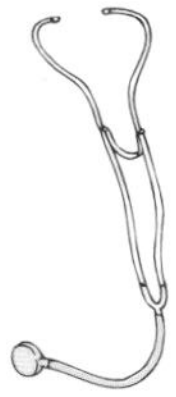

Bruits are systolic ' rushing' sounds due to turbulent blood flow. These are usually due to narrowings caused by atheromatous plaques, but also occur with other causes of narrowing such as aortic coarctation, or with abnormal connections (fistulae) between arteries and veins. Listen for bruits with a diaphragm of the stethoscope over the carotid ateries, the aorta, and the femoral arteries.

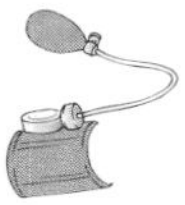

The blood pressure (properly, the arterial pressure) cannot be assessed simply by feeling the pulse. Blood pressure is measured with a sphygmomanometer which applies a variable pressure to the upper arm to find out how much is needed to impair blood flow.

Fat arms take more compressing than thin ones, so a record made in a fat arm may give a spuriously high value for the blood pressure. For this reason large cuffs should be used in fat people.

Practical Point

Ensure that the whole of the arm is surrounded by the inflatable part of the cuff.

To measure the blood pressure:

- Place the cuff fairly tightly round the upper arm.
- Ensure that the brachial artery is at the same level as the heart.
- Find the brachial pulse by palpation at the elbow.
- Inflate the cuff until the brachial pulse can no longer be felt.
- Place the diaphragm of the stethoscope over the position of the brachial pulse.
- Reduce the pressure in the cuff slowly, by not more than 2 mm per heart beat. The pressure in which the pulse can first be heard is the systolic pressure, the highest pressure generated by the heart.
- Continue to reduce cuff pressure slowly. The intensity of the pulse sound will increase and then change character, becoming 'muffled'. Reducing the pressure by a few more mm of mercury will lead to the pulse sound becoming inaudible.

The different sounds heard during the measurement of blood pressure were first described by Korotkoff, who thought there were five different sounds or phases. Korotkoff's first sound is the first that can be heard as the pressure of the sphygmomanometer cuff is reduced, and corresponds to the systolic pressure. The second and third sounds are of no clinical value and are now only of historic interest. Only the fourth, the point of muffling and the fifth, the disappearance of the sound, are of practical value.

The point of disappearance is closer to true diastolic pressure and furthermore it is the more reproducible of the two measurements. The point of disappearance should therefore be recorded as diastolic pressure.

Practical Point

Phase V is closer to true diastolic pressure, is reproducible and is the preferred diastolic pressure.

Examination of the venous circulation

In the clinical examination the important features of the venous circulation are:

- The peripheral veins.
- The jugular venous pulse.
- The size of the liver, which becomes enlarged as the venous pressure rises.
- The presence of peripheral oedema.

As with the examination of the arterial part of the circulation, it is best to think of the venous features as a set and group these physical findings together.

The peripheral veins

Superficial peripheral veins can usually be seen in the hands and feet. In the legs, superficial veins may be unusually prominent, tortuous and enlarged and they are then called 'varicose'. These abnormal veins may become thrombosed due to inflammation and this is called 'superficial phlebitis': the affected vein can be seen as a tender red cord under the skin. Phlebitis is usually associated with peripheral swelling, or oedema (fluid collecting in the interstitial tissues). Varicose veins can bleed into the skin and can ulcerate; patients who have had varicose veins for years may have a brownish discoloration of the skin due to repeated bleeding.

The deep veins of the legs are within the main muscle mass and therefore cannot be seen or felt. They can become thrombosed at times when the blood is hypercoagulable and the patient is immobile – typically after surgical operations, childbirth or trauma when the leg is immobilized in plaster. The physical signs of a deep vein thrombosis (DVT) are extremely unreliable. However, for what they are worth the signs are:

Swelling of the leg Symmetrical swelling of both legs is likely to be due to heart failure or a low plasma albumin level, but when the legs are a different size a DVT becomes more likely. The circumference of the thigh and calf should be measured with a tape measure, the thigh at a defined distance above the anterior tibial tubercle, and the calf at the point of maximum circumference.

Pain When the muscle mass containing the affected vein is squeezed the patient complains of unusual pain. In the presence of a venous thrombosis of the calf, sharp dorsiflexion of the foot will be painful (Homan's sign). Eliciting this sign is not comfortable, can be dangerous and should be avoided.

Warmth Comparison of the legs will usually reveal that the leg with a DVT is warmer to touch than a normal leg. This is because the returning venous blood is diverted through the superficial veins which become more prominent.

Discoloration A leg with a DVT is usually bluish in colour, though when the thrombosis is very severe marked swelling may prevent arterial flow into the leg and this can cause a 'white leg'.

Although DVT usually affects the legs, the major veins of the arms can also be thrombosed, particularly after trauma or when invaded by a tumour in the axilla or mediastinum.

The jugular venous pulse

The jugular veins show a pulsation that is important for two reasons:

- Their positions reflect the pressure within the right atrium.
- The wave form of the pulsation helps in the diagnosis of a variety of quite different conditions.

The abbreviation JVP is sometimes used to mean 'jugular venous pulse' and sometimes to mean 'jugular venous pressure'.

Because there is no valve between the jugular veins and the right atrium, the veins in the neck act as a dynamic manometer: the height of the column of blood above the heart measures right atrial pressure and the pulsations reflect pressure changes in the right atrium.

There are two jugular veins on either side of the neck, internal and external. (Fig. 4.6).

The internal vein runs deeply from the sternoclavicular joint upwards and laterally to the angle of the jaw, thus passing underneath the external jugular vein running from the midpoint of the clavicle upwards to cross the sternomastoid muscle obliquely. Although easily seen when distended, the external vein may give a false idea of the right atrial pressure because venous blood flow may be obstructed

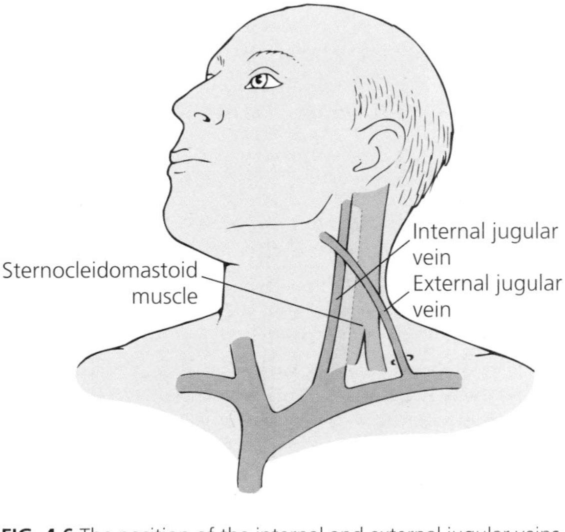

FIG. 4.6 The position of the internal and external jugular veins in relation to the sternocleidomastoid muscles.

as the vein passes through the fascia under the clavicle. For this reason the internal jugular vein should be identified whenever possible.

The jugular veins can be identified more easily by asking the patient to perform a Valsalva manoeuvre, a forced expiration against a closed glottis (tell the patient to 'strain as if opening the bowels'). The increased intrathoracic pressure raises right atrial pressure and the jugular veins become distended.

The jugular venous pressure

The measurement of any pressure requires a reference point and in the case of the jugular venous pressure this should properly be taken as the centre of the right atrium. The right atrium cannot, of course, be approached directly by clinical examination but its centre lies 5 cm vertically below the manubriosternal angle whatever the position of the subject (Fig. 4.7). The right atrial pressure can therefore be measured (in cm of blood) by adding 5 cm to the vertical height above the manubriosternal angle to which the jugular veins are distended. The normal right atrial pressure is 5 or 6 cm of blood so this is usually discounted and the jugular venous pressure is measured using the manubriosternal angle as the reference point.

It is essential to appreciate the importance of measuring the *vertical height* of the jugular venous pressure above the manubriosternal angle. In a normal subject the right atrial pressure is such that the jugular veins are not distended at all on sitting upright, but on lying down the veins may be filled for the whole of their length. On the other hand, in a patient with severe heart failure the right atrial pressure may be so high that the jugular veins are distended up to the angle of the jaw or above even when the patient sits upright. There is therefore *no set position* for the patient in which the venous pressure should be measured: the patient should simply be asked to recline at whatever angle makes the top of the column of blood in the jugular veins most obvious.

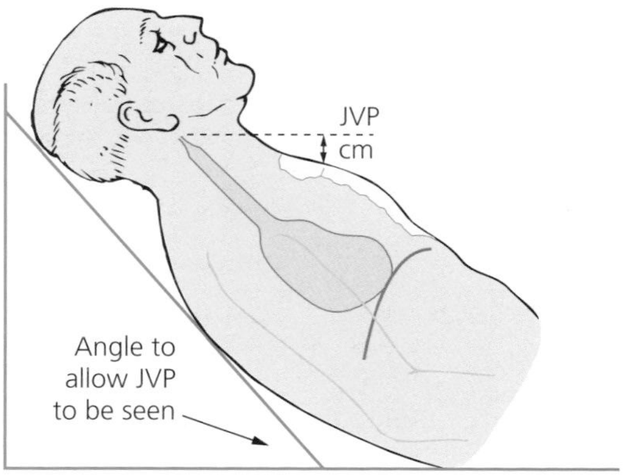

FIG. 4.7 The height of the jugular venous pulse.

> **Practical Point**
>
> *Assessing jugular venous pressure*
>
> Put patient in a reclining position (not necessarily 45 degrees) so that you can best see the top of the venous column.
>
> Measure the vertical height of the JVP above the manubriosternal joint.
>
> Use the internal jugular vein.
>
> View the pulsation obliquely.

Jugular venous pulsation

The jugular venous pulsation reflects the sequence of pressure changes within the right atrium, but the waveform of the venous pulse is complicated by transmission of a pulse from the carotid artery that runs adjacent to the internal jugular vein. The venous pulse therefore has three components (Fig. 4.8).

- The 'a' wave is due to atrial contraction: it is accentuated when right atrial pressure is high as in pulmonary hypertension and it is lost when atrial activity is disorganized by atrial fibrillation
- The 'c' wave is transmitted from the carotid artery
- The 'v' wave occurs while the tricuspid valve is shut and is therefore associated with atrial filling. It may in part be caused by upward doming of the valve as the right ventricle contracts. When the tricuspid valve is incompetent, the blood flow due to right ventricular systole is partly ejected back into the right atrium, and the 'v' wave

is accentuated. Because the mechanism of the 'v' wave is different under these circumstances it is sometimes called a 'systolic wave'.

The fall in venous pressure after the 'a' wave is called the 'x' descent and that after the 'v' wave is called the 'y' descent.

The pulsation in the jugular vein can most easily be appreciated at the top of the distended part of the vein. As with the measurement of the jugular venous pressure, it is important to place the patient *in whatever position makes this most obvious*. Examination can be markedly helped by arranging a light to fall tangentially across the neck.

The pulsation in the jugular vein can easily be confused with carotid artery pulsation because these structures are adjacent. The various pulsations can be distinguished in the following ways:

- An arterial pulsation can be felt, unlike venous pulsation which is usually impalpable except in tricuspid regurgitation (see below).
- Gentle pressure just above the clavicle will readily obliterate a venous pulsation and the vein will fill above the point of pressure. An arterial pulsation will not be affected.
- Jugular vein pulsation is best seen at the limit of venous distention, so its position in the neck will change when the patient sits up or lies down.

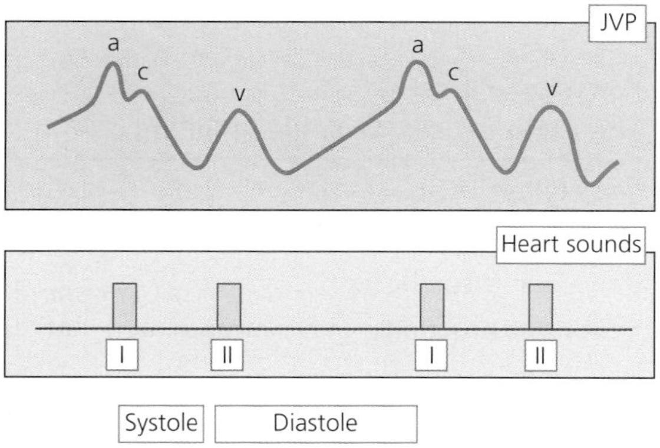

FIG. 4.8 The components of the jugular venous pulsation. Only the 'a' and the 'v' waves are detectable clinically.

- Deep inspiration reduces intrathoracic and therefore right atrial and jugular venous pressures. The position of the venous pulsation therefore moves downwards in the neck on inspiration and upwards on expiration. The position of an arterial pulse is unaffected.
- There are no valves between the superior vena cava, the right atrium, the inferior vena cava and the hepatic veins. Thus if pressure is applied over the liver just below the ribs, blood will be expressed from the liver and the right atrial pressure will rise with a consequent rise of the jugular venous pressure and pulsation. This is called 'hepatojugular reflux'.
- The pulse waveform in the carotid artery is a simple 'up and down', but that of the jugular venous pulse is more complex. Even though it can be difficult to identify the *individual* components of the venous waveform it is usually quite easy to make out rapid oscillations at the top of the venous column.

Conditions that can be diagnosed from the jugular venous pulse

Heart failure If the jugular venous pressure is greater than 6 or 7 cm above the middle of the right atrium (that is more than 2 or 3 cm above the manubriosternal angle), the filling pressure of the right atrium is abnormal and 'heart failure' may be present. When making this diagnosis it is important to ensure that the jugular veins are pulsating and that the height of the jugular venous pressure is affected by position and expiration. If this is not so the distension of the jugular veins may not reflect right atrial pressure and may be due to obstruction to venous return by a mediastinal tumour, such as lung cancer.

Tricuspid regurgitation A prominent 'v' wave which collapses due to a deep 'y' descent indicates tricuspid incompetence. A systolic wave is also generated by the right ventricle in the inferior vena cava and hepatic veins, so causing liver distension and pulsation.

Heart block In complete heart block the atria contract independently of the ventricles, so the 'a' waves in the jugular venous pulse are not regularly followed by 'c' or 'v' waves. At times the right atrium will by chance contract against a closed tricuspid valve, and when this happens the whole of the right atrial stroke volume will be expelled up the superior vena cava. This will cause a sudden and marked single pulsation in the neck called a 'cannon wave'.

Practical Point

Cardiac conditions that may be diagnosed from the JVP

Diagnosis	Effect on JVP
Heart failure	Raised JVP.
Tricuspid regurgitation	Prominent 'v' wave which collapses due to a deep 'y' descent.
Heart block	Cannon wave.
Pulmonary hypertension	Prominent 'a'wave.
Constrictive pericarditis	JVP rises instead of falls on inspiration.

Pulmonary hypertension High pressure in the pulmonary artery due, perhaps, to recurrent pulmonary emboli, causes a rise in right ventricular pressure and so a rise in right atrial pressure. The 'a' wave is then prominent and can be seen as a regular 'flick' in the jugular pulse. The same appearance is seen when right atrial pressure is high independently of the right ventricular pressure, for example in tricuspid valve stenosis or rarely when an atrial tumour or myxoma occludes the tricuspid valve.

Constrictive pericarditis The pericardium is usually a thin structure that has no influence on the performance of the heart. In some chronic diseases, typically tuberculosis but also with collagen disease or after viral inflammations of the pericardium, the pericardium becomes thickened and stiff. On inspiration the pericardium is pulled down by the diaphragm, and the heart is compressed. Instead of the usual fall in venous pressure on inspiration the jugular venous pressure rises, and at the same time the reduced inflow to the heart reduces left ventricular output and systemic pressure falls. These abnormal responses to inspiration are called venous and arterial paradox.

The liver as part of the venous circulation

The back pressure from a high right atrial pressure will be transmitted to the liver via the inferior vena cava and the hepatic veins. The liver becomes engorged (congested) with blood and is enlarged. In health, the liver lies entirely beneath the ribs on the right side and cannot be felt. In the presence of chest disease the diaphragm is pushed down, making the liver edge palpable. Percuss the chest to define the upper margin of the liver. In heart failure this will be in the normal place. The degree of liver enlargement should be expressed as a number of centimetres below the right costal margin.

A congested liver is tender and this is one characteristic feature that distinguishes hepatic enlargement due to heart failure from that of most primary liver diseases. Congestion of the liver can cause an ache in the upper abdomen, particularly in long-standing tricuspid regurgitation. Prolonged heart failure can be a cause of jaundice and in extreme cases there may be splenic enlargement.

Peripheral oedema

A combination of raised venous pressure and the hydrostatic pressure due to the height of

Revision Panel 4.5

The main causes of ankle swelling

Immobility.

Venous insufficiency (varicose veins).

Deep vein thrombosis.

Venous obstruction – pelvis or abdomen.

Lymphatic obstruction.

Low plasma albumin.

Heart failure.

Idiopathic oedema (mainly in women).

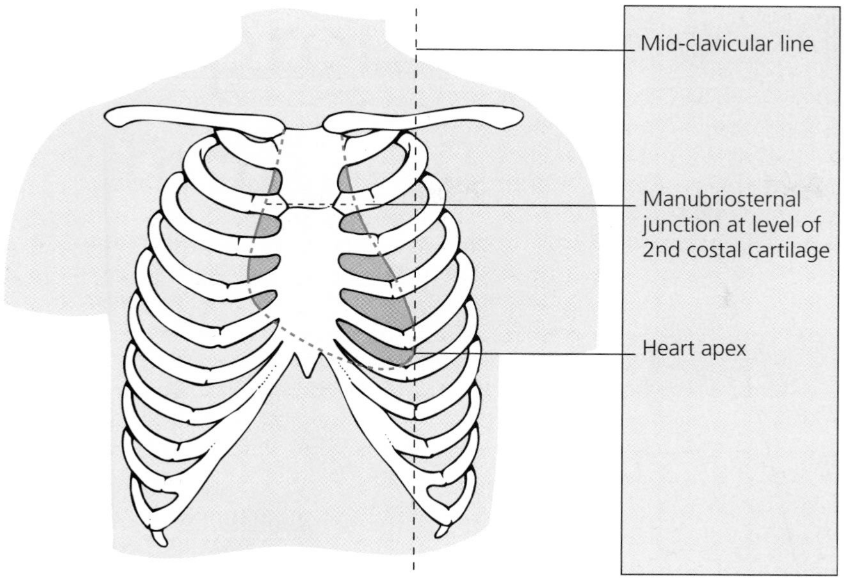

FIG. 4.9 The position of the heart in the chest (anterior view).

the heart above the feet means that in patients with heart failure fluid collects first around the ankles. The ankles are swollen and on moderately firm pressure an imprint of the fingers is left which gradually fills in. The ankle swelling of heart failure is symmetrical, unlike that resulting from venous obstruction in the leg. When patients lie in bed the most dependent part of the body is the sacrum and buttocks and fluid may collect here as readily as round the ankles. However, you should remember that most patients with ankle swelling do not have heart disease (Revision Panel 4.5).

The lungs as part of the circulation

One of the early manifestations of heart failure is a rise in the left atrial pressure. This causes an increase in the pulmonary capillary pressure and so to an engorgement and stiffening of the lungs, leading to breathlessness and sometimes an audible soft wheeze. With increasing left atrial pressure the oncotic pressure of the blood may be exceeded and fluid will then leak into the alveoli. This produces *crackles*, initially at the lung bases but spreading throughout the lung fields as heart failure increases. These crackles must be differentiated from those due to pneumonia or fibrosing alveolitis; the best way of making this distinction is from other evidence of cardiovascular disease in the history or from the examination.

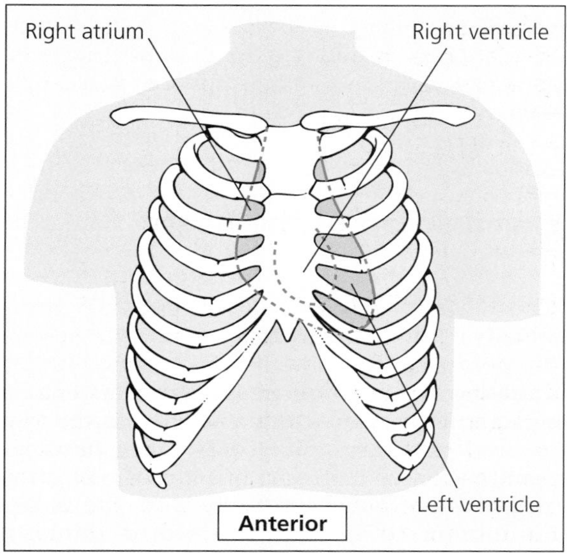

FIG. 4.10 The position of the chambers on the front of the heart.

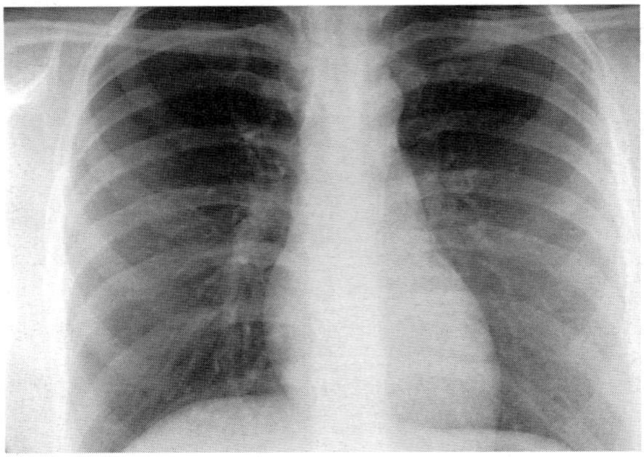

(a)

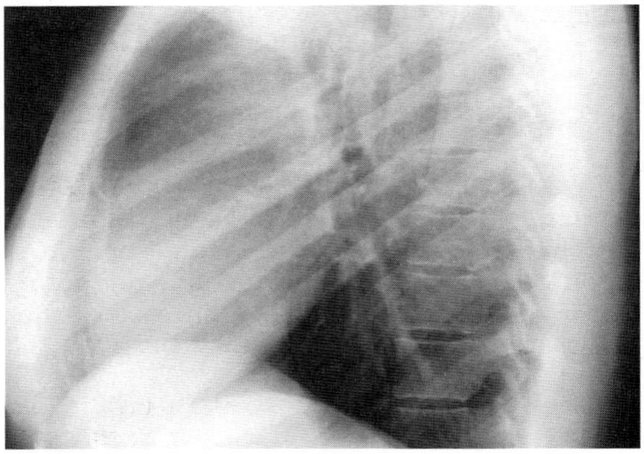

(b)

FIG. 4.11 Posterior anterior (a) and lateral (b) X-rays of the heart.

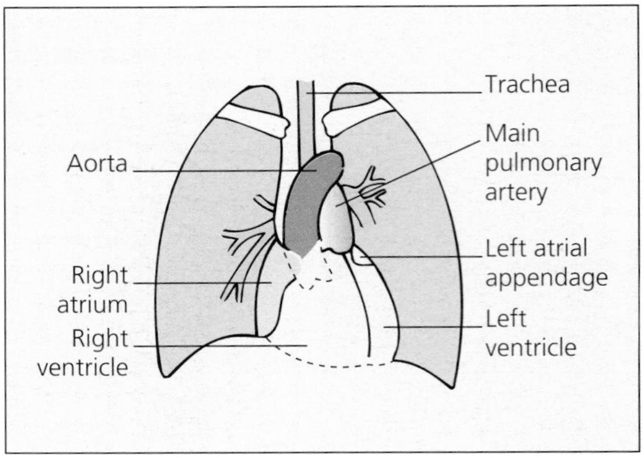

(a)

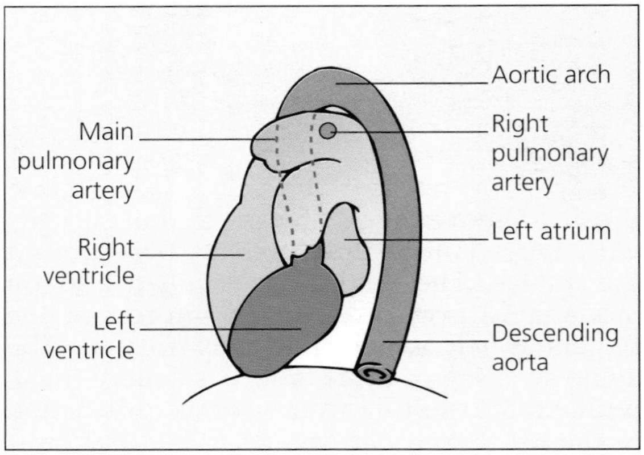

(b)

FIG. 4.12 Outlines of the chambers of the heart from the postero-anterior (a) and lateral (b) X-rays.

Examination of the heart

The position of the heart in the chest

Knowing the position of the heart, its chambers and its valves within the chest is the key to understanding not only the physical examination of the heart but also the electrocardiogram, the chest X-ray and the echocardiogram. It is therefore worth thinking about basic anatomy before discussing the physical signs in the heart that can be detected on clinical examination.

Seen from the front, the heart is roughly triangular in shape. The heart lies mainly beneath the sternum, with its base projecting just to the right of the sternum and the apex being in the left side of the chest directly below the mid-point of the clavicle (the 'mid-clavicular' line). The cardiac apex is usually in the fifth rib interspace (Fig. 4.9).

The cardiac apex forms the most important single physical sign in the cardiovascular system as its position indicates the size of the heart. The cardiac apex beat is defined clinically *as the furthest point out from the mid-line and the furthest point downwards where the heart beat can be felt*; this point corresponds reliably

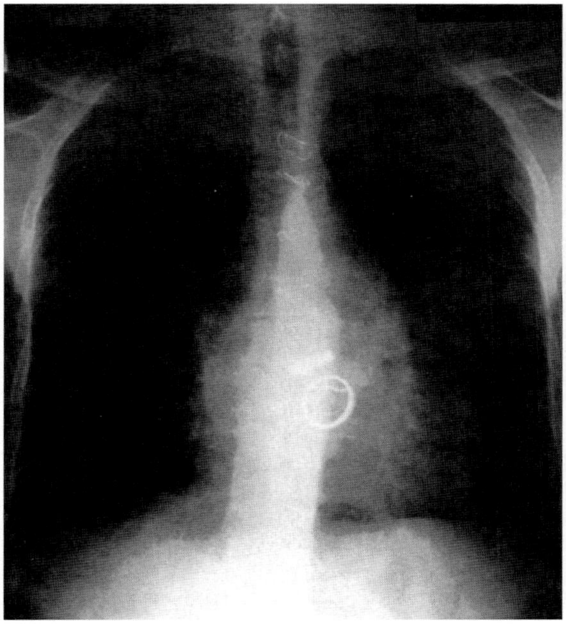

(a)

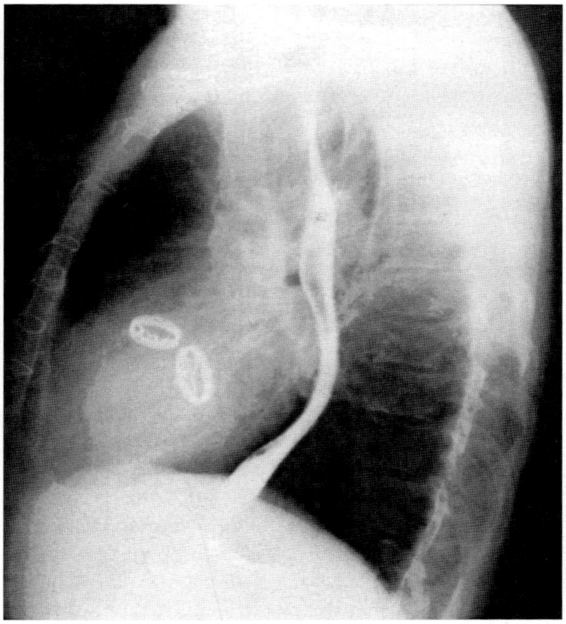

(b)

FIG. 4.13 The position of the mitral (lower) and aortic (upper) valves demonstrated by an X-ray of artificial valves. Note the presence of barium in the oesophagus which outlines the left atrium. Posteroanterior (a) and lateral (b) films.

with the position of the true cardiac apex. Note that it is not necessarily the same point where the cardiac impulse can most easily be felt: this is sometimes called the 'point of maximum impulse' but this is not useful as it does not necessarily identify heart size.

The cardiac apex is normally formed by the left ventricle. (Fig. 4.10). The left ventricle lies to the left of, and behind, the right ventricle. *Left ventricular enlargement* shifts the cardiac apex outwards and downwards, making the apex beat forceful and easy to localize. The right ventricle occupies most of the front of the heart and lies beneath and just to the left of the sternum. *Enlargement of the right ventricle* pushes the cardiac apex outwards and so brings the heart more into contact with the sternum. This can be felt to lift with each heart beat.

The right atrium forms the right border of the heart as seen from the front, but even when enlarged it seldom projects much to the right of the sternum. The left atrium lies at the back of the heart and does not form part of the cardiac silhouette seen from the front. In the side view it forms the upper part of the posterior heart border and is adjacent to the oesophagus.

Figure 4.11 shows a chest X-ray from the front (a) and the side (b). The plain X-ray does not allow separation of the different heart chambers nor does it show the valves, but in Fig. 4.12 (a,b) the position of the chambers is outlined. The position of the valves is most graphically demonstrated in an X-ray (Fig. 4.13a,b) of a patient with artificial heat valves. The aortic and mitral prostheses lie close to the middle of the heart, seen from the front, and both are beneath the sternum.

The position of the ventricles, the left atrium and the aortic and mitral valves are readily seen by echocardiography. One of the standard views is the 'long axis' which makes a slice of the heart from base to apex. Figure 4.14 shows the right ventricle in front and the left ventricle and left atrium behind. The close proximity of mitral and aortic valves is clearly seen.

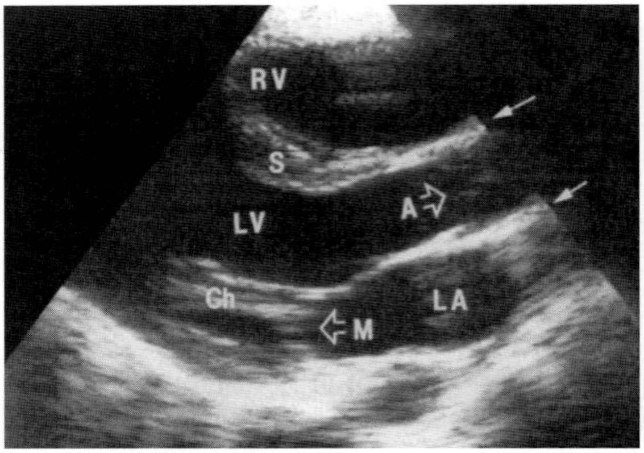

(a)

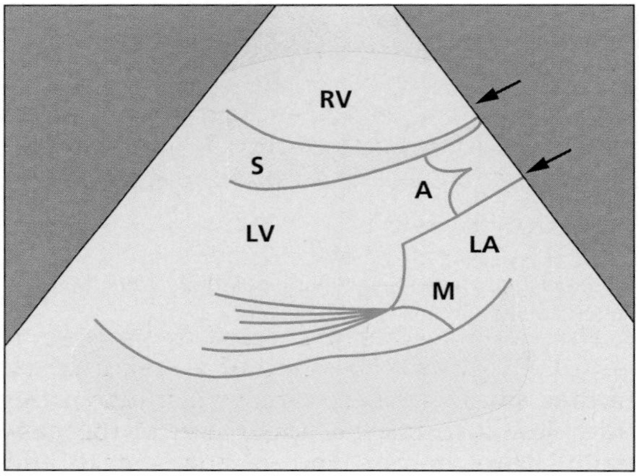

(b)

FIG. 4.14 (a) Echocardiogram showing the long axis of the heart. RV and LV: right and left ventricles; S: septum; Ch: chordae. Open arrows indicate aortic (A) and mitral (M) valves. The slim arrows indicate the walls of the aorta. (b) Diagram of Fig. 4.14(a).

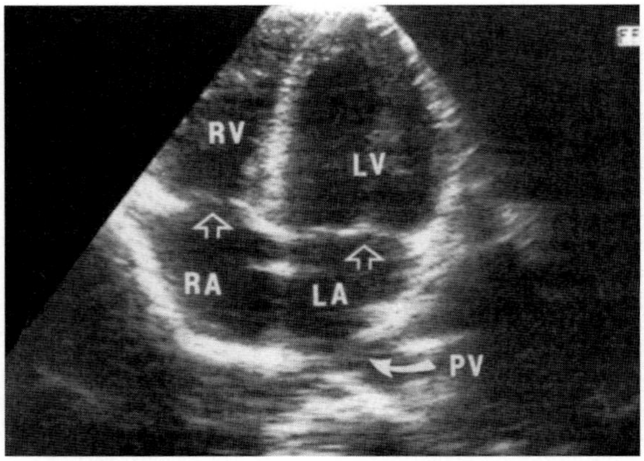

(a)

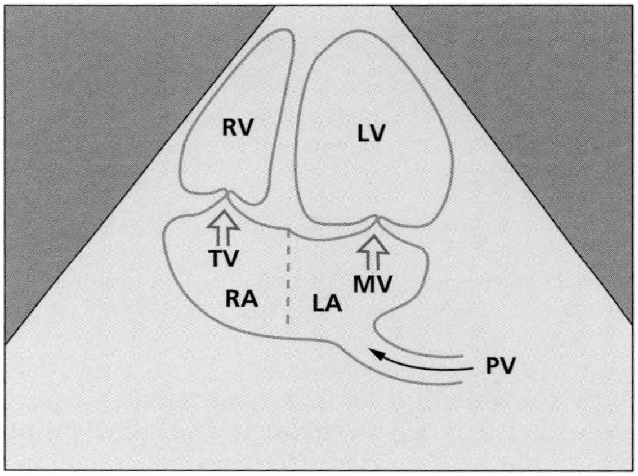

(b)

FIG. 4.15 (a) Echocardiogram viewing the heart from the apex. RA and LA: right and left atria; RV and LV: right and left ventricles; PV: pulmonary veins. (b) Diagram of Fig. 4.15(a). Open arrows indicate tricuspid valve (TV) and mitral valve (MV).

Another standard echocardiographic view with the echo probe at the cardiac apex produces a horizontal 'slice' through the heart showing the four chambers and the mitral and tricuspid valves. This view does not include views of the aortic or pulmonary valves (Fig. 4.15).

Magnetic resonance imaging (MRI) can also be used to demonstrate the position of the chambers of the heart (Fig. 4.16a). The diagonal position of the septum, with the anterior position of the right ventricle, also explains the positions used for the chest leads of the ECG: leads Vl and V2 'look at' the right ventricle, leads V3 and V4 'look at' the septum, and leads Vs and V6 the left ventricle (Fig. 4.16b).

How to examine the heart

Inspection and percussion

Usually the heartbeat cannot be seen so any visible pulsation is probably abnormal. It is

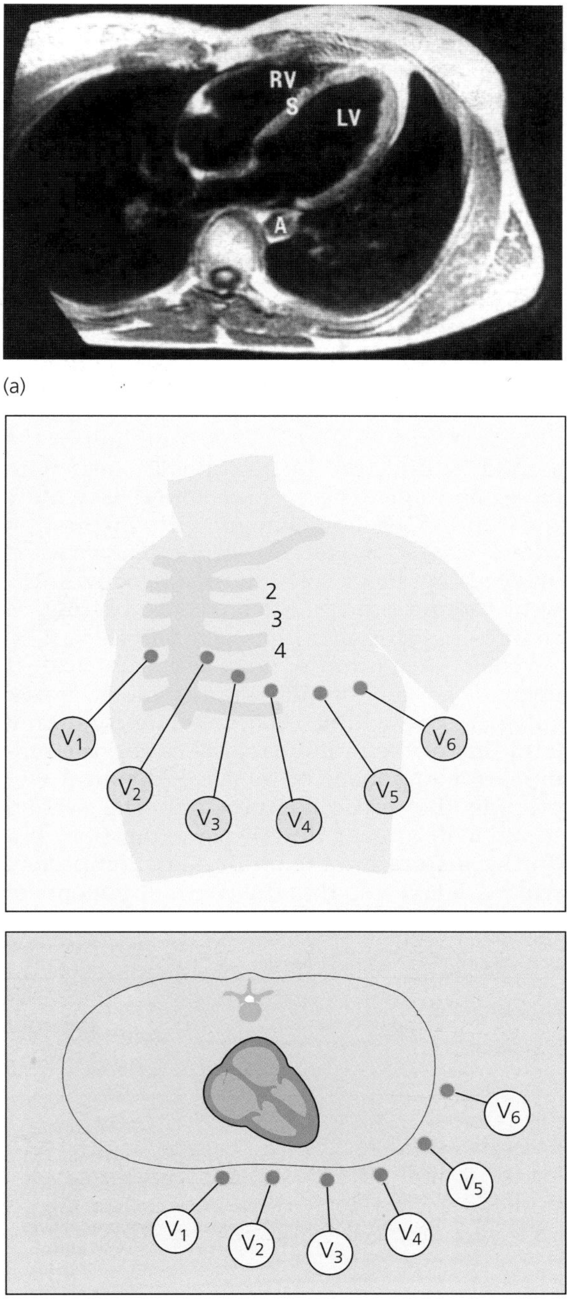

FIG. 4.16 (a) MRI scan showing the position of the chambers of the heart *viewed from below*. A: aorta. (b) Positions of the chest leads over the heart. Note that leads V1 and V2 face the anterior R ventricle, V3 and V4 the septum and V5 and V6 the L ventricle.

very difficult to demonstrate the size of the heart by percussion because it lies behind the sternum with lung in front of at least part of it. However, dullness to the right of the sternum may indicate right atrial enlargement or a pericardial effusion.

Palpation

The most important part of palpation is the identification of the cardiac apex, but it is important to feel over the whole precordium for abnormal movements. Loud murmurs will cause vibrations that can be felt on the chest wall. These are called 'thrills'.

If the cardiac apex is difficult to feel, ask the patient to turn on the left side; this brings the apex more into contact with the chest wall without changing the position of the heart.

The apex beat may be displaced from its normal position in the fifth rib interspace in mid-clavicular line by three abnormalities:

- Mediastinal shift.
- Left ventricular hypertrophy.
- Right ventricular hypertrophy.

The whole mediastinum may move when it is pulled towards the side of a collapsed or fibrotic lung, or when it is pushed away from the side of a large pleural effusion or a tension pneumothorax. In each case the trachea will deviate from the mid-line in the suprasternal notch and it is important to check this in any patient whose apex beat is displaced.

Rarely the heart may lie on the right side of the chest (*dextrocardia*) and the apex will then be in the right fifth interspace in mid-clavicular line.

The apex beat is displaced downwards and outwards by *left ventricular hypertrophy*. Its position should be described either as being a certain number of centimetres beyond mid-clavicular line or it may be related to the anterior axilliary line (a line below the anterior border of the axilla formed by the pectoralis major).

Right ventricular hypertrophy also causes an outward shift of the cardiac apex, but the apex beat is usually more diffuse. The important sign is a *lifting* or *heaving* motion felt best if the flat of the hand is placed on, or just to the left of, the sternum.

The precordial impulse may feel abnormal in the presence of a *left ventricular aneurysm*; this feels like a diffuse rocking movement between the sternum and the apex.

> **Practical Point**
>
> *Precordial impulse is abnormal in:*
>
> Right ventricular hypertrophy felt on, or just to the left of, the sternum as a *lifting* or *heaving* motion.
>
> Left ventricular aneurysm, felt as a diffuse rocking movement between the sternum and the apex.

When the first heart sound is very loud, as in *mitral stenosis*, it can actually be felt as a sharp 'tap' at the cardiac apex.

Auscultation

The identification of heart sounds and murmurs with a stethoscope is often thought of as the main art of cardiology, but its importance is overrated. A good history and recognition of other cardiac signs such as cardiac rhythm, heart size, jugular venous pressure and heart failure are usually much more important.

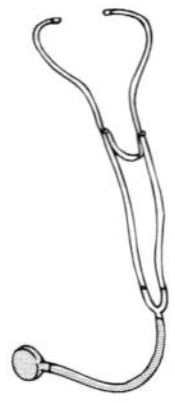

The heart sounds

These are associated with the opening and the closing of the valves, but the actual sound is made by sudden changes of velocity in the bloodstream. *High-pitched* sounds are best heard with the diaphragm of the stethoscope and *low-pitched* sounds are best heard with the bell.

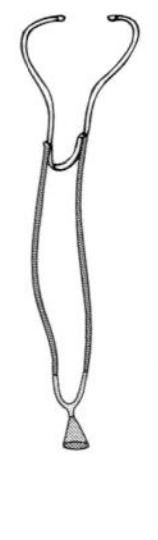

> **Practical Point**
>
> *Auscultation of heart sounds*
>
> High-pitched sounds are best heard with the diaphragm.
>
> Low-pitched sounds are best heard with the bell.

With a little practice the characteristics of sounds and murmurs become sufficiently distinct for them to be differentiated with ease.

The first sound is associated with closure of the mitral and tricuspid valves at the beginning of systole. The mitral and tricuspid components of the first sound can often be heard separately and may be confused with fourth and first sounds.

The second sound is associated with closure of the aortic and pulmonary valves. In young people valve closure is usually simultaneous on expiration, but on inspiration pulmonary closure is delayed as blood is sucked into the chest and right ventricular output is increased (see Fig. 4.17). This doubling of the second sound on inspiration is lost with increasing age. The second sound is widely split and does not change with inspiration when excitation of the right ventricle is delayed by block of conduction down the right bundle branch. Such 'fixed splitting' is characteristic of an *atrial septal defect*.

When excitation of the left ventricle is delayed by left bundle branch block, aortic valve closure will be relatively late compared with that of the pulmonary valve and the pulmonary component of the second sound will precede the aortic components. The second sound will appear double on expiration, but during inspiration the pulmonary component will be delayed so that the two components of the second sound coincide and the sound

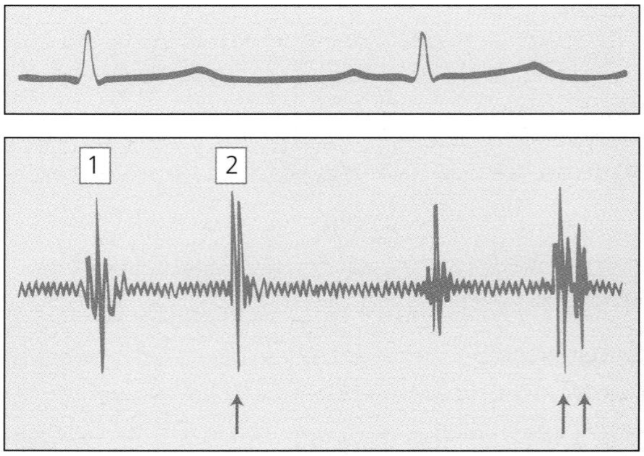

FIG. 4.17 Phonocardiogram showing the splitting of the 2nd heart sound on inspiration and timing of heart sounds in relation to the ECG.

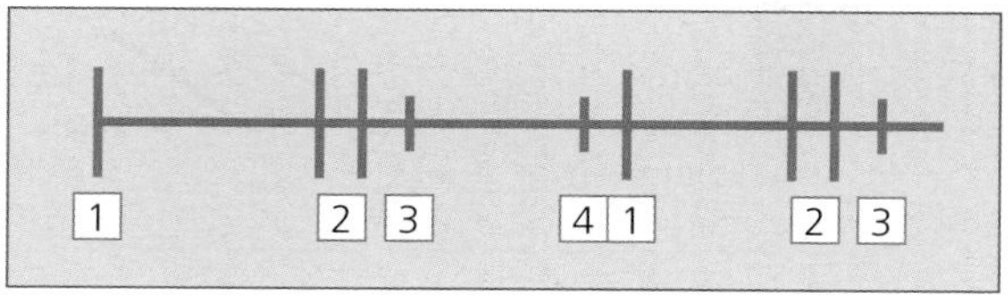

FIG. 4.18 Diagram of the phonocardiogram showing heart sounds.
1st sound: closure of mitral and tricuspid valves occurring almost or simultaneously; 2nd sound: closure of aortic and pulmonary valve; 3rd sound: occurs during ventricular filling; 4th sound: this is associated with atrial contraction.

becomes single. This is called 'reverse splitting'.

The third heart sound is associated with ventricular filling and is heard soon after the second sound (Fig. 4.18). It is dull and low pitched and is nearly always localized to the cardiac apex. A soft third sound may be normal, especially in young people, but in older patients it is usually an indication of heart failure. Most third sounds originate in the left ventricle, but occasionally right ventricular sounds can be identified because they become louder on inspiration.

The fourth heart sound is associated with atrial contraction and therefore occurs at the end of diastole, just before the first sound. When audible it is nearly always pathological and indicates heart failure. Like the third sound, it is low pitched and is localized to the cardiac apex.

In addition to the main heart sounds a variety of sharp, high-pitched clicking noises may sometimes be heard.

Systolic clicks (Fig. 4.19) may be single or multiple. A single early click is characteristic of *congenital aortic stenosis* or *congenital pulmonary stenosis* and is probably due to 'doming' of the valve before it opens. Such clicks are followed by an ejection murmur (see below). Late clicks, single or multiple, are often associated with *mitral valve prolapse*, when one or both cusps of the valve balloon back into the left atrium as the left ventricle contracts. They are usually accompanied by the murmur of mitral regurgitation that is characteristically late in systole.

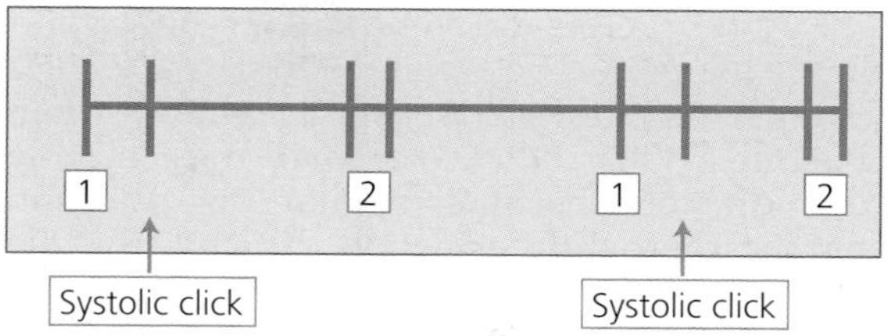

FIG. 4.19 A systolic click (arrowed).

> **Practical Point**
>
> *Auscultation of heart sounds*
>
> Systolic murmurs are usually louder than diastolic.
>
> Third and fourth heart sounds are low pitched.
>
> Systolic clicks and opening snaps are high pitched.

The 'opening snap' is the classical sharp, high-pitched extra sound of diastole.

It indicates *mitral stenosis* and precedes the characteristic diastolic murmur (see below). Although best heard at the apex it is usually also audible at the left sternal edge and this, together with its high pitch, differentiates it from a third sound. It occurs earlier in diastole than a third sound would be heard.

Heart murmurs

A murmur is due to turbulent blood flow. Murmurs arise when:

- A valve is thickened and fails to open properly (stenosis).
- A valve fails to shut properly and leaks (incompetence or regurgitation).
- There is an abnormal communication between the heart chambers due to a congenital or acquired abnormality such as a post-infarct ventricular septal defect.
- An abnormally large amount of blood flows past a normal valve as in pregnancy.

Murmurs may occur in systole or diastole and identifying these parts of the cardiac cycle is an essential prelude to determining the cause of the murmur.

'Systole' refers to ventricular contraction and is the period between the first and second sounds; its interval is usually shorter than diastole. With increasing heart rate systole and diastole become similar in duration making their differentiation difficult. Systole corresponds to the apical impulse and to the pulse in the carotid artery so you can time systole by feeling the carotid at the same time as listening to the heart. This takes a little practice.

Systolic murmurs occur when the ventricles are contracting: the aortic and pulmonary valves should be fully open and the mitral and tricuspid valves should be completely shut. Failure of the aortic and pulmonary valves to open fully (*valve stenosis*) or leakage of the mitral and tricuspid valves (*incompetence or regurgitation*) therefore cause a systolic murmur. Systolic murmurs are nearly always louder than diastolic murmurs.

Diastolic murmurs occur when the ventricles are relaxing and blood is flowing into them from the atria. The mitral and tricuspid valves should be fully open and the aortic and pulmonary valves shut. Stenosis of the mitral or the tricuspid valves, and incompetence of the aortic or pulmonary valves, therefore cause a diastolic murmur.

Murmurs also occur when there is an abnormal communication between the heart chambers due to a congenital defect. For example, if there is a ventricular septal defect (VSD) blood will flow across it in systole, when the pressure in the left ventricle is higher than in the right. This bloodflow is turbulent and causes a systolic murmur. With a patent ductus arteriosus blood can flow through the defect in both systole and diastole, leading to a 'continuous' murmur.

Types of murmur

In *valve stenosis*, the intensity of the murmur increases to a peak as resistance to blood flow becomes maximal and then decreases. Aortic and pulmonary stenosis are *ejection* murmurs (Fig 4.20a).

Valve incompetence begins the moment the valve shuts so these murmurs are 'early'. Aortic and pulmonary incompetence begin early and then decrease, causing a 'decrescendo' murmur. Mitral and tricuspid regurgitation tend to persist throughout most of systole and so cause 'pansystolic' murmurs (see Fig. 4.20b).

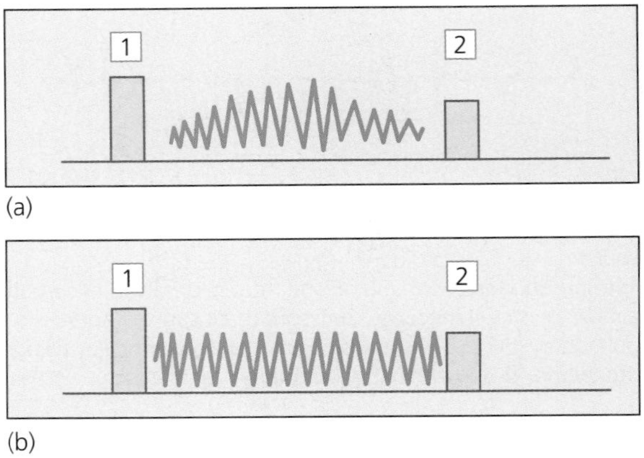

FIG. 4.20 Diagrams to show how notes might be annotated to demonstrate whether murmurs are of ejection type (a) or pansystolic (b).

Where to listen for murmurs

Some old books describe 'mitral', 'aortic', 'pulmonary' and 'tricuspid' *'areas'*, but these are meaningless and inaccurate. To have the best chance of hearing murmurs, listen to the heart with the diaphragm and the bell in four places:

- The cardiac apex.
- The upper left sternal edge – in the second rib interspace.
- The lower left sternal edge – in the fifth rib interspace.
- The right sternal edge – in the second rib interspace.

The murmurs of **mitral stenosis and regurgitation** are usually best heard at or near the apex. Those of **tricuspid stenosis and regurgitation** are often best heard at the lower left sternal edge and at this point the murmur of a VSD is also loudest.

Pulmonary stenosis causes a murmur best heard at the upper left sternal edge. The murmurs of **aortic and pulmonary incompetence** are best heard somewhere down the left sternal edge.

The murmur of aortic stenosis is best heard at the upper right sternal edge.

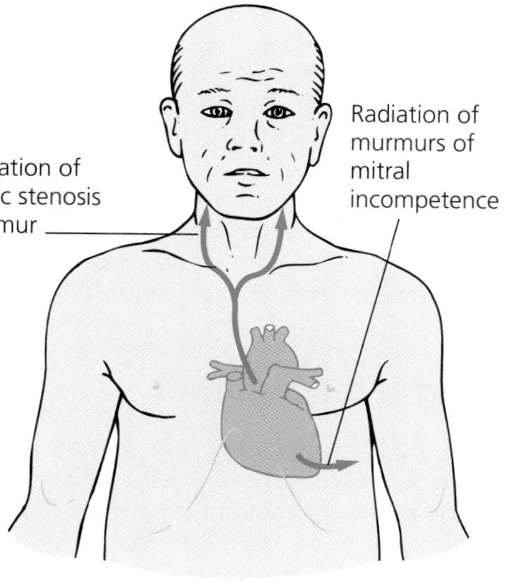

FIG. 4.21 The radiation of murmurs.

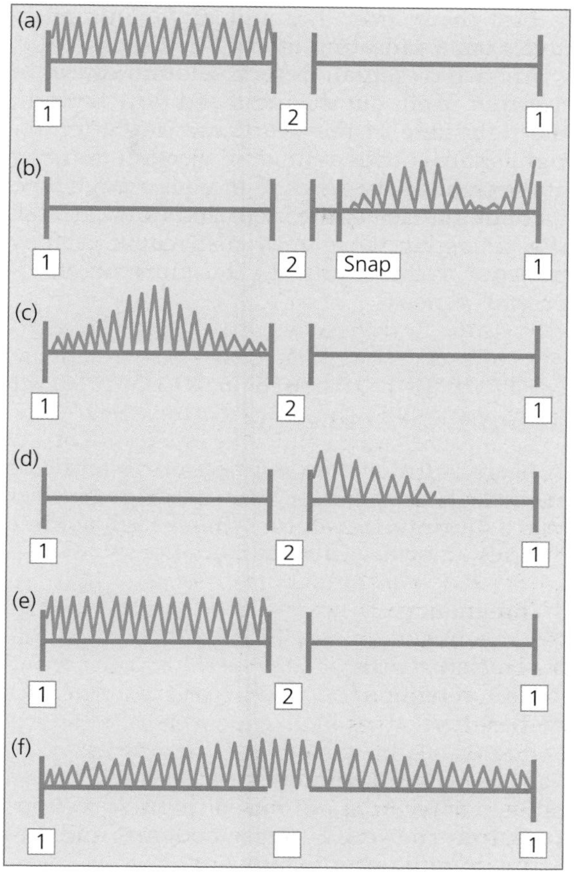

FIG. 4.22(a–f) Characteristics of cardiac murmurs in relation to heart sounds 1 and 2.
(a) Pansystolic murmur of mitral regurgitation (best heard at apex).
(b) Diastolic murmur of mitral stenosis with presystolic accentuation and an opening snap (the opening snap is often best heard to the left of the lower sternum).
(c) Ejection type murmur of aortic stenosis.
(d) Early diastolic murmur of aortic regurgitation.
(e) Murmur of ventricular septal defect or tricuspid incompetence (often heard best at lower left sternal edge).
(f) Continuous murmur of patent ductus arteriosus.

The murmur of aortic regurgitation is best heard with the diaphragm, with the patient sitting up, leaning forward and breathing out. The murmur of mitral stenosis is best heard with the bell, with the patient lying on his left side.

Some murmurs have characteristic 'radiations': the sound spreads in the direction in which the blood is flowing. Thus the murmur of **mitral regurgitation** radiates to the axilla and round to the back. That of **aortic stenosis** radiates to the carotid arteries in the neck. A murmur of **ventricular septal defect** often radiates up the left sternal edge. Murmers of **mitral stenosis, tricuspid stenosis and incompetence** tend to be localized (Fig. 4.21).

The characteristics of individual murmurs are summarized in Figs 4.22 (a–f).

Making a heart murmur easier to hear

Murmurs from valvular disease on the right side of the heart are loudest when the patient breathes in, increasing flow through the right side of the heart. This helps differentiate the murmurs of **pulmonary stenosis** and **regurgitation** from those of **aortic stenosis** and **incompetence**. The murmurs of **tricuspid stenosis** and **regurgitation** are also best heard on inspiration. The murmur of **tricuspid regurgitation** can be hard to differentiate from that of **mitral regurgitation** but the diagnosis is best made from the jugular venous pulse and from a pulsating liver.

An atrial septal defect seldom causes a murmur itself, but the increased flow through the right side of the heart due to the left-to-right shunt causes a 'flow' or ejection murmur at the pulmonary valve. If there is a large flow through the defect the increased flow through the tricuspid valve may also cause a flow murmur there, similar to the murmur of tricuspid stenosis.

Some important points to remember about heart murmurs

A heart murmur does not necessarily indicate intrinsic heart disease. You should remember that a murmur may occur when a high volume crosses a normal valve as in:

- Pregnancy.
- Anaemia.
- Thyrotoxicosis.
- CO_2 retention.
- Beri-beri.

These conditions may be associated with a sinus tachycardia, a raised jugular venous pressure and mild ankle oedema and are termed 'high output states'.

Some heart murmurs are of no consequence at all and are sometimes simply labelled 'benign'. These can be recognized by the following features:

- Lack of symptoms.
- No cardiac enlargement.
- Always systolic.
- Usually soft.
- Usually ejection in quality.

These murmurs may be due to minor aortic valve abnormalities, to trivial pulmonary stenosis or to mitral valve prolapse.

Pericardial rubs Inflammation of the pericardium causes a 'friction rub'. Rubs vary from soft shuffling sounds to scratchy noises in time with the cardiac cycle. They are often influenced by respiration when they are called 'pleuropericardial'. A friction rub can only be identified with confidence if it is heard in both systole and diastole.

When fluid is formed within the pericardial sac as a result of the pericarditis, the two layers of the pericardium separate and the noise disappears. Pericardial rubs are best heard with the patient lying flat as fluid drains to the back of the pericardium so that the anterior layers of the pericardial sac come into contact and the rub is accentuated.

Putting it all together

Making a diagnosis always depends more on an accurate history than on anything else. In cardiovascular disease the history will usually indicate what is wrong – angina, heart failure, an arrhythmia and so on – and the physical examination may confirm this either directly or indirectly.

Practical Point

The examination is most efficient when used to look *for* rather than *at* physical signs.

Although the examination is most efficient when used to look *for* rather than *at* physical signs, a full examination is always needed as sometimes the history can be misleading.

You should remember that a full diagnosis includes the underlying pathology. For example, angina must be due to something such as coronary disease, aortic stenosis, or anaemia or a combination of these; heart failure is not in itself a diagnosis but must be due to something such as ischaemic disease, valve disease, or cardiomyopathy. The history and examination together should indicate the most efficient ways of using investigations to confirm or refute a clinical diagnosis.

Think about putting the history and physical examination together with the underlying pathology by considering in turn the main symptoms of which patients with cardiovascular disease complain. To give you the general idea, described below are three patients referred by the General Practitioner to a cardiac clinic.

EXAMPLES

Case 1

Referral with chest pain

If the history suggests that chest pain is due to cardiac ischaemia, look for:

- Evidence of risk factors:
  - Smoking (nicotine stained fingers).
  - Hypercholesterolaemia (xanthelasmata).
  - Hypertension.
  - Obesity.
- Evidence of other vascular disease:
  - Absent pulses in the legs.
  - Femoral or carotid bruits.
  - Signs of previous stroke.

Consider causes of cardiac ischaemia other than coronary disease:

- Valve disease (especially aortic stenosis).
- Anaemia.
- Arrhythmia.

If the history suggests some other cause of chest pain, look for the following signs:

- Aortic dissection:
  - High blood pressure.
  - Blood pressure lower in the left than right arm.
  - Absent peripheral pulses.
  - Aortic regurgitation (due to distorted aortic root).
  - Pericardial rub (leak of blood into the pericardium).
  - Pleural effusion (leak of blood into the pleural space).
- Pericarditis:
  - Pericardial rub.
  - Raised jugular venous pulse.
  - Evidence of pericardial tamponade.
  - Jugular venous pulse increases on inspiration.
  - Systolic BP falls on inspiration.
- Pleuritic pain:
  - Asymmetrical chest movement.
  - Normal percussion note.
  - Abnormal breath sounds.
  - Pleural rub.
- Oesophageal pain:
  - Few physical signs, though pain may be produced by pressure in the epigastrium.
- Musculoskeletal pain:
  - Spinal deformity.
  - Bone tenderness.
  - Pain on pressure on the chest wall.

Case 2

Referral with breathlessness

There will usually be signs of congestive cardiac failure (i.e. right heart failure resulting from left heart failure) when breathlessness is due to cardiac disease. These include:

- Orthopnoea.
- Crepitations at the lung bases.
- Raised jugular venous pulse.
- Distended liver.
- Ankle swelling.
- Evidence of heart disease such as:
  - Enlarged heart.
  - Third or fourth heart sound.
  - Heart murmurs.

If breathlessness is due to lung disease the heart will usually be normal, but remember that right heart failure can be the result of lung disease (*cor pulmonale*) and the physical signs can be remarkably similar to those of congestive failure:

- Raised jugular venous pulse.
- Distended liver.
- Ankle swelling.
- Crepitations in the lung due to lung disease rather than pulmonary oedema.
- Right ventricular enlargement but the heart may be normal.

Practical Point

If a diagnosis of heart failure is made remember that this is a description of a collection of symptoms and signs which are the result of some specific cardiac disease. A cause for heart failure must be established and the main causes are:

Ischaemic heart disease.
Valve disease (rheumatic or congenital).
Hypertension.
Arrhythmias.
Heart muscle disease – cardiomyopathy.

Case 3

Referral with valve disease

Having identified the cause of a heart murmur (valve stenosis or regurgitation, a septal defect etc) you must next diagnose the underlying cardiac pathology.

- Mitral stenosis is nearly always rheumatic (NB: atrial myxomas can cause a similar murmur by obstruction of the valve orifice).
- Mitral regurgitation may be seen after rheumatic fever, myocardial infarction, valve prolapse, cardiomyopathy (due to valve ring dilatation), infective endocarditis.
- Aortic stenosis: Congenital valve disease, calcification in the elderly, especially with a congenitally biscupid valve.
- Aortic regurgitation: rheumatic fever, aortic dissection, infective endocarditis, ankylosing spondylitis and other collagen diseases, inflammatory bowel diseases.
- Ventricular septal defects: Congenital, post-myocardial infarction.

How patients with respiratory disease present

5

Respiratory disease is a very common reason for a patient to seek medical help, accounting for about a fifth of all consultations in general practice. Taking a good history, characterizing symptoms and their relationship to other symptoms and a detailed occupational history are of key importance.

THE HISTORY

Patients usually present with one or more of three main respiratory symptoms:

- Breathlessness (a better term than 'dyspnoea'). (See also Chapter 24.)
- Cough.
- Chest pain.

Breathlessness

This very common medical complaint is an uncomfortable awareness of the need to breathe. The sensation of breathlessness that healthy people get on strenuous exertion is probably similar to that experienced by patients on mild exertion or at rest.

Three basic mechanisms can lead to breathlessness, acting singly or jointly (Revision Panel 5.1).

In asthma, for example, airflow obstruction increases the work of breathing, hyperinflation impairs diaphragm function and anxiety increases neurological drive; the combination of these main factors, and others, causes breathlessness. Symptoms arise when there is an abnormal drive to breathe which does not meet or exceeds requirements.

To diagnose breathlessness, cover the following key points (Revision Panel 5.2):

Revision Panel 5.1
Mechanisms leading to breathlessness

Increased work of breathing	*Example*
Airways obstruction.	Asthma.
Stiff lungs.	Pulmonary fibrosis.
Stiff chest wall.	Scoliosis.
Decreased neuromuscular power	Muscular dystrophy.
Increased drive to breathe	
Chemical drive.	Hypoxia, acidosis.
Neurological drive.	Pulmonary oedema.

Revision Panel 5.2
Establishing the cause of breathlessness

Is it really breathlessness?
Timescale.
Severity of breathlessness?
How variable is it –
  spontaneous/nocturnal/postural?
Precipitating factors.
Treatment effects.
Associated symptoms.

Is it really breathlessness?

Try to define exactly what symptom your patient has. Many say they are 'short of breath' or 'short of puff' rather than 'breathless'. Patients complaining of 'chest tightness' may not necessarily mean difficulty with breathing but angina; sometimes both may occur together. Patients with pleuritic chest pain often complain of breathlessness and these symptoms may coexist in pulmonary infarction. They may, however, be referring to an inability to take normal breaths because of pain on inspiration due to fractured ribs for example.

Timescale

'How long have you been breathless?' or 'When did your breathing difficulties begin?' are vital questions, because the timescale of onset of breathlessness can be very helpful in diagnosis (Revision Panel 5.3).

However, there is much overlap. Left ventricular failure (LVF) can, for example, present acutely or with increasing breathlessness over several weeks. Patients are usually poor at dating the onset of longstanding breathlessness. You should press them on this, as patients who say they have been breathless for several months often later recall deteriorating exercise tolerance over many years.

Revision Panel 5.3
Timing of onset of breathlessness[a]

Seconds/minutes
Left ventricular failure.
Pulmonary embolism.
Pneumothorax.
Asthma.

Hours/days
Left ventricular failure.
Pneumonia.
Asthma.
Acute exacerbation of chronic obstructive pulmonary disease.
Adult respiratory distress syndrome.
Allergic alveolitis.
Pleural effusion.

Weeks
Left ventricular failure.
Anaemia.
Asthma.
Pleural effusion.

Months/years
Chronic obstructive pulmonary disease.
Asthma.
Anaemia.
Pulmonary fibrosis.

[a]There is much overlap between categories. This list is by no means exhaustive.

Severity of breathlessness

Systems for grading the severity of breathlessness exist but a simpler clinical approach is to consider how your patient's lifestyle is affected by asking some general questions such as:

- 'How far can you walk on the flat without stopping?'
- 'Can you get upstairs in one go?'
- For a housewife – 'Can you do your cleaning?'
- For a retired man – 'Can you still dig the garden?'

Be careful with patients with multiple pathology; the exercise tolerance of an elderly woman with arthritic knees and a man with intermittent claudication may be reduced more by leg pain than breathlessness.

Practical Point

Assess the severity of breathlessness by asking to what extent your patient's lifestyle is affected.

Variability

Variability of breathlessness is an important clue, and occurs in different ways:

Spontaneous breathlessness This may be fairly constant or slowly progressive as in chronic obstructive pulmonary disease (COPD) or episodic and varying daily as in asthma.

Nocturnal breathlessness Waking during the night occurs in two conditions which are sometimes difficult to distinguish: pulmonary oedema and nocturnal asthma. In pulmonary oedema due to left ventricular failure or valvular heart disease, patients are woken abruptly by breathlessness ('paroxysmal nocturnal dyspnoea') but get relief by sitting up or getting out of bed, manoeuvres which reduce capillary hydrostatic pressure. In poorly controlled asthma (a more common problem), breathlessness also occurs around 2 or 3 am but accompanied by cough and wheeze, reflecting an exaggeration of the normal circadian variation in airway calibre.

Postural breathlessness Becoming breathless when lying flat (orthopnoea) is not just a feature of heart failure. This may be particularly marked in bilateral diaphragmatic paralysis. Relief of breathlessness on lying down (platypnoea) is rare and seen in various types of arteriovenous shunts.

Precipitating factors

Breathlessness related to an environmental factor, identifiable or not, is usually due to asthma. Some asthmatics, for example, become breathless when exposed to cats, or to a particular perfume or have seasonal symptoms when pollen counts are high. Breathlessness is almost always worse *during* exertion, but exercise-induced asthma often occurs *after* exercise. Acute breathlessness may be due to allergic alveolitis rather than asthma; farmers or pigeon-breeders may develop symptoms 4 to 12 hours after exposure to relevant antigens. Occupation is particularly important; ask all patients with breathlessness how it relates to their work. Two questions identify most patients with occupational asthma. 'Is your breathing (or wheeze or cough) better at the weekends?' and 'Is it better when you are on holiday?'

Treatment effects

Breathlessness which is relieved by diuretics suggests pulmonary oedema. Marked improvement over several days with steroids strongly suggests asthma or, less commonly, parenchymal disease such as allergic alveolitis. Rapid relief with a bronchodilator supports a diagnosis of asthma.

Associated symptoms

The inter-relationship of symptoms is important. Breathlessness in a smoker with haemoptysis and weight loss suggests collapse or effusion due to cancer while breathlessness with wheeze in a young person is usually asthma. Breathlessness is a common symptom of hyperventilation, often unrelated to exertion and occurring with other symptoms such as palpitations, tingling in the arms, dizziness, chest pain and sighing respiration. Such patients often complain of 'being unable to take a deep enough breath' or 'can't get enough air into my chest'.

Wheeze This whistling or musical sound which occurs with breathing is important because it indicates airflow obstruction. Principal causes are:

- Asthma
- COPD (chronic bronchitis and emphysema).
- Fixed airway obstruction e.g. due to tumour.

You may have to explain what a wheeze is, as not all patients will understand what it means. The important diagnostic features of wheeze are the same as breathlessness; thus, variability in wheeze, spontaneously or with exercise, allergens, occupation, drugs (e.g. beta-blockers, aspirin), or nocturnal wheeze, suggests asthma.

Cough

This may vary from a mild irritation to a distressing symptom. It is common in respiratory disease but rarely of diagnostic help by itself. Cough is a forced expiratory effort against a closed glottis that suddenly opens with an explosive release of air and respiratory secretions. The cough reflex is initiated by receptors in the larynx and major airways which are stimulated both by material within the airway (such as sputum, foreign bodies or inhaled irritants) and events in the airway wall (such as inflammation or sudden changes in thoracic volume).

Points about cough

Many smokers and people in industrial areas regard cough as a normal part of life. Their response to 'Do you have a cough?' may therefore often be 'no' or 'just the usual'. In this case you must find out what your patient considers is normal, whether the cough has changed recently and in all cases the following features:

Duration Try to establish how long the cough has been present. A morning cough for many years productive of white sputum is characteristic of chronic bronchitis while a cough of a week or two is usually due to the common cold.

Variability Nocturnal cough may occur in asthma. Though often combined with breathlessness and wheeze, it may be the sole presenting symptom of childhood, and occasionally adult, asthma. Daytime cough is variable in asthma, but persistent cough over a few weeks or months in a smoker raises the possibility of bronchial carcinoma.

Precipitating factors Cough related to meals or lying down may be due to aspiration of oesophageal contents. Cough may be related to particular dusts or fumes.

Sputum production A longstanding, highly productive cough suggests bronchiectasis.

Associated symptoms The commonest causes of a longstanding undiagnosed cough are:

- Postnasal drip.
- Occult asthma.
- Gastro-oesophageal reflux.

It is imperative, therefore, to ask about nasal blockage, rhinorrhoea, and sinusitis; other symptoms of asthma; heartburn and indigestion. Inhalation of foreign bodies such as a peanut, which may cause cough, is often unnoticed in children.

Type of cough If your patient coughs during the examination you may confirm that it is productive. Otherwise the character of the cough is rarely of diagnostic help. With unilateral vocal cord paralysis (as in recurrent laryngeal nerve palsy from malignant mediastinal invasion) the cough may be prolonged and has been likened to the lowing of cattle (hence 'bovine' cough). Laryngitis, especially in children, leads to a harsh 'croupy' cough. A weak cough occurs in bilateral cord palsy, respiratory muscle weakness, severe illness of any cause and when cough causes pain.

Sputum Ask about 'phlegm' rather than 'sputum', a term that means nothing to most patients. About 100 ml of secretion is produced daily by the normal respiratory tract and this is usually swallowed. With a productive cough it is useful to know roughly how much is being produced, though some patients swallow the increased phlegm. Sputum volumes of, say, an eggcupful or cupful a day are often found in bronchiectasis, sometimes more in lung abscess. A general point about history taking is worth making here. When asking about, for example, the amount of phlegm or the number of episodes of chest pain 'in a day', you will usually be referring to a 24-hour period, while the patient often assumes you mean the 'daytime' as opposed to the 'night time'. Keep on the same wavelength as your patient.

Sputum colour and consistency Clear or white (grey in industrial areas) sticky or mucoid sputum is typical of bronchial mucus gland hypersection, as in chronic bronchitis. When sputum is yellow or green (purulent), often thick, it contains white cells indicating infection, though in asthma green sputum may be due to eosinophils. Coal workers may cough up black sputum (melanoptysis). Asthmatics often have viscid, stringy sputum ('I can't seem to get it out' is a common comment) and less commonly cough up small bronchial casts (Curschmann's spirals) which may be brown in bronchopulmonary aspergillosis. Frothy, sometimes pink, sputum is seen in severe acute pulmonary oedema. The copious secretions of alveolar cell carcinoma are rare. Foul-smelling sputum suggests anaerobic infection, as in a lung abscess or empyema with bronchopleural fistula.

Haemoptysis (see also Chapter 38) Coughing up blood causes patients and doctors to worry about cancer, though this is the cause in only about 3% of cases. Faced with a patient coughing up blood, two questions need to be answered:

Is it really haemoptysis? You should remember that blood might be produced from outside the respiratory tract. Haematemesis is usually easy to exclude, but bleeding from the nasopharynx may be difficult to distinguish. If there is nose bleeding or blood just appears in the mouth, a nasopharyngeal source is likely, whereas if the blood definitely comes up with coughing or is mixed with or streaked in sputum then the chest is the likely source. Blood from the chest is usually red, not brown.

How severe is haemoptysis? The volume of blood is a guide to the seriousness of the problem and is important in management. Haemoptysis of over 200 ml per 24 h has a high mortality.

A cause for haemoptysis (see Revision Panel 5.4) is found in only about half of all patients. Clues come from the history and examination.

Frank haemoptysis with pleuritic pain, breathlessness and sometimes a pleural rub is seen in pulmonary infarction, or with fever, purulent sputum and signs of consolidation in pneumonia. Recurrent haemoptysis over several years is common in bronchiectasis. In a smoker aged 40 years or more, bronchial carcinoma must always be considered. Haemoptysis should never be ascribed to 'bronchitis' before serious causes have been excluded, and even if they have, it is better to be honest and say that the cause is unknown.

> Revision Panel 5.4
> **Causes of haemoptysis**
>
> *Common*
> No cause found.
> Acute respiratory infection.
> Bronchiectasis.
> Lung cancer.
> Tuberculosis active/inactive.
> Chest trauma.
>
> *Uncommon*
> Pulmonary vasculitis.
> Arteriovenous malformations.
> Benign tumours.
> Foreign body.
> Mitral stenosis.
> Clotting disorders.

Chest pain (see also Chapter 25)

The lung itself has no pain fibres so parenchymal diseases such as fibrosing alveolitis or cancer do not cause chest pain. The parietal pleura is very sensitive, however, and pleuritic chest pain can be very severe. Typically this is sharp, stabbing and worsened by breathing in or coughing. Patients may say 'it catches me when I breathe'. Pleuritic pain occurs in inflammation of the pleura (pleurisy), or with musculoskeletal causes, because chest wall pain (e.g. from a fractured rib) can closely mimic pleurisy (Revision Panel 5.5).

The main diagnostic difficulties revolve around infection *versus* infarction *versus* musculoskeletal causes. Associated fever and purulent sputum suggest infection, breathlessness and haemoptysis support infarction and a history of trauma and pain reproduced by tenderness at the site of the pain favours a musculoskeletal cause. Central diaphragmatic pleurisy causes pain referred to the shoulder since the pain fibres from this part of the diaphragm run with the phrenic nerve (C3,4,5) while pleurisy involving the outer part of the diaphragm causes pain referred to the lower chest and upper abdomen. The extremely severe pleuritic pain of the Coxsackie viral disease epidemic myalgia (Bornholm disease or 'devil's grip') in which the intercostal muscles are extremely tender, is fortunately rare. Pain radiating round from

Revision Panel 5.5

Causes of pleuritic chest pain

Pleural
Infective e.g. pneumonia.
Pulmonary infarction/embolus.
Neoplastic – primary or secondary.
Connective tissue disease
 systemic lupus erythematosus[a]
 rheumatoid arthritis.[a]
Asbestos-related pleurisy.[a]

Musculoskeletal
Rib fracture (trauma, cough or pathological).
Muscular strain.
Herpes zoster.[a]
Bornholm disease.[b]

[a]Uncommon. [b]Rare.

the thoracic spine from vertebral collapse sometimes has a pleuritic quality and may be exacerbated by coughing.

Other respiratory chest pains

Large pleural effusions often cause a dull heavy sensation. Characteristically, mesothelioma causes constant, often severe pain. Pneumothorax sometimes causes pleuritic pain but patients more often describe a dragging or drawing sensation. Pain and swelling over sternocostal junctions bears the name Tietze's syndrome but it is far more common to find pain on palpation over the sternocostal junctions without swelling. Tracheitis, and occasionally mediastinal or hilar lymphadenopathy, as in sarcoidosis, can cause an uncomfortable central chest ache often described as a 'raw feeling'. Any persistent coughing may lead to chest soreness and, occasionally causes rib fracture.

Checklist of other important points in the history

The following are points of particular importance:

Ankle oedema Peripheral oedema in patients with chronic lung disease may signify cor pulmonale (right heart disease secondary to lung disease) and indicates a poor prognosis.

Arthritis and arthralgia Connective tissue diseases (e.g. rheumatoid arthritis) are associated with several respiratory problems including fibrosing alveolitis and pleural effusion. Pain in the wrists and ankles from hypertrophic osteoarthropathy (Fig. 5.1) suggests lung cancer.

Practical Point

Hypertrophic osteoarthropathy occurs at the ends of the long bones (wrists, ankles and sometimes knees); don't expect to see it at the ends of the fingers and toes.

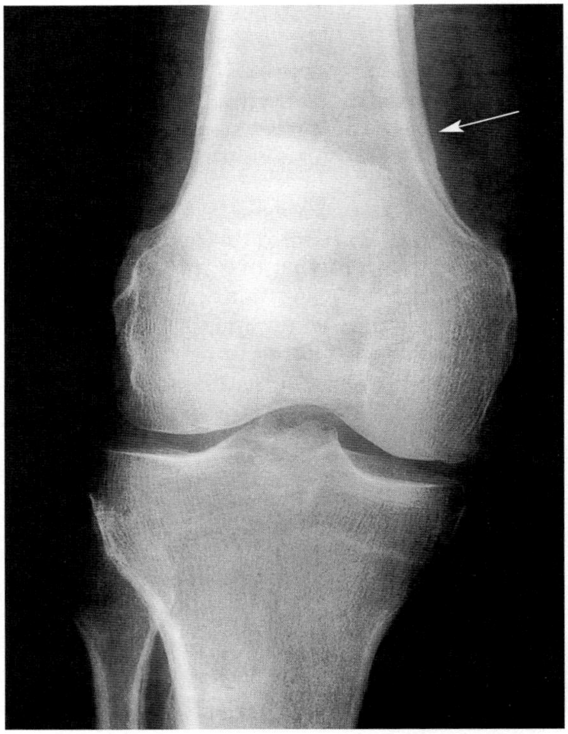

FIG. 5.1 Hypertrophic pulmonary osteoarthropathy. Arrow points to subperiosteal new bone formation. The knee is a relatively unusual site for this complication.

Rashes Sarcoidosis causes many skin signs, of which erythema nodosum (See Fig. 11.1) is self-limiting and may have resolved by the time you see your patient. Rashes due to vasculitis may also be transient and only discovered during the history.

Daytime sleepiness and nocturnal apnoea Daytime sleepiness occurs in hypercapnic respiratory failure, or in obstructive sleep apnoea when it may be associated with obesity, upper airway obstruction, large collar size and high alcohol intake.

Smoking You should ascertain how much your patient smokes and, if he has given up, how long ago that was. In the absence of a history of smoking COPD is very uncommon, while wheeze in a lifetime non-smoker is usually asthma. The smoker's risk of lung cancer declines after stopping smoking, coming close to the non-smoker's risk after 15 years.

Occupation A full occupational history is often vital, particularly in asthma, pulmonary fibrosis or pleural disease. Job titles such as engineer mean little; it is the processes involved that are important. The list of causes of occupational asthma is growing but some important causes are:

- Isocyanates (used in paint spraying).
- Flour (used in baking).
- Epoxy resins (used in adhesives).
- Colophony (used in solders).

Coal workers' pneumoconiosis is increasingly rare but in pulmonary fibrosis or pleural disease you must enquire about asbestos exposure (e.g. in laggers, shipworkers, joiners and in many other trades).

Practical Point

A single year's exposure to asbestos may be the cause of mesothelioma 50 years later.

Drugs Aspirin and other non-steroidal, anti-inflammatory drugs may cause or worsen airflow obstruction. Many drugs cause pulmonary eosinophilia. Nitrofurantoin, amiodarone and busulphan are among many drugs associated with pulmonary fibrosis.

Hobbies Budgerigars and pigeons may cause extrinsic allergic alveolitis. The former are associated with insidiously progressive breathlessness, while the latter more often cause acute disease.

Immunodeficiency You must be alert to the possibility of human immunodeficiency virus (HIV) disease or other immunodeficient states particularly with unexplained respiratory symptoms or chest X-ray abnormalities. A history of haematological malignancy, or cytotoxic and steroid therapy is usually clear, but you may need to enquire specifically about HIV risk factors (see Chapter 21).

Practical Point

Always ask when and where previous chest X-rays were taken. Much time and many investigations may be saved if old X-rays are available for comparison.

Past medical history Ask about past tuberculosis and its treatment, or contact with the disease, and about past or current malignancy and cardiac disease.

Family history A family history of cystic fibrosis or of emphysema at a young age (as in α-1-antitrypsin deficiency) is important.

THE PHYSICAL EXAMINATION

Extrathoracic signs

Finger clubbing

When all the signs of clubbing are present recognition is easy. Less obvious cases engender arguments on ward rounds as to whether clubbing is present, though the outcome of the discussions rarely affects management.

Signs of clubbing (Fig. 5.2) are:

- Increased sponginess of nail bed.
- Increase in angle between nail and nail bed, usually but not always to > 180°.
- Increased nail curvature in longitudinal *and* lateral axes.
- Ends of fingers become bulbous.

It is reasonable to recognize three categories i.e. clubbing is either definitely present, definitely absent or possible.

The pathogenesis of clubbing remains unknown. There is increased bloodflow through the fingers and a neurogenic component seems likely as vagotomy can abolish clubbing. Many conditions are associated with clubbing (Revision Panel 5.6), the most common respiratory cause being bronchial carcinoma. Clubbing occurs more frequently in Black people in the absence of any underlying pathology. Patients are often unaware of the changes in their fingers or toes, probably because clubbing usually develops slowly.

Hypertrophic pulmonary osteoarthropathy causes pain and sometimes swelling over the ends of the long bones above the wrists and ankles symmetrically. It usually occurs with clubbing, most cases being associated with squamous carcinoma of the lung. X-Rays show subperiosteal new bone formation on the shafts of the long bones (Fig. 5.1).

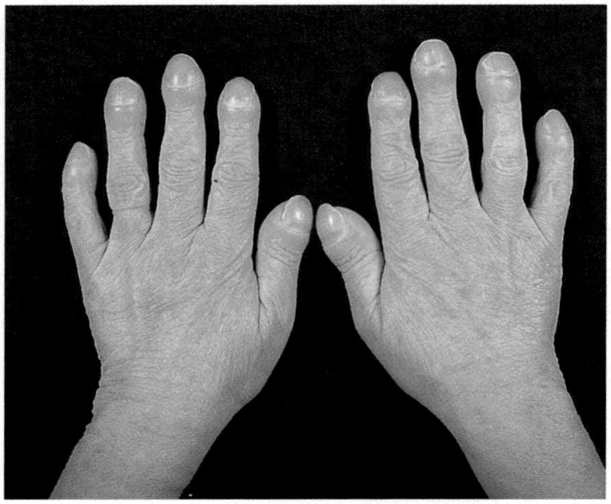

FIG. 5.2 Clubbing of the fingers.

Revision Panel 5.6
Causes of clubbing

Congenital

Lung
Bronchial carcinoma.
Fibrosing alveolitis, asbestosis.
Chronic pulmonary sepsis e.g. bronchiectasis, cystic fibrosis, lung abscess.

Heart
Infective endocarditis.
Cyanotic congenital heart disease.

Gut
Ulcerative colitis, Crohn's disease.
Cirrhosis of liver.

Other
Many other rare causes e.g. pleural fibroma.

Cyanosis

Look at the tongue, lips and nails for the blue discoloration of cyanosis. If cyanosis is seen in all these three sites it is 'central' (Revision Panel 5.7) and if just in the nails, it is 'peripheral'.

The ability to recognize cyanosis varies widely among doctors but cyanosis should be detectable when the arterial oxygen saturation

Revision Panel 5.7
Common causes of central cyanosis

Acute
Severe pneumonia.
Acute asthma.
Left ventricular failure.
Pulmonary embolus.
Hypoventilation due to respiratory depression e.g. opiate overdose.

Chronic
Severe chronic obstructive pulmonary disease.
Pulmonary fibrosis.
Right-to-left cardiac shunt.

is 80–85%. As an approximate guide, it indicates that the blood contains at least 1.5 g/dl of reduced haemoglobin. Cyanosis is easy to detect in polycythaemia but may be absent in anaemia despite severe hypoxaemia. Peripheral cyanosis is usually due to increased oxygen extraction with a slow-moving circulation, as in cold weather, Raynaud's phenomenon, or peripheral vascular disease.

Superior vena caval obstruction

This is most often due to:

- Bronchial carcinoma and/or associated mediastinal glands.
- Lymphoma.
- Mediastinal fibrosis and other rare causes.

Of these, only bronchial carcinoma is common.

Patients may complain of headache or worsening breathlessness as well as a puffy face. The resulting signs vary in severity:

- Dilated veins on anterior chest wall (Fig. 5.3).
- Engorged, fixed, non-pulsatile jugular veins.
- Swollen face, neck and (sometimes) arms.
- Conjunctival oedema.

The dilated veins on the chest wall represent the collateral circulation bypassing the obstructed superior vena cava and returning to the heart via the intercostals and azygos system. The engorged neck veins may be impossible to see if the neck itself is swollen.

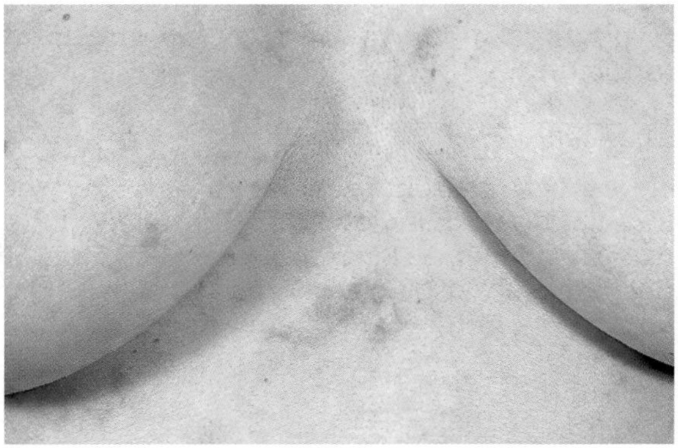

FIG. 5.3 Superior vena caval obstruction. Note dilated veins on chest and upper abdomen; this subtle physical sign can be easily missed.

Other signs

Always examine the supraclavicular fossae for enlarged glands frequently found in bronchial carcinoma, lymphoma, tuberculosis and sarcoidosis.

Inspection of the chest

Make sure your patient is comfortable, sitting at about 45° and in a good light. A great deal is gleaned by simple observation (Revision Panel 5.8). Ask yourself whether the chest wall

Revision Panel 5.8
Inspection of the chest

Appearance of the chest wall
General shape.
Chest deformity.
- Pectus carinatus.
- Pectus excavatus.
- Scoliosis.
- Kyphosis.
- Thoracoplasty.
- Chest wall lesions.

Breathing
Rate.
Breathing pattern.
- Shallow.
- Kussmaul.
- Cheyne–Stokes.
- Sighing.
- Pursed-lip.
- Orthopnoea.

Chest wall movement
Expansion.
- General reduction.
- Unilateral reduction.

Paradoxical movement.
- Flail chest.
- Intercostal recession.
- Indrawing ribs.

Use of accessory muscles

itself is normal, before looking at the pattern of breathing and movements of the chest.

Appearances of the chest wall

General shape

Note the general shape of the chest. An increase in the anteroposterior axis of the chest causes patients to look *barrel chested*. You will see this in patients with longstanding hyperinflation of the lungs, as in emphysema, and sometimes in kyphosis (see below).

Chest deformity

Pectus carinatus and pectus excavatus

There are various deformities of the chest: mild forms of pectus carinatus (pigeon chest) and pectus excavatus (funnel chest) (Fig. 5.4) are quite common. *Pectus carinatus*, with its prominent sternum and costal cartilages, may be congenital or secondary to severe childhood asthma, rickets or congenital heart disease. When the cause is asthma, Harrison's sulci – horizontal grooves at the bottom of the rib cage in children caused by persistent indrawing of the ribs – may also be present. *Pectus excavatus* is congenital and not secondary to lung disease. The lower end of the sternum is depressed, though when severe the whole sternum and costal cartilages are sunken.

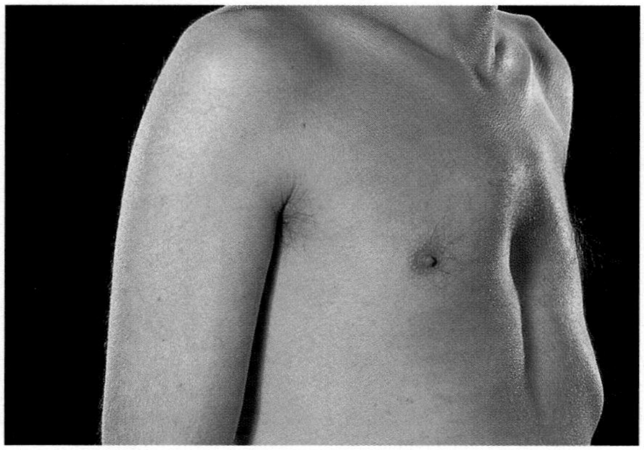

FIG. 5.4 Pectus excavatus.

Practical Point

Pectus excavatus may cause:

- Displaced apex beat.
- Cardiac murmur.
- Apparent cardiomegaly on chest X-ray.
- Abnormal lung function if very severe.

Scoliosis

Scoliosis (Revision Panel 5.9) (see also Chapter 20) is a lateral curvature of the spine. At the apex of the curve, the vertebral bodies are rotated and the ribs protrude backwards to cause a posterior hump (see Fig. 20.11).

Revision Panel 5.9
Causes of scoliosis

- Idiopathic – commonest.
- Congenital.
- Neuropathic e.g. poliomyelitis.
- Myopathic e.g. muscular dystrophy.
- Traumatic.

Kyphosis

This is an increased anteroposterior curvature of the spine seen most frequently in the elderly with osteoporosis (Figs 5.5, 5.6), or in men with ankylosing spondylitis. Both deformities, especially scoliosis, can cause serious respiratory disability and sometimes respiratory failure.

Thoracoplasty

Note any *scars* from previous chest surgery or trauma. Before chemotherapy for tuberculosis was available, a *thoracoplasty* consisting of pushing in part of the ribcage to collapse the underlying lung was sometimes performed. A thoracoplasty may cause respiratory failure in later life.

Other chest wall lesions

Look carefully at the skin (see Fig. 2.15). Assess any *lumps* in the usual way and

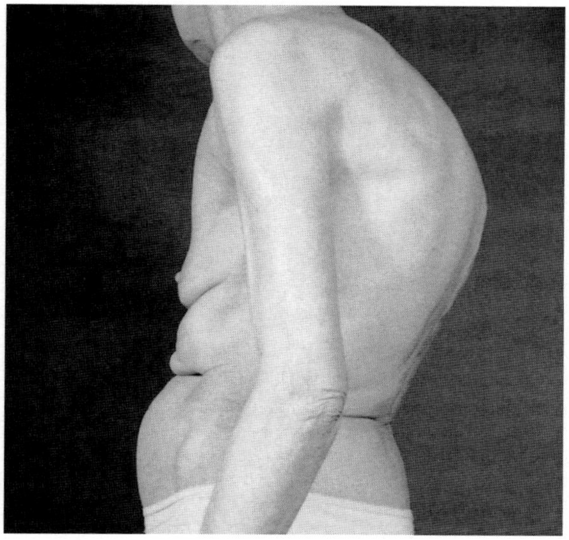

FIG. 5.5 Kyphosis due to multiple collapsed vertebrae in osteoporosis. Note the transverse abdominal crease indicating trunk shortening.

remember that chest wall lumps (e.g. lipomata) may cause a chest X-ray shadow simulating an intrapulmonary lesion. Feel for the crackling sensation of *subcutaneous emphysema* in pneumothorax or chest trauma. Is there any *local tenderness*? *Dilated veins* on the chest wall should prompt you to look for other signs of superior vena caval obstruction (Fig. 5.3).

Observing respiration

Rate

The normal respiratory rate is about 10–15 breaths a minute, over 20 being abnormal (*tachypnoea*). Don't make it obvious that you are watching your patient's breathing since anxious patients often increase their respiratory rate while being observed. Tachypnoea is an important sign and sometimes the only clue to the presence of respiratory disease.

Almost any respiratory disease can increase respiratory rate but an increase is sometimes found with fever due to non-respiratory causes.

Practical Point

Tachypnoea is an important sign and sometimes the only clue to the presence of respiratory disease.

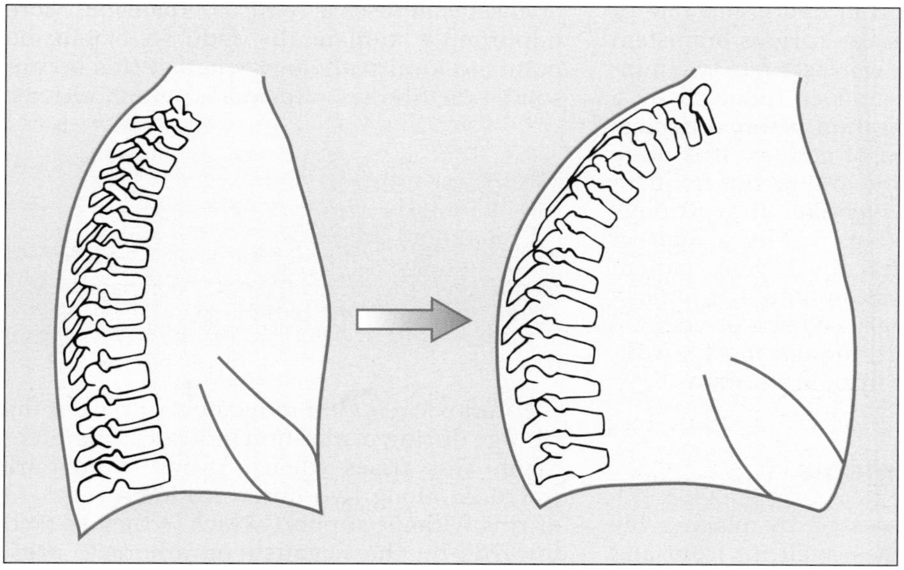

FIG. 5.6 Schematic lateral view of chest in Fig. 5.5 to show development of kyphosis due to wedging of thoracic vertebrae.

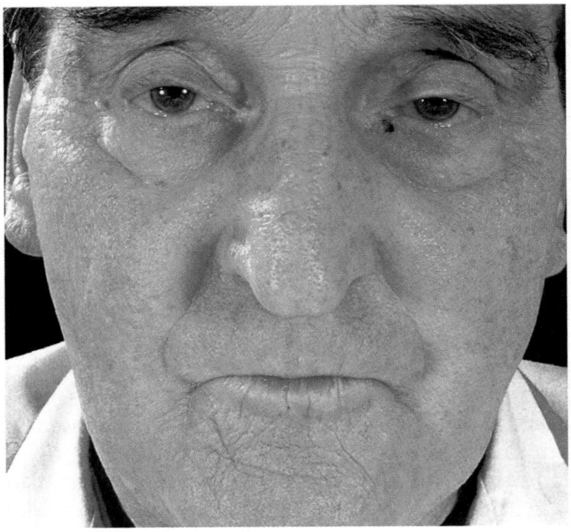

FIG. 5.7 Pursed-lip breathing.

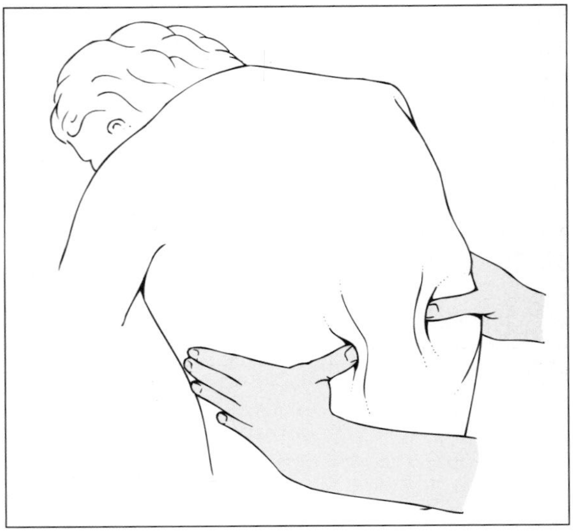

FIG. 5.8 Assessing chest expansion (see text).

Pattern of breathing

Observe the pattern of breathing. Shallow breathing is seen when breathing is restricted either by lung (e.g. fibrosis) or chest wall disease, or by pain. Metabolic acidosis, as in renal failure or diabetic ketoacidosis, causes an increased depth of respiration (Kussmaul breathing). Cheyne–Stokes breathing (a cyclical or periodic variation in depth and rate of breathing) usually indicates serious brainstem dysfunction. Each cycle can last up to two minutes, with a period of apnoea followed by a gradual return of respiration before a decline again to another period of apnoea. It is quite normal to sigh from time to time but frequent sighing suggests hyperventilation syndrome. Pursed-lip breathing (Fig. 5.7) is a sign of severe airflow obstruction. If your patient becomes more breathless on lying flat (*orthopnoea*), consider pulmonary oedema or bilateral diaphragmatic paralysis, though most breathless patients prefer the upright position.

Chest wall movements

Chest expansion is assessed by placing the hands on the lateral chest wall (in front and behind), picking up a fold of skin with the thumbs and watching the thumbs move apart in inspiration (Fig. 5.8). Normal chest expansion, at the level of the nipples, is usually not less than 5 cm. However, in routine practice it is quite sufficient to note whether expansion appears normal or reduced; exact measurement is unnecessary, being crude and of little diagnostic help since any cause of diffuse lung or chest wall disease reduces expansion. More importantly, unilaterally reduced expansion points to local pathology whether this is consolidation, fibrosis, effusion or pneumothorax.

Practical Point

If you cannot decide which is the abnormal side from minor differences in the physical signs, then the side with reduced expansion is likely to contain the pathology.

Paradoxical *inward* movement of part of the ribcage during inspiration indicates a flail segment. This arises when a group of ribs are fractured along two lines creating a segment of ribs without support which is then sucked inwards by the negative intrathoracic pres-

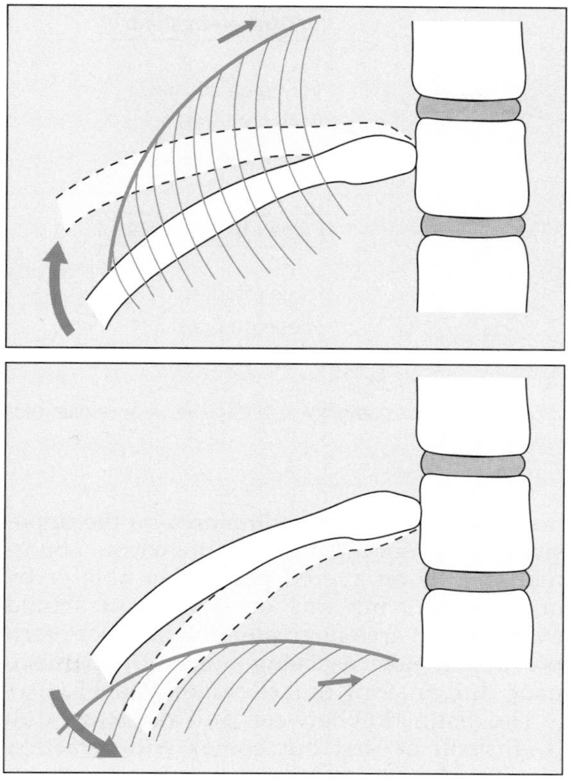

FIG. 5.9 Upper diagram: normal out and upward movement of ribs on inspiration with normal diaphragm (small arrow). Lower diagram: paradoxical upward movement of ribs when diaphragm flat as in hyperinflation.

sure during inspiration. The high negative pressure created by airflow obstruction can similarly lead to intercostal recession on inspiration. Normally during inspiration the lower ribs move outwards but with hyperinflated lungs in airflow obstruction the diaphragm becomes flat and causes indrawing of the ribs (Fig. 5.9). Watch abdominal movement during respiration. Normally the abdomen moves out due to diaphragmatic descent as the rib cage expands; inward or asynchronous abdominal movement suggests diaphragmatic paralysis or fatigue. Finally, in severe airflow obstruction, you may see the accessory muscles, scalenus anterior and sternomastoid, helping in the work of breathing. Such patients also use their arms to fix the shoulder girdle to increase the effectiveness of the accessory muscles.

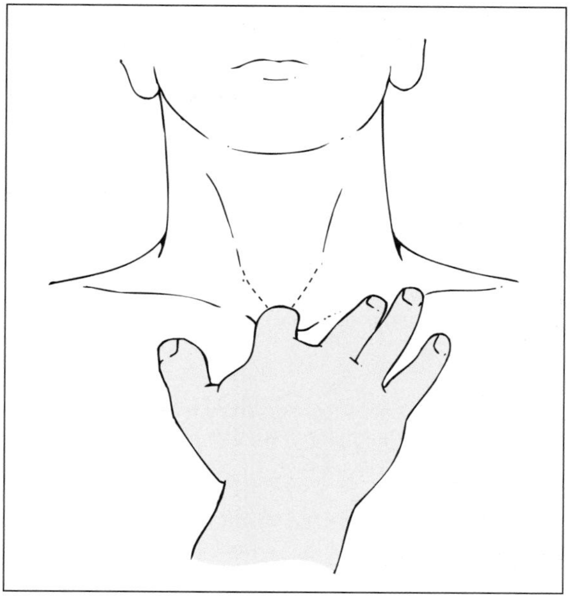

FIG. 5.10 Palpation of trachea.

Palpation of the trachea

Next, assess whether the trachea is central. There are several methods, the easiest being to put your index finger centrally in the suprasternal notch and gently move it backwards until the tip of your finger meets the trachea (Fig. 5.10), feeling then whether it is central or deviated. This is a crude test, which detects only major degrees of tracheal shift. Further information about the position of the mediastinum is gained from the position of the apex beat, the displacement of which is, however, more commonly due to cardiac than respiratory disease (Fig. 5.11).

Percussion of the chest

Percussion requires practice but should become second nature. If you are right-handed put the middle finger of your left hand flat on the chest wall and strike its middle phalanx smartly with

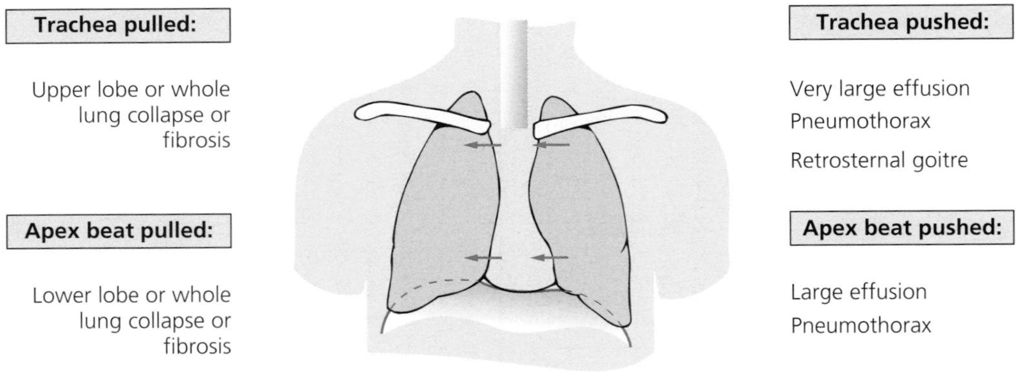

FIG. 5.11 Movement of the mediastinum (trachea and heart) as the result of various pathologies. The trachea may remain central despite collapse/effusion if fixed by mediastinal cancer.

the tip of the terminal phalanx of your right middle finger (Figs 5.12 and 5.13), the movement in your right hand coming from the wrist. You should assess the percussion note by both the pitch of the noise produced and the vibrations detected under your left middle finger. Percuss the clavicle directly with your right middle finger. Percuss over the sites in Fig. 5.14, the key point being to compare the percussion note over the corresponding area on the opposite side. If your attention is drawn to an abnormal area by an altered percussion note or by other local symptoms or signs, you should examine that area in greater detail. Assess each percussion note as being normal, hyperresonant, dull or stony dull (Revision Panel 5.10).

The distinction between dull and stony dull is difficult at first but comes with practice.

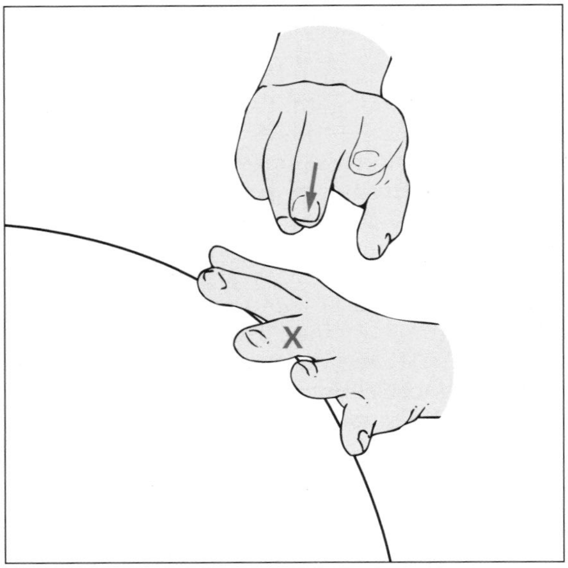

FIG. 5.12 Technique of percussion. The middle phalanx of the left middle finger (X) is struck at right angles by the terminal phalanx of the middle finger of the right hand.

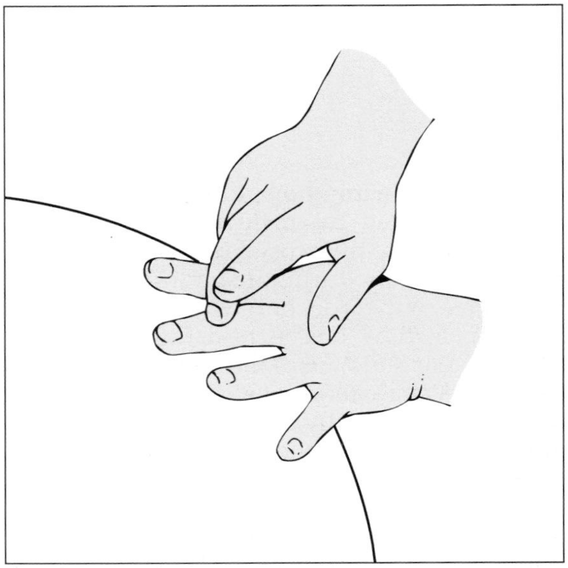

FIG. 5.13 Technique of percussion. Note that the movement in percussion is at the wrist.

Revision Panel 5.10
Percussion note

Hyperresonant
Hyperinflation e.g. emphysema/asthma.
Pneumothorax.
Very thin individuals.

Dull
Consolidation/collapse/fibrosis.
Obesity.

Stony dull
Pleural effusion.

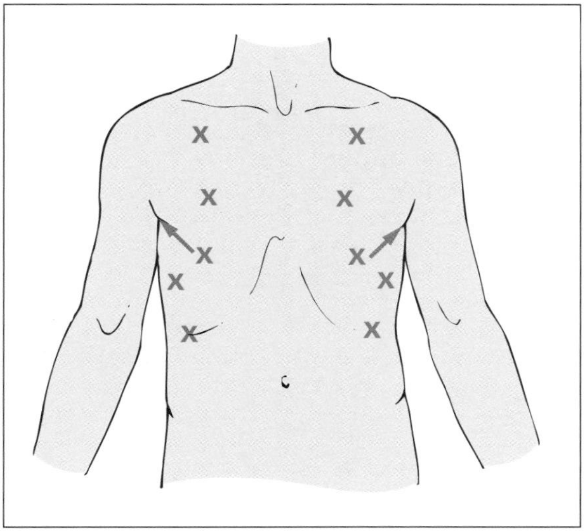

FIG. 5.14 Approximate sites for routine percussion (posterior similar).

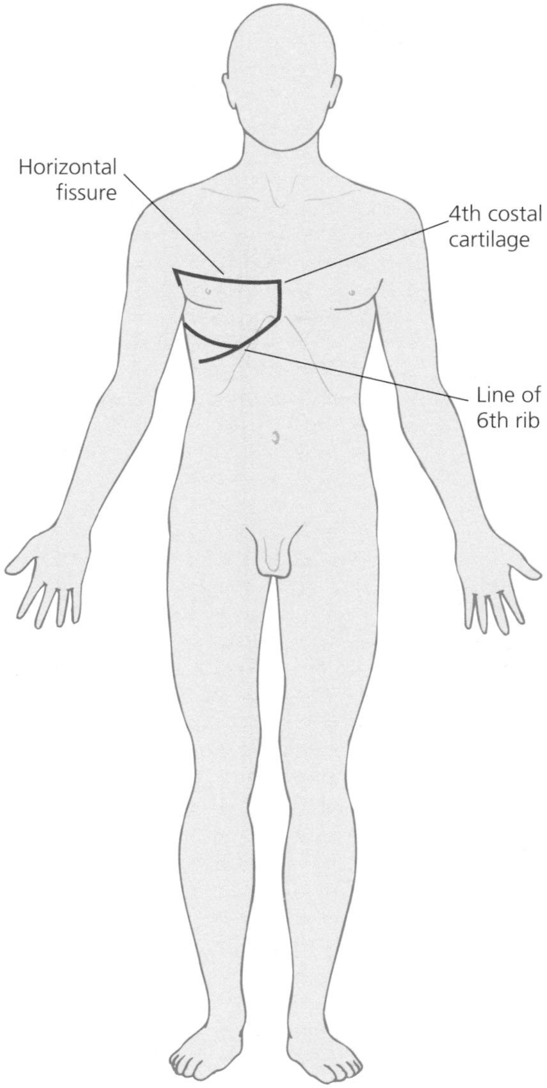

FIG. 5.15–5.17 Surface anatomy of right lung. Oblique fissure follows a line from T2 posteriorly to the sixth rib in the mid-axillary line. Horizontal fissure follows lower border of fourth rib to meet the oblique fissure in the mid-axillary line. Surface anatomy on the left is similar but there is no horizontal fissure.

Remember that if the percussion note on one side is different from the other side, there is likely to be an abnormality, either hyper-resonance on one side or dullness on the other side.

If, however, you find the same apparent abnormality on both sides, it is less likely that there is a significant problem. Thus bilateral basal dullness may be due to bilateral pleural effusions, but may simply be due to obesity. Diaphragmatic movement is difficult to detect by percussion but right basal dullness sometimes reflects a raised right hemidiaphragm and left basal hyperresonance reflects a raised left hemidiaphragm.

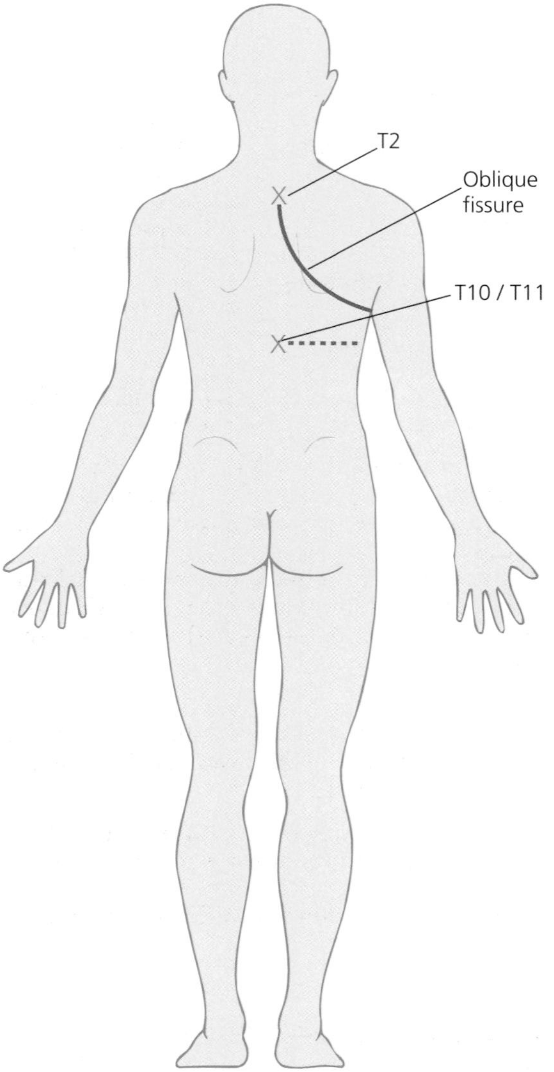

FIG. 5.16 Surface anatomy of right lung.

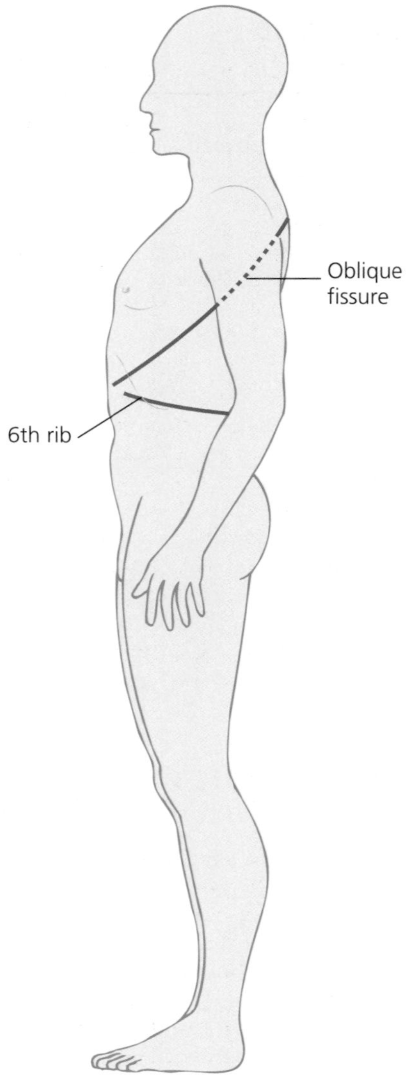

FIG. 5.17 Surface anatomy of left lung.

Surface anatomy

Keep in mind what part of the lung you are examining (Figs 5.15–5.17) and Revision Panel 5.11.

Dullness to percussion due to the liver is usually detected below the level of the 6th rib in mid-clavicular line although the upper border of the liver extends to just above the level of the 5th rib. Hyperinflated lungs push this upper border of liver dullness to a lower.

The breath sounds

Sounds heard at the mouth

In a healthy person at rest, you should not be able to hear the breath sounds at the mouth.

Revision Panel 5.11

A simple guide to surface anatomy of the lung

Right	Anterior	Upper chest.	Upper lobe
		Below horizontal level of 4th costal cartilage.	Middle lobe
	Posterior	All apart from apex.	Lower lobe
Left	Anterior	Almost all apart from lateral basal.	Upper lobe
	Posterior	All apart from apex.	Lower lobe

By contrast, in airways obstruction (COPD or asthma) breath sounds are often easily heard; in general the worse the airway narrowing the more noisy the breathing. These sounds arise from increased turbulence of air flow in the main airways. Noisy breathing should be considered separately from wheeze though the two may co-exist. Stridor is a harsh, sometimes musical, note heard at the mouth, most marked on inspiration. It denotes major airway obstruction (see below).

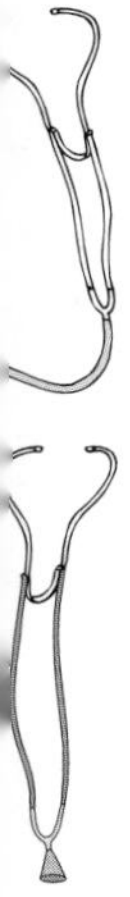

Auscultation

How to listen Ask your patient to 'take some deep breaths in and out with your mouth open'.

The diaphragm of the stethoscope is better suited to listening to high-frequency sounds and the bell to lower-frequency sounds. Many prefer to use the diaphragm to listen to the breath sounds but the bell can be useful in patients with hairy chests (to reduce crackling sounds produced by movement of hair) or in very thin patients in whom it may be difficult to flatten the diaphragm on the chest wall.

Make sure the pattern of breathing is otherwise normal but be gentle with patients with pleuritic pain who may be unable to take deep breaths.

Where to listen Auscultate over the same sites you percussed (see Fig. 5.14), comparing the sounds at each position with those heard in the corresponding position on the opposite side. Listen more than 2–3 cm away from the midline to listen over lung rather central airways. The number of sites at which you listen and the number of breaths you listen for at each site depends on experience and the likelihood of a respiratory problem:

- For a preoperative assessment for herniorrhapy in a fit young male it is sufficient to listen to three or four positions on both sides.
- More careful auscultation for a pleural rub is essential in a young woman with chest pain and breathlessness and who takes the contraceptive pill.

What to listen for Train yourself to listen through the full respiratory cycle, asking yourself at each site:

- Are breath sounds of normal intensity?
- Are breath sounds normal in character, or bronchial?
- Are there any added sounds on inspiration or expiration?

Practical Point

What to listen for on auscultation

Breath sounds
Normal or reduced/absent.
Bronchial (see Fig. 5.18).

Added sounds
Wheeze.
Crackles.
Rub.

With practice and concentration, ear and brain automatically answer these questions.

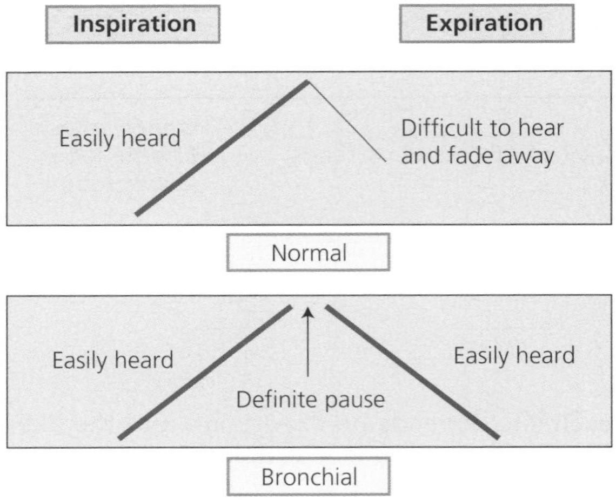

FIG. 5.18 Normal and bronchial breath sounds.

Revision Panel 5.12
Bronchial breathing (BB)

Absence of BB never excludes consolidation. If main bronchus obstructed, BB will *not* be heard over LOWER lobe consolidation or collapse.

If main bronchus obstructed, BB may be heard over UPPER lobe consolidation or collapse due to tracheal sounds transmitted across adjoining lung.

Normal and bronchial breath sounds

Normal breath sounds These are the sounds you hear over normal lung. Sometimes they are termed 'vesicular' but 'normal' is preferable. The sounds probably arise from turbulent airflow in major airways rather than movement of air in alveoli. They are transmitted across intervening lung to the chest wall, with resulting loss of the higher frequencies. The sounds increase in inspiration but fade soon after expiration begins (Fig. 5.18).

Breath sounds may be:

- Reduced or absent if there is a barrier to their transmission as in pleural effusion or pneumothorax, or when airflow is reduced locally to part of the lung, as in collapse.
- Quiet bilaterally in obesity, hyperinflation and when respiration is depressed as in an unconscious patient.

It is sometimes difficult to be sure if the breath sounds are quite normal but if they are similar on both sides they most likely are normal.

Bronchial breath sounds When the lung between the large airways and the chest wall is relatively solid, breath sounds are transmitted more readily than normal. The sounds resemble those heard by listening directly over the larynx or trachea. You will hear this 'bronchial breathing' over consolidation, collapse and sometimes fibrosis (but see Revision Panel 5.12 and Fig. 5.19).

The breath sounds in bronchial breathing are distinguished from normal (Fig. 5.18) since:

- They are harsher with their higher frequencies preserved.
- They have a definite pause between inspiration and expiration.
- They can be heard throughout expiration.

Added sounds

The classification of added sounds is now straightforward. Concentrate on three sounds: wheezes, crackles and rubs.

Wheezes Wheezes are musical sounds produced by airway walls oscillating between the open and nearly closed positions. They usually occur in expiration but also in inspiration in severe airway narrowing. Wheeze indicates airway narrowing which may be:

- Generalized as in asthma (Revision Panel 5.13) in which wheeze is composed of sounds of many different pitches (polyphonic). In very severe airflow obstruction, wheeze may be absent.
- Localized, of single pitch unaltered by coughing (monophonic or fixed). This strongly suggests large airway obstruction, most commonly due to tumour.

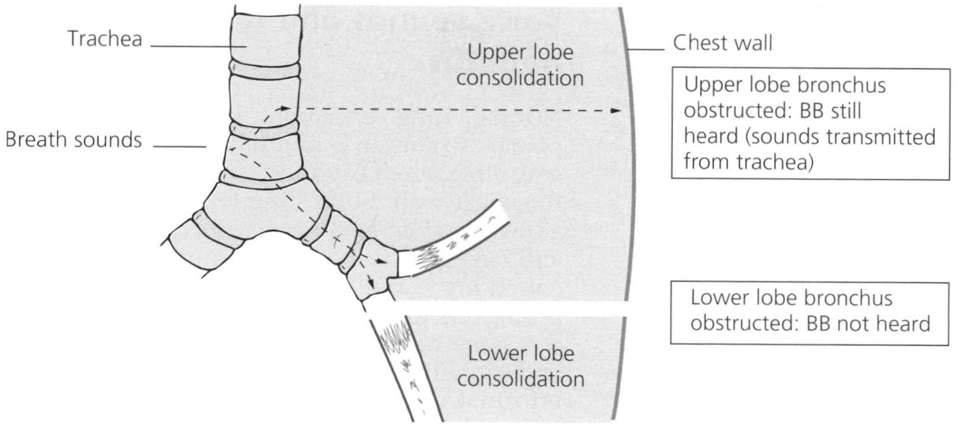

FIG. 5.19 Transmission of breath sounds when central airways obstructed. BB: Bronchial breathing.

Revision Panel 5.13
Causes of wheeze on auscultation

Generalized	*Localized*
Asthma.	Tumour.
COPD.	Foreign body.[b]
Left ventricular failure.[a]	

[a]Common.
[b]Rare.

Wheeze or stridor? Stridor is a loud, mainly inspiratory noise, usually heard at the mouth. It is produced by potentially serious laryngeal, tracheal or major airway obstruction and must therefore be recognized. Like wheeze, stridor can be a musical noise and difficult to recognize in patients with co-existing generalized airway narrowing. Always suspect stridor if wheeze is louder on inspiration than expiration.

Crackles Crackles are most often due to the sudden opening of lightly occluded airways when gas passes through, though may sometimes be produced by secretions in main airways. Note the position of crackles in the respiratory cycle and whether they are localized to a certain area in the lung (Revision Panel 5.14).

Be careful as crackles may be produced by hair moving under the stethoscope. Distinguishing fine from coarse crackles often adds little diagnostically, though certain crackles are characteristic – e.g. those of fibrosing alveolitis sound like unfastening Velcro.

Revision Panel 5.14
Causes of crackles

Late inspiratory (typically bilateral and basal)
Pulmonary oedema (e.g. left ventricular failure).
Fibrosing alveolitis.
Asbestosis.

Early inspiratory/expiratory
Bronchiectasis *(localized)*.
Chronic bronchitis *(scanty)*.

Inspiratory (localized)
Pneumonia.

Pleural rub This is a coarse, creaking sound probably produced by the movement of inflamed visceral and parietal pleurae on each other. You may hear it both in inspiration and expiration but rarely if a substantial pleural effusion is present. Any cause of pleural inflammation can cause a rub (commonly infection, pulmonary infarction or pleural trauma, including biopsies).

Practical Point

Always suspect stridor if wheeze is louder on inspiration than expiration.

Other added sounds A bruit is likely to be due to an arteriovenous communication such as an aneurysm. Listen carefully for a bruit if the patient has a rounded opacity on the chest X-ray of uncertain aetiology, particularly before biopsy. Clicks may be heard over a left-sided pneumothorax but are of little significance. Squeaks, rather than wheezes, are sometimes heard in small airway inflammation such as in acute extrinsic allergic alveolitis.

Voice sounds and tactile vocal fremitus

Normal lung transmits higher frequencies poorly, so speech is unintelligible and whisper inaudible when listening with a stethoscope at the chest wall. Solid lung (e.g. consolidation) allows higher frequencies to be transmitted and so speech becomes intelligible ('bronchophony') and whispering audible ('whispering pectoriloquy'). These two signs share the same mechanism, are only present when bronchial breathing is present, add no further information and are redundant.

The transmission of voice sounds to the chest wall is palpable as low-frequency vibra-

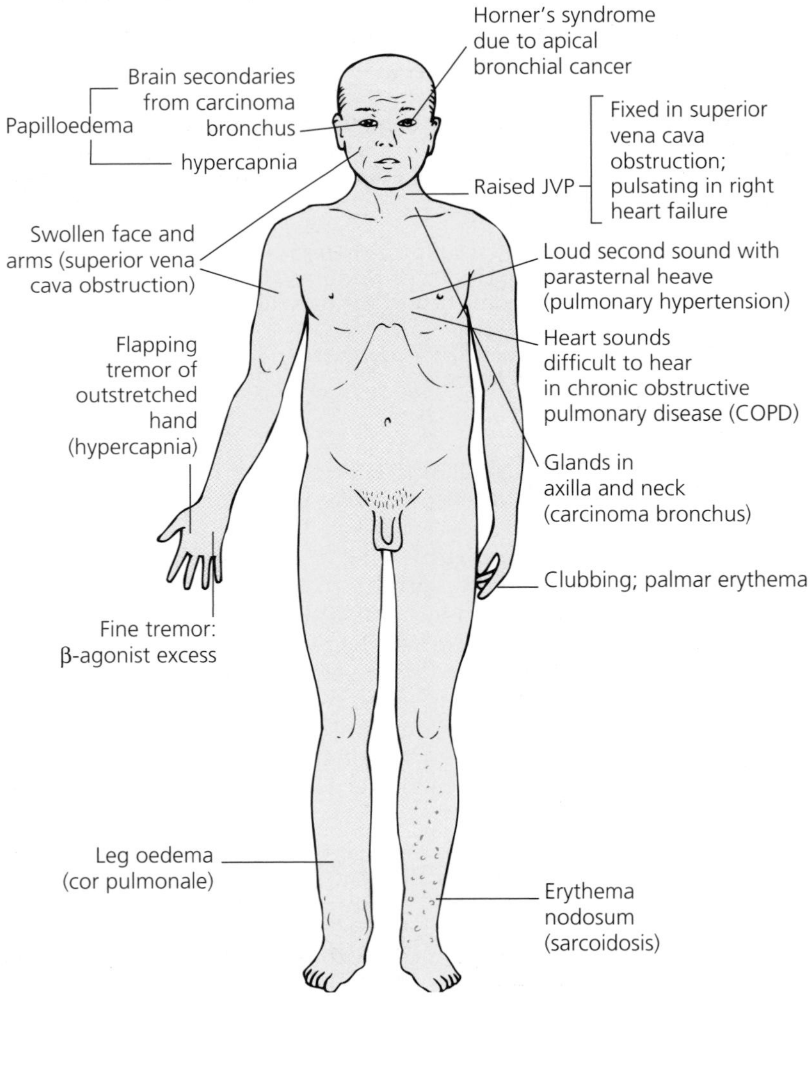

FIG. 5.20 Extrathoracic signs associated with respiratory disease. JVP: Jugular venous pressure.

Practical Point

Don't waste time with voice sounds and tactile vocal fremitus in the routine examination of the chest if there are no significant abnormalities otherwise.

tion. This is tactile vocal fremitus (TVF) and, as always, the key is comparison of the two sides, preferably simultaneously. Put the sensitive part of the palms of both hands on the chest wall and ask your patient to say 'Ninety-nine'. TVF is palpable over normal lung and remains palpable or increased over consolidation, but is always reduced over an effusion.

The present-day value of the voice sounds and TVF is doubtful. However when you find a reduced percussion note for which the reason is unclear, either because there is no bronchial breathing or the breath sounds are only slightly reduced, then a reduction in voice sounds or, especially, TVF strongly favours pleural effusion or thickening.

Other signs

Since lung disease, such as cancer, may have widespread systemic effects and systemic diseases frequently involve the lungs, you should complete a full examination with particular reference to the signs in Fig. 5.20. Examine your patient's sputum if available. Urine analysis is vital – haematuria, for example, may give the important clue to vasculitis being the cause of diffuse chest X-ray shadowing. If you suspect airflow obstruction (see Fig. 5.21), measure your patient's peak expiratory flow rate (PEFR) using a peak flow meter.

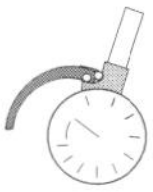

Putting it all together: physical signs in common respiratory conditions

The next few pages bring together these physical signs. The principal signs of the following respiratory conditions are shown in Figs 5.21–5.26.

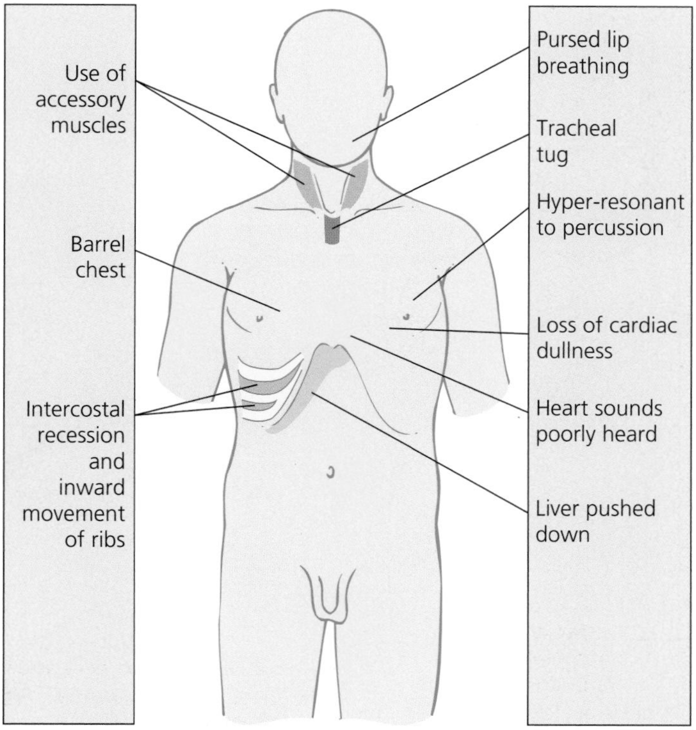

FIG. 5.21 Diagram of signs seen in airflow obstruction.

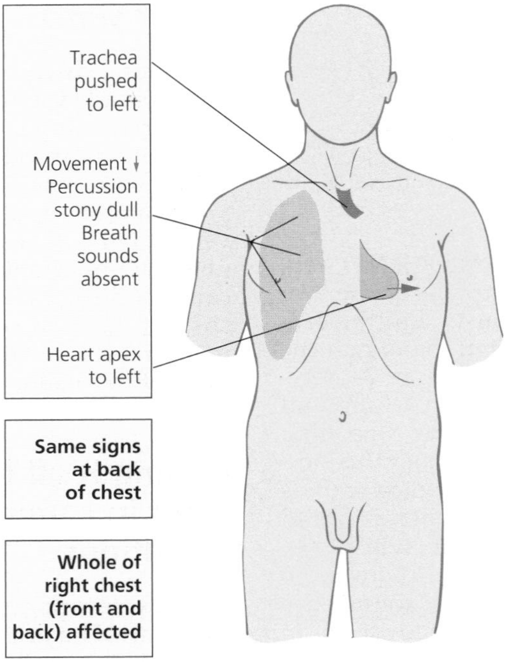

FIG. 5.22 Signs of a massive right-sided pleural effusion.

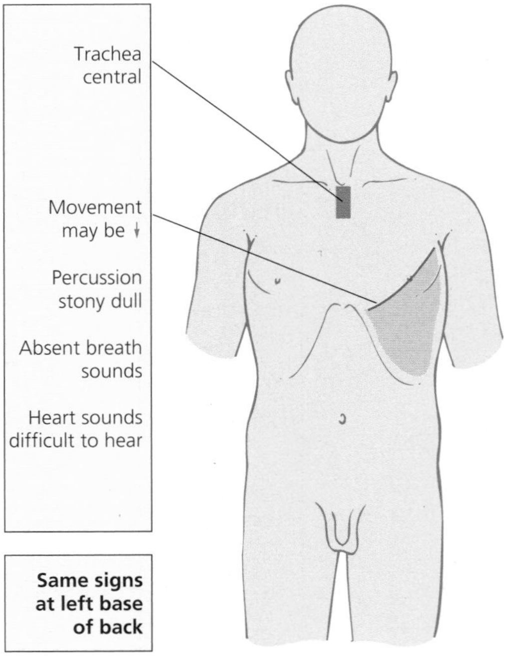

FIG. 5.23 Signs of a moderate left-sided pleural effusion.

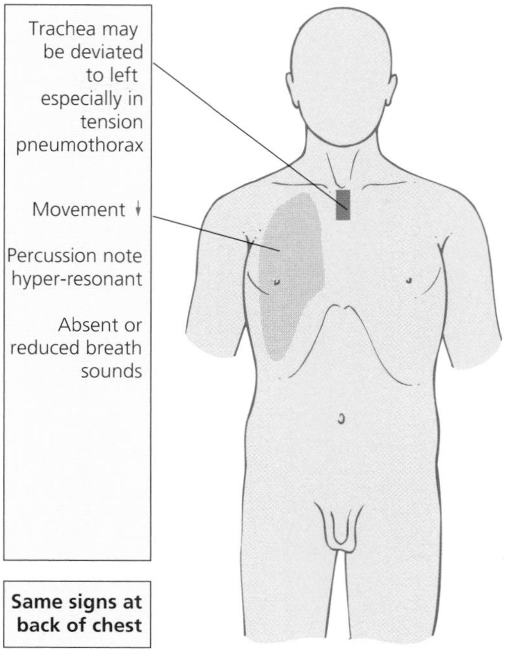

FIG. 5.24 Signs of a right-sided pneumothorax.

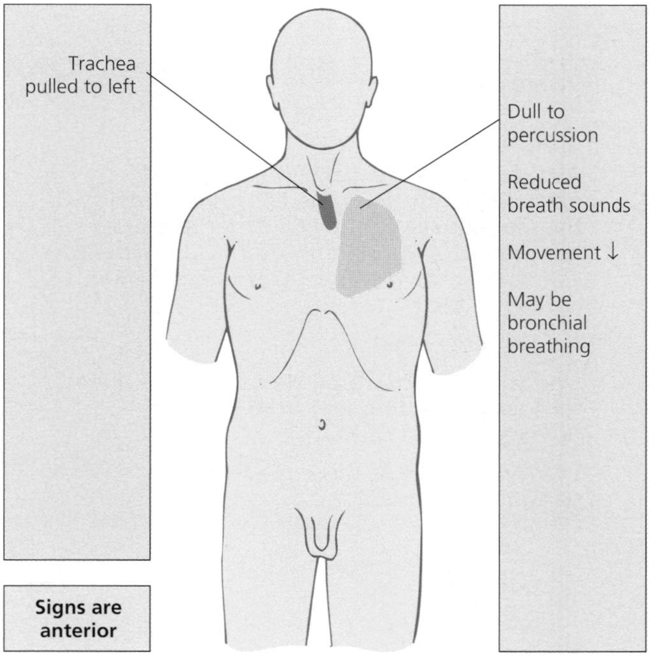

FIG. 5.25 Signs of collapse of the left upper lobe.

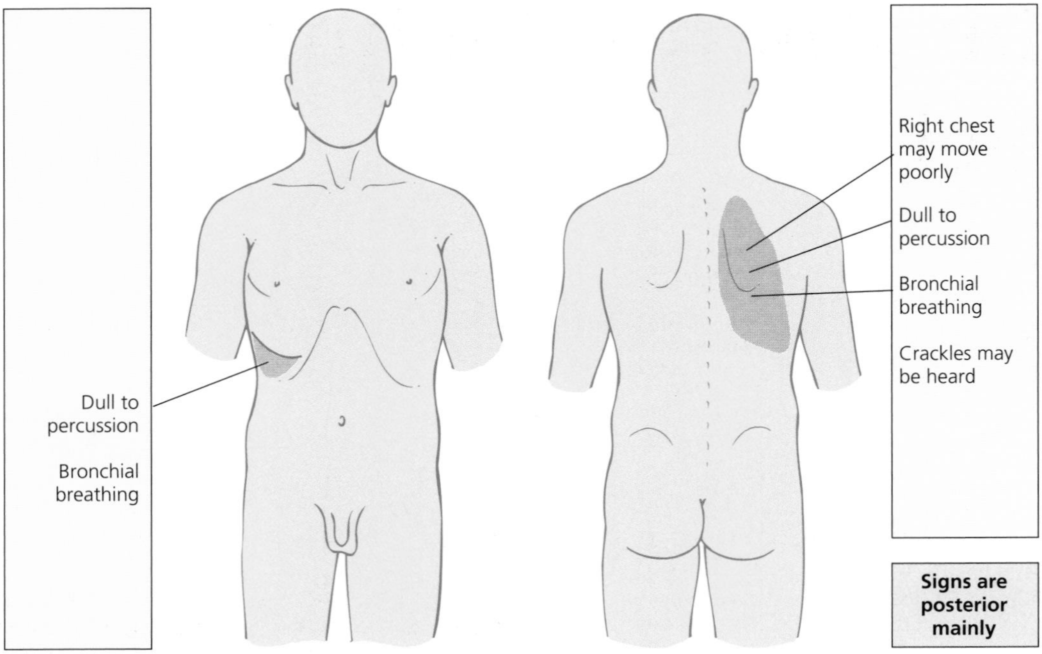

FIG. 5.26 Signs of consolidation of the right lower lobe.

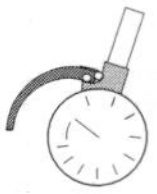

Practical Point

Measuring peak flow

Ask your patient to take in the biggest possible breath, close the lips tightly round the mouthpiece of the PEF meter and blow out as hard as possible. A short sharp blow is essential as the meter records the maximum airflow in the first 10 ms.

Record three readings.

Find your patient's predicted value (calculated for height, sex and age) from tables of predicted values of PEFR.

Express the best of three readings as a percentage of predicted.

The gastrointestinal tract

6

In this section we deal with the gastrointestinal tract, from mouth to anus, including the liver and pancreas.

SYMPTOMS

Here you have to be patient and question closely; many of the terms used by your patients are vague, imprecise and often frankly confusing. They will know what they mean but that doesn't necessarily mean that you will. Some confusing terms include:

Indigestion This may mean anything from pain to anorexia.
Heartburn True acid reflux or angina?
Wind Does it come up or down? Or is it merely gurgling in the belly?
Sickness Malaise, fever, nausea or true vomiting?

Find out what your patient really means.

> **Practical Point**
>
> The factory worker who develops burning substernal pain coming on whilst hurrying back to his bench after his midday meal at the canteen may not be suffering from simple heartburn as he supposes. It could well be angina coming on after food.

Pain

Pain is a common symptom in gastrointestinal disease and a few minutes of history-taking may save hours of unnecessary, expensive and uncomfortable investigations. First of all try to establish what sort of abdominal pain you are dealing with (see Revision Panel 6.1). Is the pain visceral, parietal or referred? This may be quite difficult but knowledge of the embryology does help to explain the site of the pain.

Visceral pain arises as the result of stretching or contractions of hollow organs such as gut, gallbladder or uterus. As these organs are midline structures embryologically the pain is felt in the midline. In contrast, pain from the ureters is unilateral. Unlike the visceral peritoneum the parietal peritoneum contains pain

> Revision Panel 6.1
> **Types of abdominal pain**
>
> *Visceral*
> As in gut colic.
>
> *Parietal*
> Localized peritoneal inflammation.
>
> *Referred*
> Shoulder tip pain in diaphragmatic irritation.

fibres. When it is inflamed it causes pain immediately over the affected area which is aggravated by moving or stretching the peritoneum. This gives rise to guarding and pain after sudden release of pressure over the inflamed area (*release pain*). An example of the combination of both visceral and parietal pain is seen when a patient gets biliary colic due to a stone in the common bile duct. This produces midline visceral pain. If, as is often the case, the gallbladder distends and becomes secondarily inflamed the overlying parietal peritoneum is responsible for localized pain in the right upper quadrant.

Referred pain occurs when pain in one area is felt in another area, which has the same sensory supply. The best example of this in the abdomen is shoulder tip pain which occurs with subdiaphragmatic irritation as with a perforated peptic ulcer.

Get into the habit of asking questions about abdominal pain in a set sequence (see Revision Panel 6.2).

Revision Panel 6.2

Questions to be asked about abdominal pain

How long? Hours, days or months?

Constant, progressive or recurring?

Position, radiation and aggravating factors?

Relation to food?

Change in bowel habit?

Associated weight loss?

Nausea and/or vomiting?

More details are given in Chapter 27 which helps you to sort out the various types of abdominal pain seen in practice.

Anorexia, nausea and vomiting

Anorexia encompasses a wide range of symptoms extending from mild loss of appetite to intense distaste of food. It is a non-specific symptom and occurs in many acute and chronic non-gastrointestinal illnesses. In acute gastrointestinal disease it is a highly disagreeable feature of the prodromal phase of infectious hepatitis and in chronic disease it is a prominent symptom in carcinoma of the stomach. The disease of teenage girls, *anorexia nervosa*, has already been alluded to in Chapter 2. They lose much weight as the result of denial of food but curiously rarely complain of a poor appetite.

Many patients will complain that they 'feel sick' when they just feel generally unwell. Nausea as an isolated symptom, without vomiting, is more likely to be due to depression or neurosis than gastrointestinal disease. When nausea is associated with vomiting you must first, in middle-aged and older patients, consider upper gastrointestinal problems such as carcinoma of the stomach or peptic ulceration. There is likely to be associated anorexia and weight loss. With gastric outlet obstruction the vomits are likely to be huge containing undigested food taken many hours, or even a day or so, previously.

The vomiting of blood, *haematemesis*, is nearly always due to ulcerative lesions of the gastrointestinal tract as far down as the second part of the duodenum, or to bleeding varices secondary to portal hypertension. Brisk bleeding usually causes vomiting of fresh blood but slower bleeding into the upper gastrointestinal tract may not necessarily be vomited but continues on through the gut to be passed as black diarrhoea or *melaena*. Repeated vomiting, as after an alcoholic binge, may tear the gastro-oesophageal junction. The bleeding from this source is not usually severe and is referred to as *Mallory–Weiss* bleeding after the two doctors who first described it.

Substernal burning, commonly termed heartburn, is characteristic of gastro-oesophageal reflux; this is aggravated by heavy meals, smoking, sitting in a slumped position or working bending over as in gardening. Burning fluid, sometimes called waterbrash, often regurgitates into the mouth but is rarely vomited.

As with anorexia, not all nausea and vomiting is due to disease of the gastrointestinal tract. Recurrent and profuse vomiting may occur with:

- Migraine in children and young adults; ask carefully about any associated headaches, which may be mild and may not be considered by the patient to be of any great significance.
- Hypercalcaemia.
- Uraemia.
- Drug toxicity e.g. digoxin.
- Raised intracranial pressure.

Problems with swallowing

Patients will tell you that they have pain on swallowing or food sticking in the throat. The latter symptom must always be taken seriously. Doctors tend to use the term dysphagia rather loosely. Strictly speaking it means 'difficulty in swallowing' and it is better to restrict its use to this and to the sensation of food sticking. If you have to use a long word to describe pain on swallowing use the term *odynophagia*.

Pain on swallowing is usually due to oesophagitis. Ask about symptoms of reflux of acid fluid on bending or lying down. Patients will often call substernal pain 'heartburn'. Make sure that you know what they are actually describing. A common, and potentially serious error, is to confuse this with angina precipitated by heavy meals.

In the second half of life patients who complain, for the first time, of increasing difficulty in swallowing are likely to have a serious cause such as carcinoma of the pharynx, oesophagus or gastro-oesophageal junction. There has to be quite significant narrowing before the symptom of dysphagia is felt and the severity of this symptom often increases rapidly over the next few days.

Practical Point

Patients who complain of increasing difficulty in swallowing must be investigated urgently.

Chronic and/or intermittent dysphagia is more likely to be due to a benign stricture or achalasia of the cardia (see Revision Panel 6.3). The latter disease usually becomes evident during the first half of life and is due to spasm at the lower end of the oesophagus; it is said that patients experience more difficulty in swallowing liquids than solids but this is by no means always true. With all other causes of dysphagia it is easier to swallow liquids than solids. A common symptom, encountered often in young women of nervous disposition is an apparent need to swallow frequently to overcome what seems to be an obstruction at the back of the throat. No cause is found for this symptom which is termed 'globus hystericus'. It has to be said that though nervous, these young women are by no means hysterical.

Revision Panel 6.3
Causes of dysphagia

Achalasia of the cardia.

Benign stricture (usually secondary to reflux).

Ulceration (e.g. moniliasis).

Carcinoma of the oesophagus.

Carcinoma of the cardia of the stomach.

External pressure (e.g. carcinoma of bronchus, aneurysm of the aorta).

Neurological lesions (e.g. motor neuron disease).

Bowels

Many would have us believe that the only way to achieve perfect health is to have one formed bowel action each day after breakfast. This is complete nonsense. For some people two or three bowel actions each day may be normal whereas for others two or three bowel actions each week are compatible with perfect health. Much depends on personal habits, physical activity, fluid intake and diet. Long, thin, tapered stools are rarely of significance. A flurry of two or three bowel actions on rising is often of nervous origin.

Some symptoms are certainly not normal and must be investigated properly. These are:

- Bleeding on defaecation.
- Mucus with the stools.
- Diarrhoea with blood and mucus.
- A change from a previously well established bowel habit.
- A sensation of incomplete emptying of the rectum.
- Nocturnal diarrhoea.
- Frequent large, bulky, pale stools.

The passage of blood with the stools is dealt with in Chapters 35 and 37.

Practical Point

Unexplained rectal bleeding must be fully investigated with sigmoidoscopy and colonoscopy or barium enema.

In any patient with diarrhoea associated with blood or mucus you must ask about recent travel abroad but bear in mind that parasites or infection found in the gut may not necessarily be the cause of the illness. Tropical infections such as amoebiasis or strongyloidiasis together with some other sexually transmitted diseases such as syphilis or gonorrhoea may form the 'gay bowel' syndrome encountered in male homosexuals.

Constipation is dealt with in more detail in Chapter 36 but remember that this is a common symptom with many simple causes such as prolonged immobility and bed rest, slimming diets, change in habitat, travel and dehydration.

Jaundice

Jaundice is an alarming symptom, which quickly brings patients to consult their doctors. In practical terms you can usually make a diagnosis on the history alone as to whether the jaundice is infective hepatitis, chronic liver disease or obstructive jaundice. More details are given in Chapter 39. Do not forget that drugs as medication can produce hepatitic or cholestatic type jaundice. Sharp episodes of haemolysis, as in malaria or sickle cell disease, may produce significant jaundice but, on the whole, the actual jaundice is but a minor feature of the basic disease.

If the patient is young and an infective cause is suspected you need to ask about:

- A prodromal illness of anorexia, fever and malaise.
- Contacts.
- Intravenous drugs, accidental needle stabs, blood transfusions, homosexuality (hepatitis B and C).
- Recent travel abroad.

If the patient is middle aged or elderly and an obstructive jaundice is suspected, ask about:

- Colour of stools (pale if obstruction is complete).
- Upper abdominal pain suggestive of gallstones.
- Back pain and fatty stools if pancreatic tumour is suspected.

If the jaundice is suspected to be due to cirrhosis ask about:

- Alcohol.
- Previous episodes of jaundice.
- Previous transfusions.
- Skin itching (particularly severe in primary biliary cirrhosis).

Wind

This common symptom rarely has a serious cause. Wind belched up is described as flatulence and wind passed downwards is politely described as flatus. Make sure that you know what your patients are talking about. They, and some of their doctors, confuse the two terms. If necessary resort to basic everyday speech.

Chronic belchers are usually air swallowers. Gas is not generated in the stomach unless antacids are taken – but patients are often reluctant to accept this point. However, air may be trapped in a large paraoesophageal hernia which, when expelled by belching, gives relief. Excessive flatus is produced in alactasia and is also noted by those on high fibre diets.

Abdominal bloating refers to windy distension of the abdomen often aggravated by physical inactivity and reluctance to pass flatus.

Practical Point

High fibre diets often produce windy colicky pain.

THE EXAMINATION

THE MOUTH

Do not neglect the mouth when you are examining a patient with abdominal symptoms. It is, after all, the first part of the gastrointestinal tract. Patients stick out their tongues for inspection as an expected and essential part of their clinical examination. We can, of course, gain much information from this procedure though the state of the tongue certainly cannot be used as an index of health in the way that many patients believe.

Practical Point

A dirty furred tongue does not necessarily indicate poor health.

A smooth, clean, red, depapillated tongue usually does.

When you examine the mouth remember that you need:

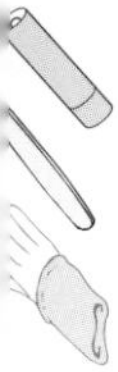

- A good light.
- A spatula to depress the tongue and to retract the cheeks.
- A pair of gloves to palpate lesions bimanually.

Examination of the mouth allows you to:

- Check the degree of hydration – but it is important to differentiate between the symptom of thirst and factors that cause dryness of the mouth (see Revision Panel 6.4).

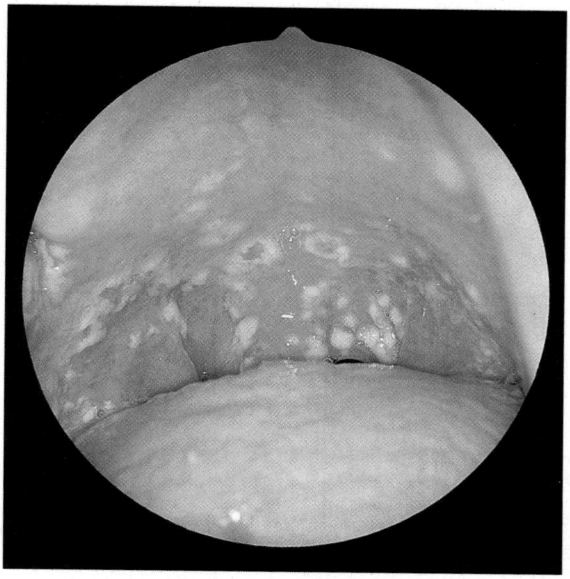

FIG. 6.1 Moniliasis of the soft palate in a man with AIDS.

- Look for specific lesions such as ulcers and lumps.
- Search for local and/or supplementary clues that may help in the diagnosis of more generalized disease e.g. the finding of moniliasis in a patient with AIDS (Fig. 6.1).

Revision Panel 6.4

Causes of thirst	Causes of a dry mouth
Diabetes mellitus.	Emotion.
Diabetes insipidus.	Drugs (e.g. atropine, inhalers, antidepressives).
Diuretic therapy e.g. frusemide.	Mouth breathing.
Hypercalcaemia.	Local radiotherapy, especially with irradiation of salivary glands.
Renal failure.	Diseases of salivary glands (e.g. Sjögren's).
Compulsive water drinking.	Old age.
Dehydration.	Dehydration.

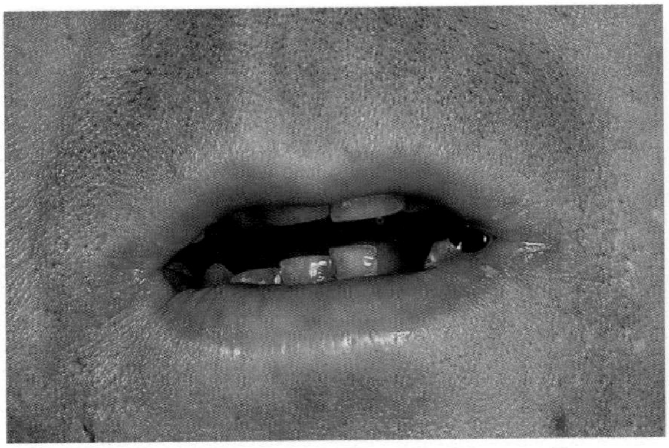

FIG. 6.2 Angular stomatitis. The cracks at the angles of the mouth often, as in this case, become infected with monilia.

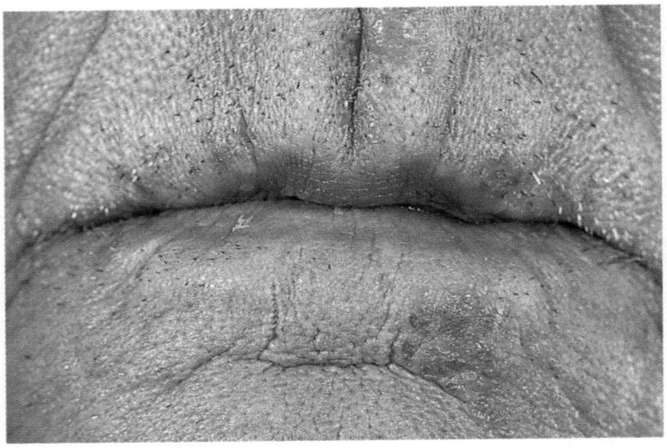

FIG. 6.3 Herpes labialis. A common viral infection complicating febrile states.

The lips

Cracks at the angles of the mouth (cheilosis or angular stomatitis) are very common. They are described in most textbooks as being due to anaemia and malabsorption. Indeed they are, but much more commonly they are caused by overlapping of the lips in edentulous patients or in those with badly fitting dentures. The overlapped skin becomes sodden and macerated and often becomes secondarily infected with monilia (Fig. 6.2).

Herpes labialis (Fig. 6.3) presents as a cluster of vesicles on the lips or surrounding skin often in an entirely well patient. Crops of lesions may be associated with febrile states, but florid and recurrent infections are common in the immunosuppressed.

Carcinoma of the lip presents as a warty growth or a thickened plaque, usually on the lower lip in men who are pipe smokers. Always feel the submental nodes for possible metastases.

Syphilitic primary chancres are rare but may appear as button-like nodules on the lip which ulcerate and crust. They are highly contagious, so wear gloves when examining a suspicious lesion.

The lesions of hereditary haemorrhagic telangiectasia (Osler–Weber–Rendu syndrome) (Fig. 6.4) are seen on the lips, tongue, buccal and nasal mucosa and on the fingertips. They may extend down the upper part of the gastrointestinal tract as far as the lower end of the oesophagus. They often bleed into the gut leading to iron-deficient anaemia. The nasal lesions commonly give rise to recurrent epistaxes.

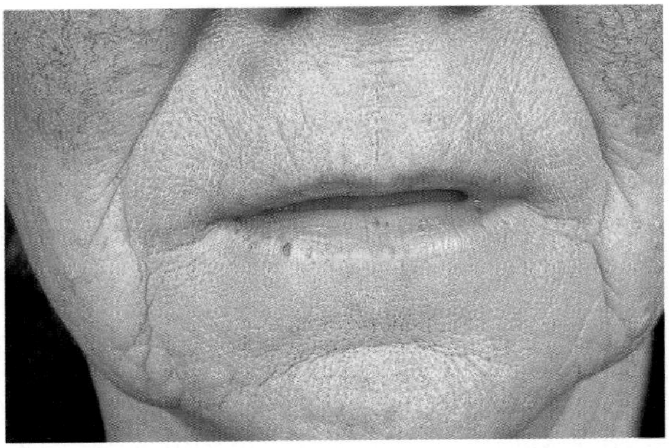

FIG. 6.4 Hereditary haemorrhagic telangiectasia. The lesions may be relatively insignificant but may extend into the pharynx and oesophagus.

The lesions of the very rare Peutz–Jeghers syndrome appear as pigmented flecks at the mucocutaneous junction or around the mouth. Their clinical importance is that they are associated with small intestinal polyps, which may cause intussception.

Teeth and gums

The condition of the teeth is often a good index of both a patient's oral hygiene and of their health consciousness. The commonest simple disorder of the gums is gingivitis, often due to irritative calculous formation, which results in swelling, redness and bleeding. Acute necrotizing ulcerative gingivitis is a painful viral infection causing swelling, sloughy inflammation and highly unpleasant halitosis.

With advancing years recession of the gum margins causes exposure of the necks of the teeth; as a result the elderly become 'long in the tooth'.

Brownish pigmentation is seen on the buccal mucosa, opposite the molar teeth, in Addison's disease. This must not be confused with the very common melanotic pigmentation on the gums in healthy Black people.

Gum swelling occurs:

- Physiologically at puberty and in pregnancy.
- As the result of chronic ingestion of some drugs including phenytoin, cyclosporin and nifedipine.
- In acute leukaemia (Fig. 6.5); the gums bleed and become infected.
- In Vitamin C deficiency (scurvy) which also causes bleeding of the gums.

The tongue

You must be aware of the variation in the appearance of the tongue in healthy people.

- A dirty tongue may be compatible with normal health but is seen in mouth breathers and smokers.
- Irregular clefts sometimes develop with increasing age, the so-called 'scrotal' tongue.
- Other normal tongues have irregular patches, denuded of papillae, producing a map-like area on the dorsum. These change from time to time and form what is termed the 'geographical' tongue.
- The black hairy tongue is caused by elongation of the filiform papillae on the dorsum. It may, but not necessarily always, follow antibiotic therapy.
- Elderly people may have varicosities on the under surface of the tongue – the 'caviar' tongue.

Whilst the coated tongue may be normal, smooth, red, depapillated ones are certainly not and may indicate iron-deficiency anaemia, pernicious anaemia, malabsorption or recent treatment with antibiotics (Fig. 6.6). Similar changes are seen with the mucositis of chemotherapy or radiotherapy.

Moniliasis is characterized by curdy, white patches on the palate and cheeks. Ill patients who are particularly vulnerable to moniliasis

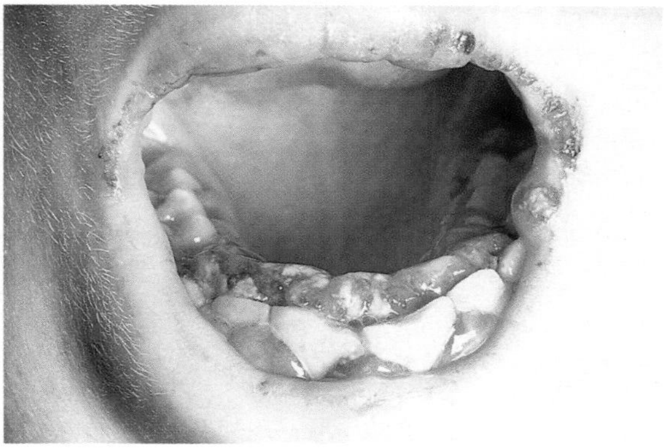

FIG. 6.5 Swollen, haemorrhagic, infected gums in acute leukaemia.

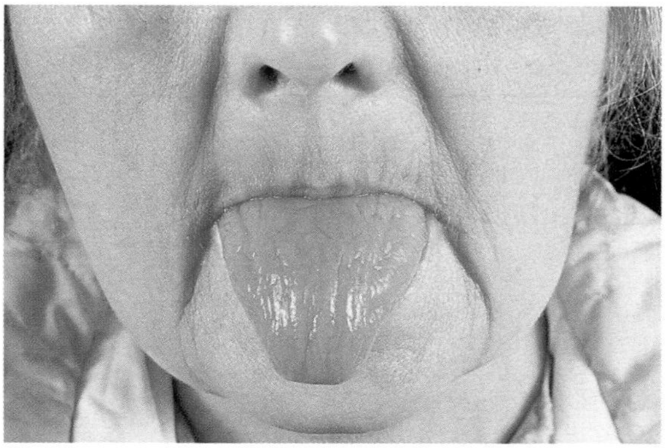

FIG. 6.6 The smooth, red tongue. Note the associated pallor; this woman had a chronic iron deficiency anaemia.

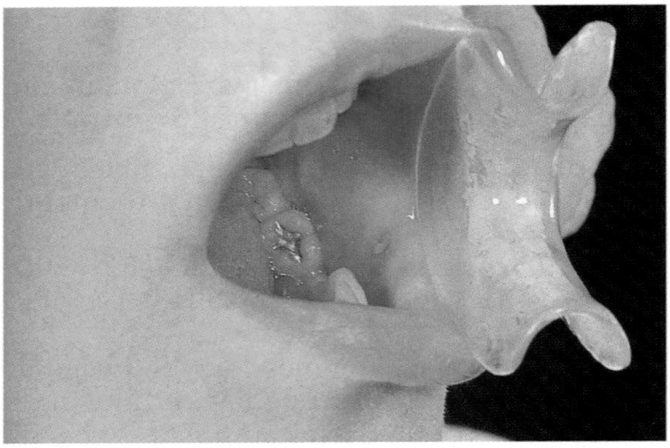

FIG. 6.7 An aphthous ulcer on inside of the cheek.

include the old and debilitated, patients taking antibiotics or undergoing chemotherapy and those with carcinoma or lymphoma. Its appearance in an apparently fit young adult should always alert you to a possible defect in immunity, quite possibly the AIDS-related complex.

Aphthous ulcers are extremely common (see Revision Panel 6.5). These very painful lesions mainly affect women and may appear in crops to coincide with periods. Each lesion starts as a tiny whitish-grey nodule, a few mm in diameter, which quickly ulcerates and then slowly heals over three or four days (Fig. 6.7). The ulcers may appear anywhere on the tongue or buccal mucosa. Coeliac disease is a possible cause in a patient with unusually severe and intractable aphthous ulceration.

Revision Panel 6.5
Ulcers of the tongue

Acute
Aphthous[a]
Herpetic
As part of a stomatitis
Traumatic[a]

Subacute or chronic
Irritative (usually from teeth)
Tuberculous
Syphilitic chancre
Carcinoma
Non-Hodgkin's lymphoma

[a]Common

Stomatitis

This covers an extremely wide range of conditions in which there may be ulceration, infection, necrosis or desquamation of the mucosa. The conditions range from the benign but painful aphthous ulceration to the potentially fatal cancrum oris (see Revision Panel 6.6).

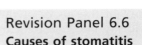

Revision Panel 6.6
Causes of stomatitis

Infective
Moniliasis.
Acute herpetic gingivostomatitis.
Glandular fever.
Vincent's infection.
Herpangina.
Hand, foot and mouth disease.

Toxic agents
Radiotherapy.
Chemotherapy.

Unknown aetiology
Behçet's.
Stevens–Johnson syndrome.
Aphthous ulceration.

Haematological
Acute leukaemia.
Agranulocytosis.
Aplastic anaemia.
Scurvy.

Drugs
Gold.
Methotrexate.
Etoposide.

Immunosuppression
AIDS.

Generalized debility
Malignancy.
Starvation.

Skin diseases
Lichen planus.
Pemphigoid/pemphigus.

SOME GENERAL POINTS ABOUT THE ABDOMEN

Abdomens, like their owners, come in all shapes and sizes. Obesity always makes clinical examination more difficult; with the abdomen, gross obesity makes the interpretation of signs well nigh impossible. Traditionally the subcostal margins and xiphoid limit the anterior abdomen above. These are easy to feel in all but the fattest patients. Below the abdomen is limited by the anterior superior iliac spines, the inguinal ligaments and the symphysis pubis (Fig. 6.8). The anterior iliac spines are usually palpable but may be overlaid by an apron of fat in obese patients. You must remember that whilst these limits are convenient they only surround a rhomboid shaped 'window' of abdominal wall through which you can palpate only some of the abdominal contents. The domes of the diaphragm, the liver, part of the stomach and the spleen extend well above the costal margins whereas much of the pelvis extends below the pubis and inguinal ligaments.

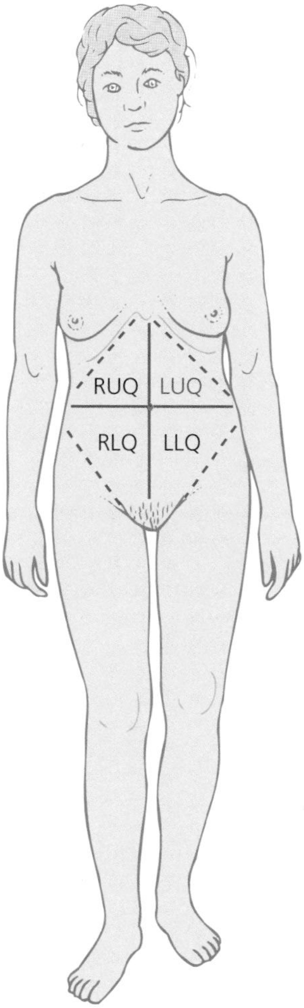

FIG. 6.8 The boundaries of the rhomboid shaped area which limits palpation of the abdominal contents. For descriptive purposes this area can be divided into four quadrants. RUQ: Right upper quadrant. LUQ: Left upper quadrant. RLQ: Right lower quadrant. LLQ: Left lower quadrant.

Short squat individuals have wide subcostal arches whereas those who are tall and slim tend to have more narrow arches. With trunk shortening, which occurs with advancing years and osteoporosis, the abdominal window becomes smaller and on standing the lower ribs ride on the iliac crests or funnel into the pelvis (Fig. 6.9).

For descriptive purposes it is helpful to draw one imaginary line from xiphoid to pubis and another across the abdomen at the level of the umbilicus to divide the abdomen into four quadrants: right upper, left upper, left lower and right lower.

It is useful to be able to correlate the positions of the abdominal organs with anterior anatomical planes and vertebral levels. Thus the xiphisternum corresponds with T9. A line midway between the sternal notch and the pubis (the transpyloric plane) is at the level of L1 and, in addition to crossing the pylorus, passes along the long axis of the pancreas and the duodenojejunal flexure. The subcostal plane is at the level of L3 and a line joining the highest points of the iliac crest corresponds to L4.

The position of the patient

Don't make your job too difficult! It is easiest to examine with the flat of the hand with the forearm horizontal. If the bed or couch is too low, kneel down to get into the optimum position. Ideally your patient should be:

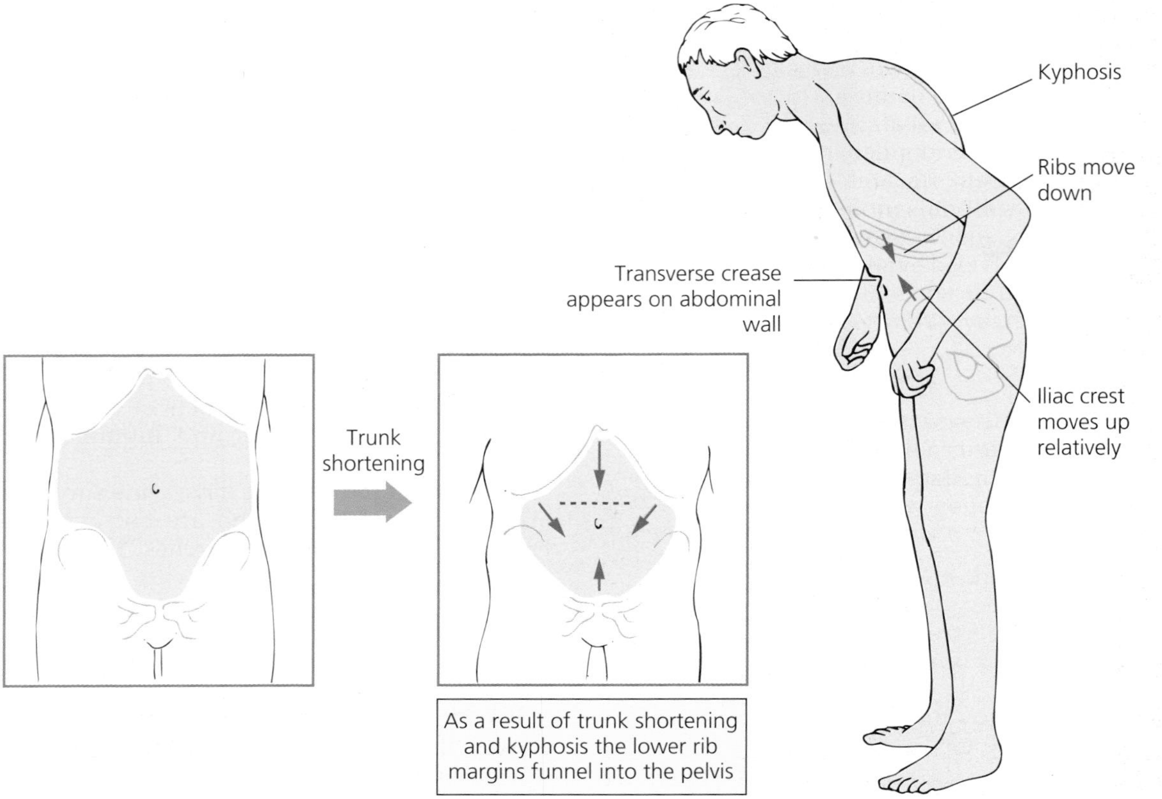

FIG. 6.9 The reduction of the rhomboid area which occurs with trunk shortening and kyphosis due to ageing and osteoporosis.

- Lying horizontally in bed or on an examination couch with one pillow under the head and arms by the side.
- Warm but with the abdomen exposed from xiphoid to pubis.
- In a good light.
- Relaxed and reassured.

In return the examining student or doctor must:

- Have warm hands.
- Enquire about sites of tenderness.
- Watch the patient's face to ensure that the examination is as painless as possible.

Inspecting the abdomen

This is often most easily done obliquely to show up subtle changes in contour and movement. A glance is not enough; you may need to watch for a minute or two to pick up visible peristalsis. Look for the following:

Changes in the contours of the abdomen Fluid within the peritoneal cavity (ascites) causes fullness in the flanks as well as generalized distension.

Abnormal veins It is not unusual to see a leash of fine veins over the costal margins in normal elderly slim patients. When the inferior vena cava is obstructed, distended collateral veins are present over the lower abdomen (Fig. 6.10) in addition to leg oedema. The blood in these veins runs towards the umbilicus. Check the direction of flow in veins by placing the tips of your two forefingers over the vein and moving them apart to empty a length of vein. By lifting one or other finger it

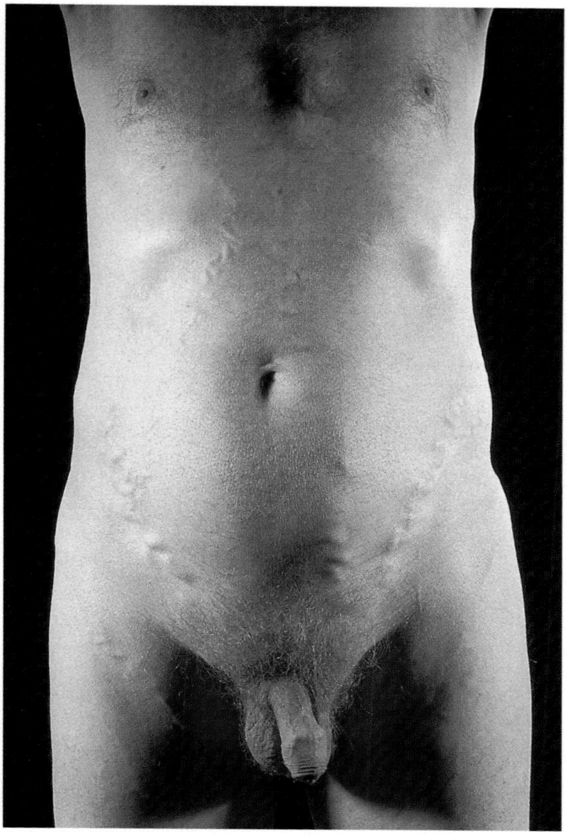

FIG. 6.10 Abnormal distended collateral veins on the abdominal wall as a result of inferior vena caval obstruction.

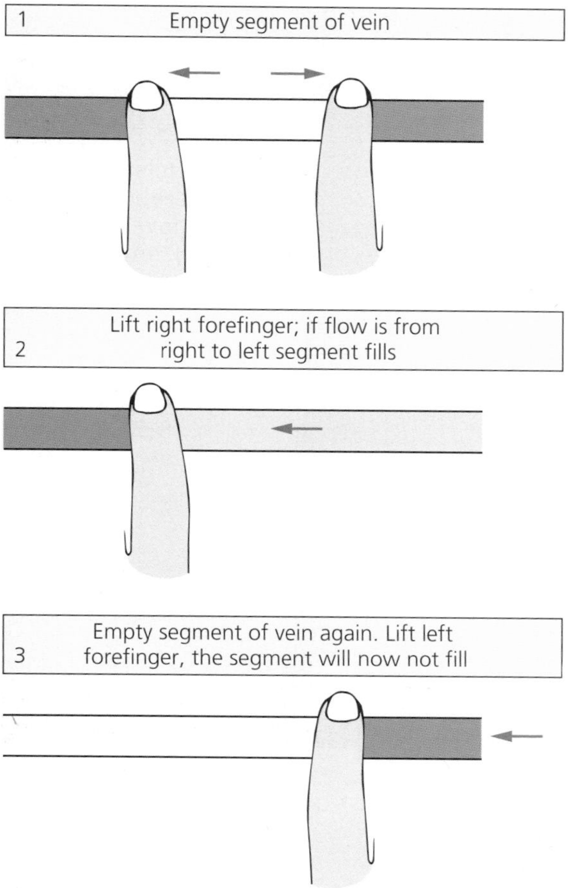

FIG. 6.11 Determining the direction of flow in superficial veins.

is possible to see the direction of filling of the empty section (Fig. 6.11). A rare physical sign is the so-called caput medusae in which large veins radiate out from the umbilicus. This occurs in portal hypertension and the veins are anastomoses between the systemic and portal circulations along the round ligament.

Scars on the abdominal wall These tell you about the patient's past surgical history and each must be accounted for. Keloid scars are exuberant scars in which the fibrous tissue extends beyond the limits of the original incision; they are particularly prone to occur in Black people.

Striae gravidarum These silvery scars are stretch marks on the abdominal wall following pregnancy. However any quick weight gain as in pubertal girls, patients undergoing steroid therapy or with Cushing's syndrome may produce striae which are initially reddish-purple but which fade to a silvery grey.

Changes at the umbilicus There may be a paraumbilical hernia in obese people. In the elderly and unwashed the umbilicus may be the site of a horny sebaceous plug. With gross distension, as with ascites, the umbilicus is stretched – 'the grinning umbilicus'. Alternatively it may be pushed out as an

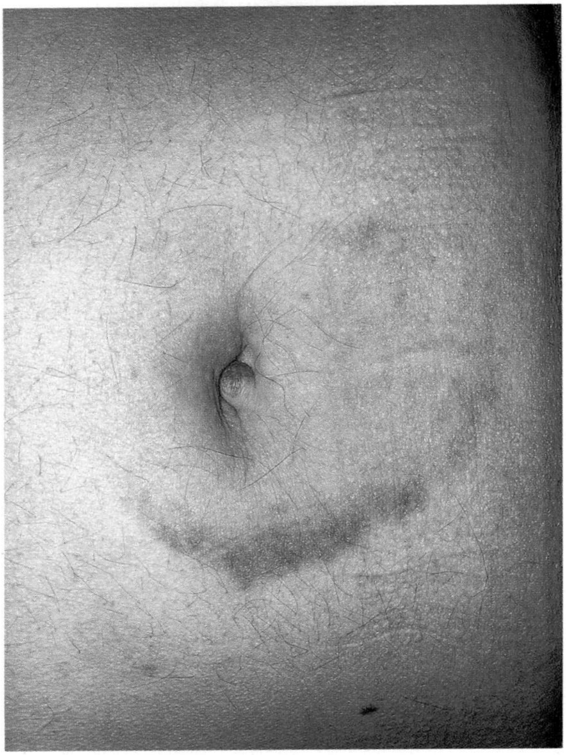

FIG. 6.12 Cullen's sign.

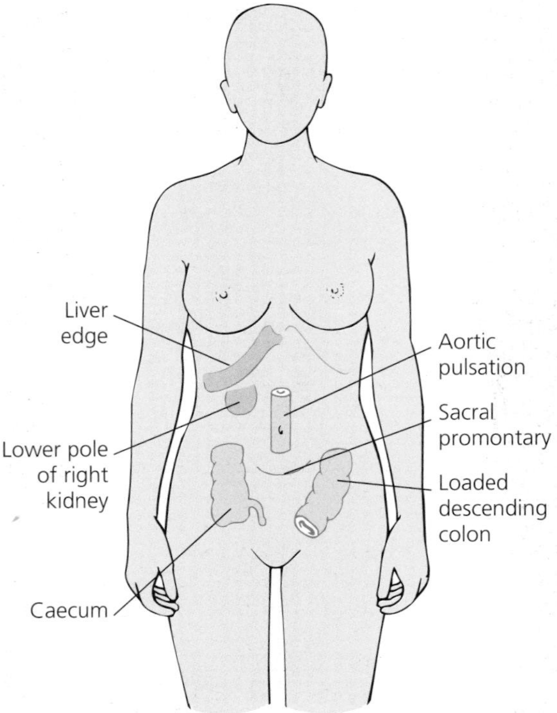

FIG. 6.13 Normal structures often palpable in the slim abdomen.

umbilical hernia. Intra-abdominal bleeding may discolour the umbilicus. Originally this was described in association with acute pancreatitis and termed Cullen's sign (Fig. 6.12).

Visible peristalsis This is best seen in an oblique light. In thin, frail, elderly patients visible peristalsis may be seen normally. With gastric outlet obstruction, visible peristalsis moves from left to right along the body of the stomach. It may take a minute or so to pick it up, so don't try to hurry; this is often a subtle physical sign. Large gut obstruction is said to move from right to left but this only occurs when it is seen along the course of the transverse colon.

Palpation

This is the most important part of the abdominal examination.

- Palpate from the right side of the patient.
- Use the whole of the hand as an extension of a horizontal forearm.
- Start your palpation well away from any painful area.
- Be gentle and give your patient confidence.
- Watch your patient's face whilst you are palpating.

There are certain structures that are often palpable in the normal slim abdomen (Fig. 6.13).

You will learn from experience that:

- It is often possible on deep inspiration to flip a normal liver edge which may be slightly tender.
- The caecum may be felt as a soft squelchy ill-defined mass in the right iliac fossa.
- The aortic pulsation is palpable in the epigastrium; this does not necessarily mean that it is aneurysmal.
- A loaded descending colon is often palpa-

ble as a cylindrical structure in the left iliac fossa.
- The sacral promontory may be felt in slim patients, particularly in women with an exaggerated lumbar lordosis.

Auscultation

This is an art neglected by physicians; surgeons are more adapt at auscultation because of its immense value in the diagnosis of the acute abdomen. In health a few low pitched gurgles are heard every few seconds. If the gut is dilated and peristalting, as with obstruction, higher pitched sounds are heard which may have a tinkling quality. When there is a paralytic ileus the abdomen is ominously silent, except for the distant heart sounds.

Vascular bruits are often heard from kinked, narrowed or roughened arteries. You cannot, on auscultation, distinguish accurately the causes or origins of these bruits and it is unwise to attach too much significance to them unless they are unusually loud and/or accompanied by a thrill.

Percussion

Percussion of the abdomen can help to:

- Confirm that distension is due to gas. The percussion note over obstructed gut is tympanitic, like a drum.
- Demonstrate shifting dullness due to ascites (see Fig. 6.26).
- Define the borders of solid organs or masses.
- Identify pockets of gas which have leaked from perforated viscera.

THE LIVER

It is important to realize that even in health the liver is variable in shape and position (Fig. 6.14). Its upper border reaches as high as 1 cm above the 5th rib in the mid-clavicular line and its lower anterior border extends to the costal margin. In slim people this lower border can be flipped on deep inspiration. In patients with overexpanded chests, as in emphysema, the liver may be as much as two rib spaces lower. The left lobe of the liver extends to just beyond the left mid-clavicular line. The commonest normal variation in liver shape is the presence of a tongue of liver extending downwards to the right iliac fossa, termed a Riedel's lobe.

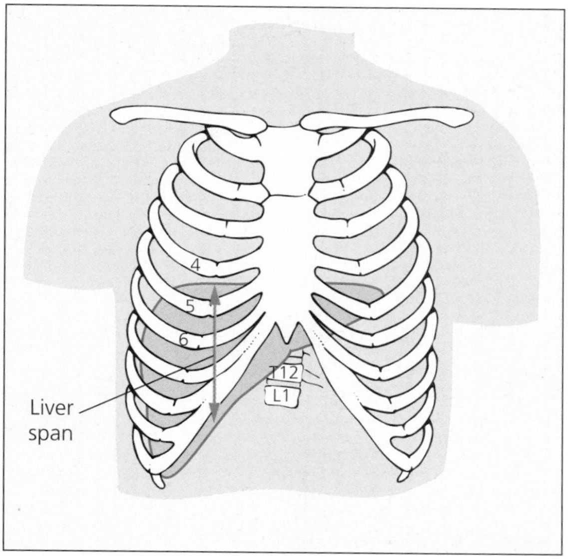

FIG. 6.14 The surface markings of the liver showing the site at which the span is measured.

The best way to pick up hepatic enlargement is to start with the flat of the right hand on the abdominal wall with the index finger parallel to the right costal margin (Fig. 6.15a) which will enable you to assess the general extent of the enlargement. This can be confirmed more accurately moving the forearm and hand parallel to the long axis of the body and using the finger tips to define the exact position of the liver edge (Fig. 6.15b). Enlargement of the liver should be expressed in centimetres below the right costal margin in the right mid-clavicular line. Do not use fingerbreadths, an old fashioned and inaccurate measure.

The fact that the liver edge is palpable below the costal margin does not necessarily mean that the liver is enlarged.

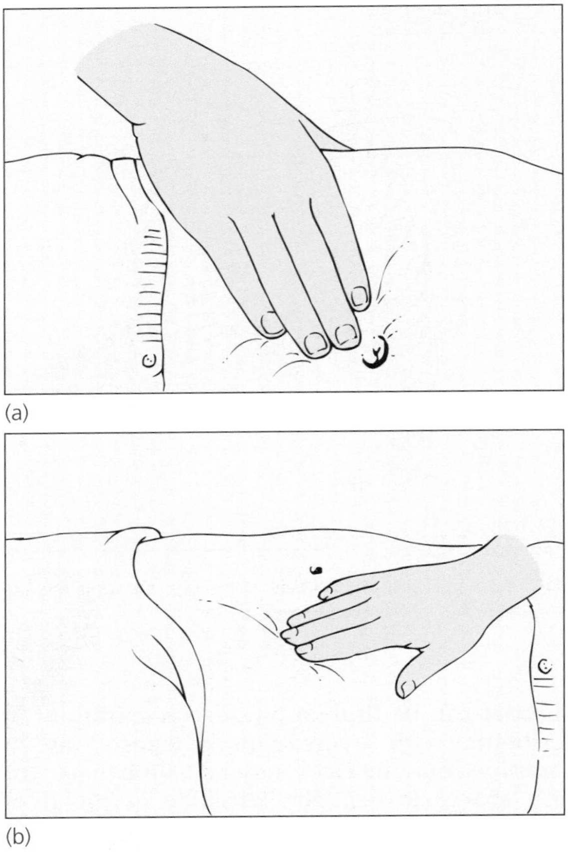

FIG. 6.15 (a) Start palpation of the liver with the index finger parallel to the lower border of the liver; this will enable you to assess the general size of the liver. (b) Define the edge more accurately with the fingers parallel to the long axis of the body.

Hyperexpanded lungs can push it down. Because of this some clinicians measure the liver span (See Fig. 6.14) which is the distance from the upper border of the liver to the costal margin in the mid-clavicular line. In health this is 8–10 cm in women and 10–12 cm in men but bear in mind that in health liver size is proportional to body size.

The gallbladder

Under normal conditions the gallbladder is not palpable. When distended with bile it can be felt as a smooth oval swelling emerging from below the right costal margin. The hemispherical fundus can often be felt through the abdominal wall as though floating in water.

Size, shape and consistency of the liver in disease

The changes in liver size and shape with various common diseases are shown opposite in Fig. 6.16a–f.

Stigmata of chronic liver disease

No examination of the liver is complete without a search for the stigmata of chronic liver disease. Many of these are common to all forms of chronic hepatitis or cirrhosis; others have specific associations with particular forms of liver disease (see Revision Panel 6.7).

- Spider naevi are small vascular lesions each consisting of a central feeding arteriole with smaller tortuous arterioles spreading outwards from it like the legs of a spider (Fig. 6.17). A few may be present in normal health, particularly in women and increasing during pregnancy. Each fades on pressure with a glass slide, but more specifically the whole lesion disappears when the feeding arteriole is compressed with a pencil point. In chronic liver disease, particularly in chronic active hepatitis and in cirrhosis complicated by hepatoma, spider naevi are distributed extensively over the upper half of the body.
- Palmar erythema. As part of generalized vasodilatation in liver disease, the hypothenar and thenar eminences are erythematous (Fig. 6.18). However, this is not an unusual appearance in plethoric and otherwise normal people.

FIG. 6.16 (facing page) Liver changes with disease. (a) Right heart failure. (b) Overinflated lungs. (c) Cirrhosis of the liver. (d) Hepatic metastases. (e) Primary hepatocellular carcinoma in an African patient. (f) Diffuse infiltration of the liver.

Right heart failure

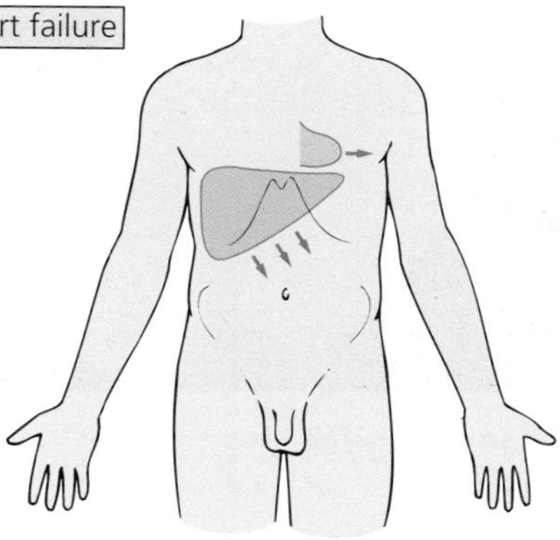

(a)

Tender enlarged liver
Cardiomegaly
Right diaphragm may be elevated
Hepatojugular reflux positive
Other signs of right heart failure
Systolic pulsation of liver if tricuspid incompetence present

Overinflated lungs

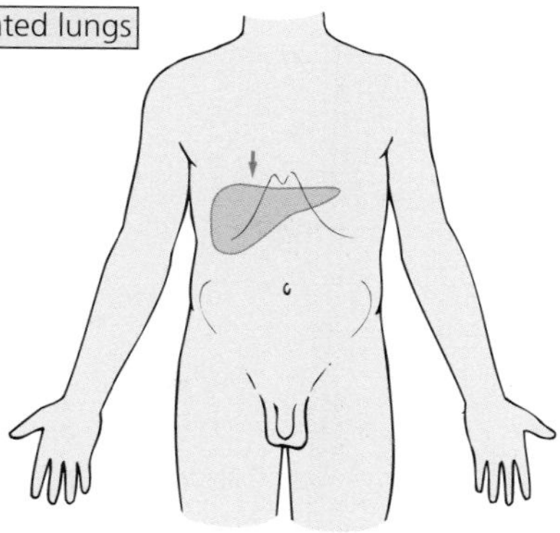

(b)

Liver edge soft and palpable per abdomen
Chest hyper-resonant with levels of liver dullness depressed

Cirrhosis of liver

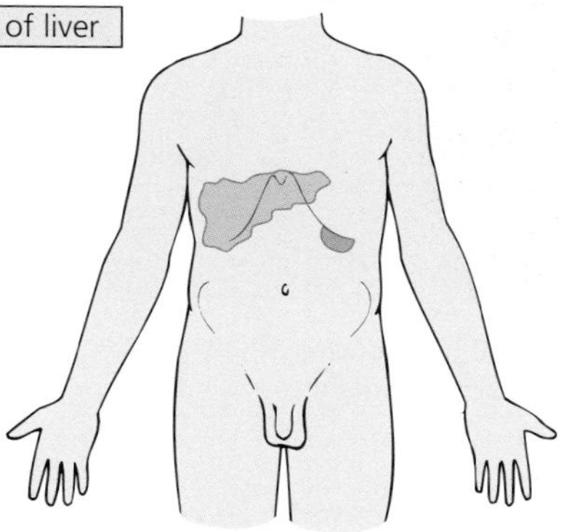

(c)

Hard irregular liver
May be small, normal or large in size
Stigmata of chronic liver disease
Splenomegaly
May be ascites

Metastases

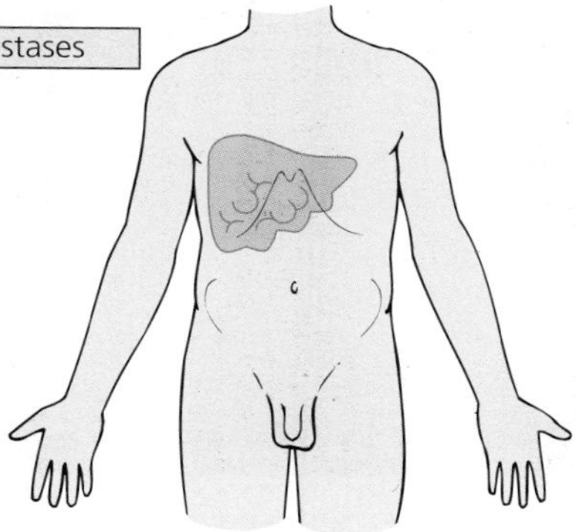

(d)

Large hard knobbly liver easily palpable per abdomen
High right diaphragm with dullness to percussion and diminished breath sounds over lower chest
Clinical signs may simulate pleural effusion at right base posteriorly

Primary hepatocellular carcinoma

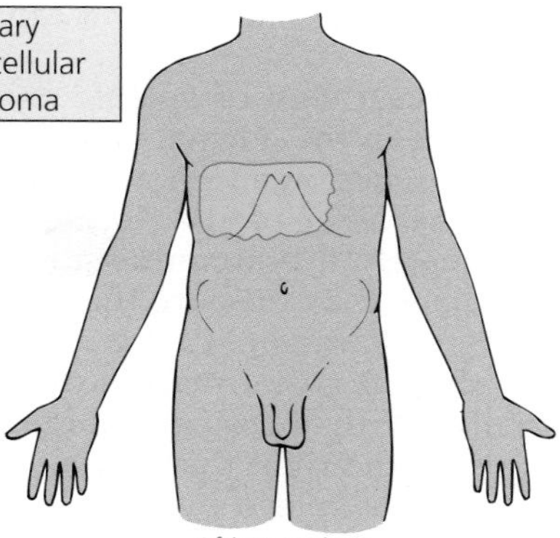

(e)

African patient
Tenderness in epigastrium
Wasting +

Diffuse infiltration

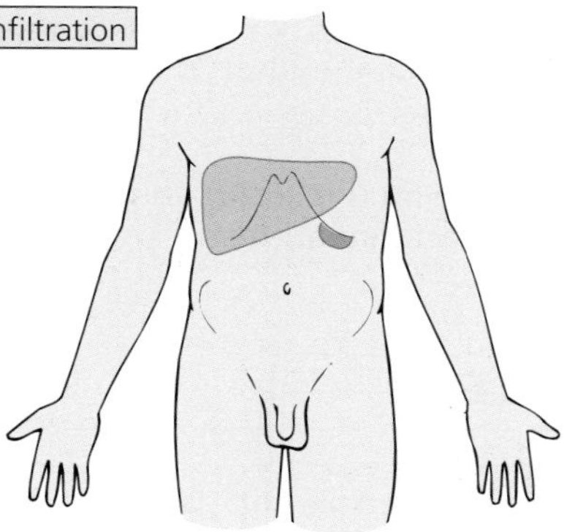

(f)

e.g. Amyloid or sarcoidosis
Generalized firm regular enlarged liver
Spleen may also be palpable

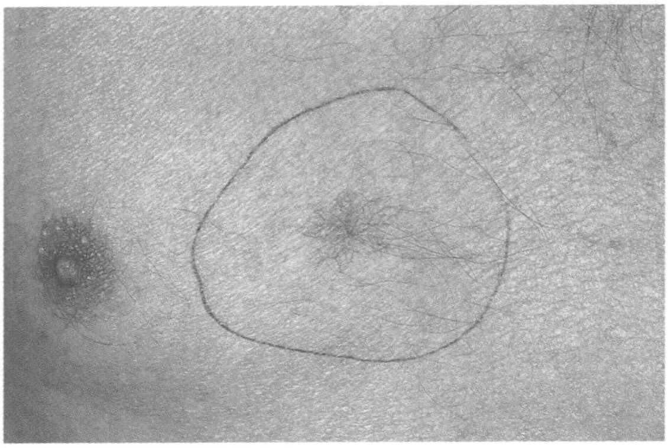

FIG. 6.17 Spider naevus.

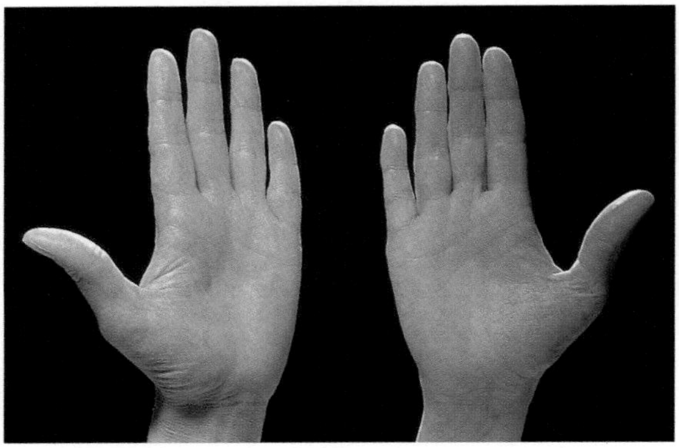

FIG. 6.18 Liver palms. The mottled appearance on the hypothenar eminences is characteristic.

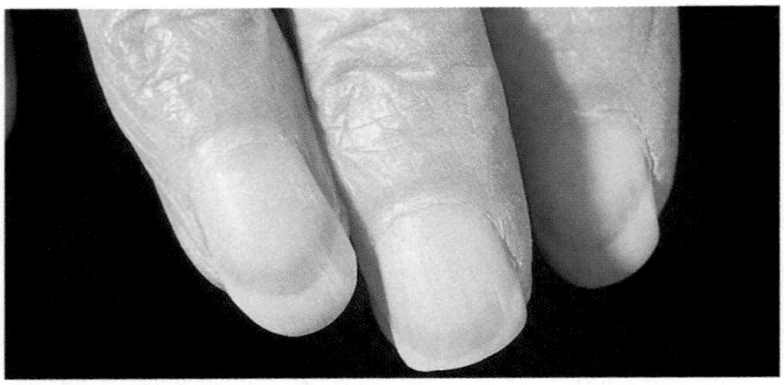

FIG. 6.19 Leuconychia.

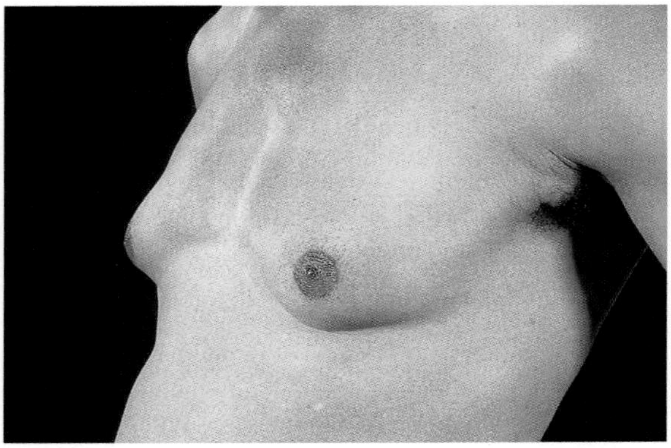

FIG. 6.20 Gynaecomastia in a West Indian patient with chronic active hepatitis.

- Clubbing is common in cirrhosis.
- Leuconychia – whiteness of the nails (Fig. 6.19). This is said to be associated with hypoalbuminaemia but the scientific evidence for this is not particularly convincing.
- Gynaecomastia (Fig. 6.20), impotence, scanty body hair and small testes in male.

THE SPLEEN

The normal spleen is not palpable. In young adults it is the size of a fist lying in the left upper quadrant of the abdomen with its long axis approximately 10 cm long and parallel to the left 10th rib. As with other lymphoid tissue, it atrophies with advancing years and by old age will have shrunken from 200 g in youth to 70 or 80 g. The oft-quoted statement that the spleen has to be enlarged two or three times its normal size before it can be detected is incorrect.

The earliest sign of splenic enlargement is an increase in the normal area of splenic dullness to percussion anterior to the mid axillary line at the level of the 10th rib (Fig. 6.21). Unfortunately a tympanitic note from gas in the stomach may obscure this sign. With progressive enlargement the spleen extends below the left costal margin downwards and medially. With massive enlargement it may even reach the right iliac fossa.

Feel for the spleen by placing the left hand under the left lower ribs and lifting them forwards. Use the right hand to feel the anterior,

Revision Panel 6.7
Stigmata of chronic liver disease

Site	*Physical sign*	*Specific association*
Face	Spider naevi, paper money sign, telangiectasia	
	Scleral icterus.	
	Cushingoid facies.	Alcoholic liver disease.
	Xanthelasma.	Prolonged cholestasis.
	Kayser–Fleisher rings (light brown rings of copper chelates at the periphery of the cornea).	Wilson's disease.
Skin	Spider naevi (see Fig. 6.17).	
	Icterus.	
	Scratch marks.	Prolonged cholestasis, particularly primary biliary cirrhosis.
	Slate grey pigmentation.	Haemochromatosis.
Hands	Clubbing.	
	White nails (leuconychia) (see Fig. 6.19).	Hypoalbuminaemia.
	Dupuytren's contracture.	Alcoholic liver disease (perhaps).
	Liver palms (see Fig. 6.18).	
	Flapping tremor.	Hepatic encephalopathy.
Endocrine system (in men)	Gynaecomastia (see Fig. 6.20).	
	Scanty body hair.	
	Atrophic testes.	
Nervous system	Tremor and athetoid movements.	Wilson's disease.

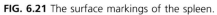

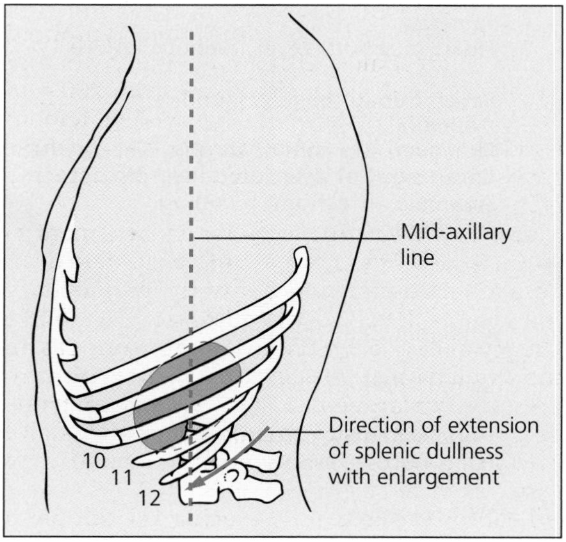

FIG. 6.21 The surface markings of the spleen.

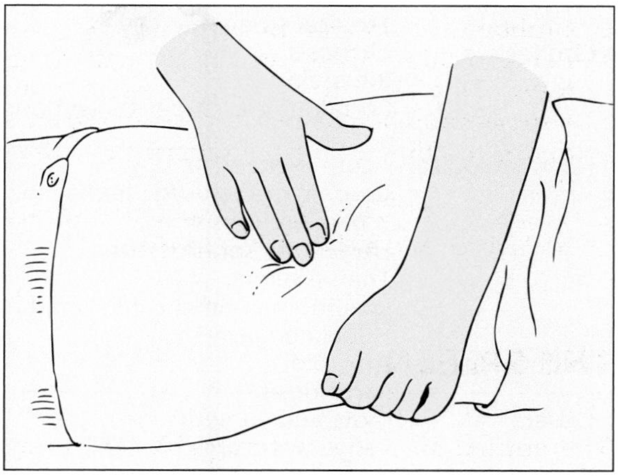

FIG. 6.22 Palpation of the spleen.

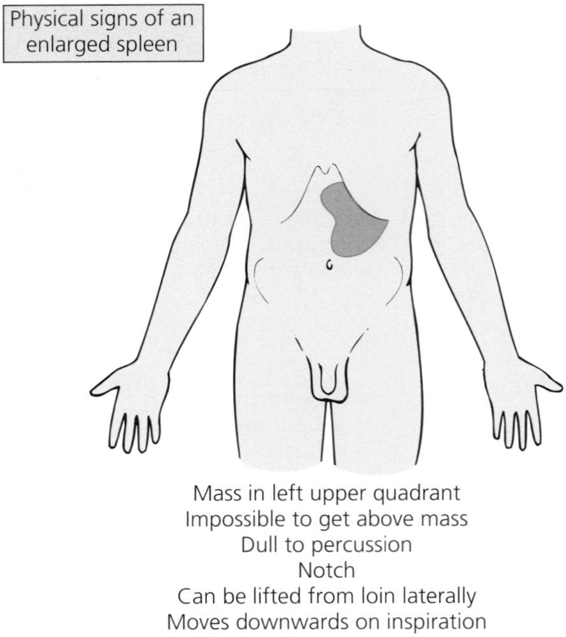

Physical signs of an enlarged spleen
Mass in left upper quadrant
Impossible to get above mass
Dull to percussion
Notch
Can be lifted from loin laterally
Moves downwards on inspiration

FIG. 6.23 The physical signs of the enlarged spleen.

lower border of the organ (Fig. 6.22). Record the size of the spleen as the number of centimetres (not fingerbreadths) that its lower border is below and at right angles to the left costal margin. The physical signs are summarized in Fig. 6.23.

Enlargement of the spleen may be confused with enlargement of the left kidney. Under these circumstances the spleen is dull; in contrast the area over the left kidney will be resonant because the enlarging kidney pushes the gas-filled splenic flexure in front of it (see Revision Panel 6.8).

MIDLINE ABDOMINAL MASSES

In this section we consider the midline abdominal masses that are seen in clinical practice. The separation between upper, central and lower abdominal masses is, of course, an arbitrary one but it allows a simple diagnostic approach. The physical signs of the

Revision Panel 6.8
Causes of splenomegaly

Aetiology	*Disease*	*Associated physical signs*
Infective	Infective mononucleosis (glandular fever).	Sore throat, mild lymphadenopathy.
	Infective hepatitis.	Jaundice.
	Subacute infective endocarditis.	Heart murmurs, fever, embolic lesions.
	Kalar-azar.[a]	
	Malaria.	Fever, hepatomegaly, jaundice.
	Tropical splenomegaly.[a]	Anaemia.
Congestive	Cirrhosis.	Firm liver, stigmata of chronic liver disease.
	Bilharzia.[a]	Often signs of associated liver disease.
	Portal and splenic V thrombosis.	Anaemia, infections, bleeding.
		Anaemia.
Haematological	Acute leukaemia.	
	Chronic granulocytic leukaemia[b] and myelosclerosis[a]	
	Hereditary spherocytosis.	Anaemia (see Fig. 40.6).
	Thalassaemia	
	Lymphoma and chronic lymphatic leukaemia.[b]	Lymphadenopathy.
Infiltrations	Amyloid.	Hepatomegaly, cardiomegaly.
	Sarcoidosis.	Lung fibrosis, iridocyclitis.
Others	Cysts and tumours.	
	Felty's syndrome.	Arthropathy.

[a]Mainly in tropics. [b]In older patients.

more common masses are summarized diagrammatically in Figs 6.24(a–d).

In the Western world a hard, irregular, fixed mass in the epigastrium is likely to be an advanced carcinoma of the stomach and the patient will have suffered from anorexia, pain and loss of weight for at least weeks and probably months. Metastases occur early to

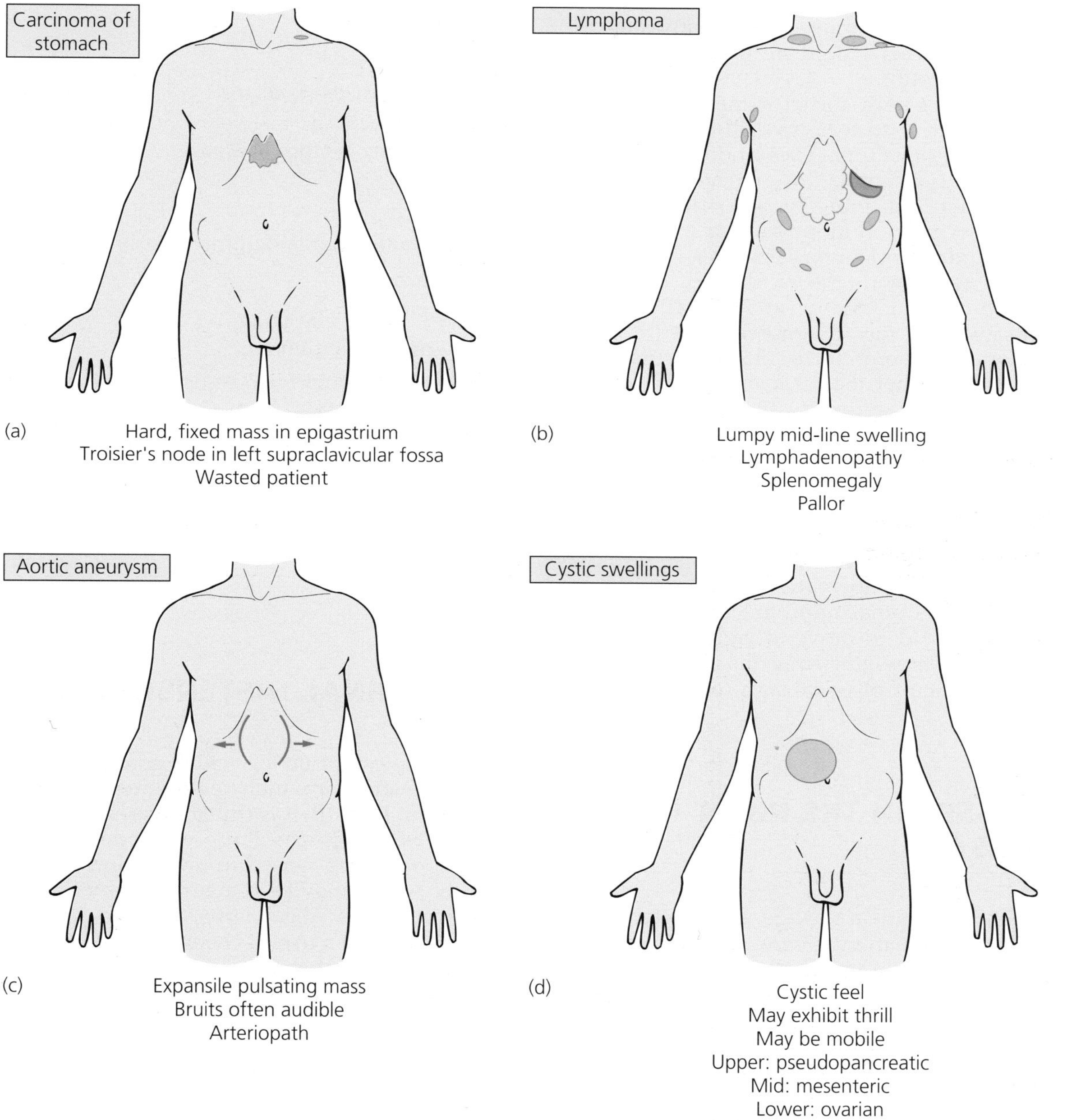

FIG. 6.24 Physical signs of abdominal masses. (a) Carcinoma of the stomach. (b) Lymphoma. (c) Aortic aneurysm. (d) Cystic swellings in the abdomen.

regional nodes and liver. If the tumour is causing gastric outlet obstruction there will be large volume vomits of undigested food. A large pancreatic tumour may be felt in this region but this is likely to be associated with obstructive jaundice. A metastasis in the left lobe of the liver may cause diagnostic difficulties but this would be expected to move with respiration.

Masses of para-aortic or mesenteric glands may give rise to a lumpy, ill-defined central abdominal swelling. These nodes are usually due to lymphoma or chronic lymphatic leukaemia but may be secondary deposits from a primary tumour such as a seminoma.

An abdominal aneurysm gives rise to a pulsatile swelling in the midline in an arteriopathic patient. Many abdominal swellings pulsate but the diagnostic feature of an abdominal aneurysm is that the pulsation is expansile rather than transmitted.

The most common cystic midline swellings in the lower abdomen are ovarian cysts – if malignant there may be associated ascites. Sometimes benign ovarian cysts are situated surprisingly high in the abdomen. Other abdominal cysts are rare, except for hydatid cysts in regions where the disease is indigenous. Pseudopancreatic cysts are situated behind the stomach and are fixed. Mesenteric cysts are said to move at right angles to the axis of the mesentery but this is a rare tumour and a difficult physical sign to demonstrate.

MASSES IN THE RIGHT ILIAC FOSSA

Much depends on the age, circumstances and race of the patient. Some of the causes are shown in Revision Panel 6.9.

A mass in the right iliac fossa in a child or young adult who has had a recent history of pain starting centrally and moving to the right is likely to be an inflammatory appendix mass. Fever, rigors and increasingly severe pain suggest abscess formation.

The differential diagnosis of these conditions is discussed later in Chapter 27.

Revision Panel 6.9
Causes of a mass in the right iliac fossa

Appendix mass[a] (common in Western world).

Appendix abscess.[a]

Crohn's disease.[a]

Carcinoma of the caecum.[b]

Amoeboma[a] (seen mainly in tropical areas).

Tuberculosis.[a]

Lymphoma[b] (less common but widespread distribution).

Psoas abscess.[a]

Mobile ovarian cyst.[b]

Retroperitoneal tumours.[b]

Malignant undescended testicle and other unusual tumours.[b]

Bony tumours.[b]

Iliac aneurysm.[b]

[a]May be seen at all ages. [b]Mainly in older patients.

ABDOMINAL DISTENSION

This is a symptom of which many patients complain and for which no obvious cause may be found. Usually it is due to overeating or an excess of gas in the large gut. Nevertheless there are some very important and serious causes which may be remembered by the five Fs-fluid, flatus (gas), fetus, fat and faeces – which provide a useful checklist (see Revision Panel 6.10). To this list may be added fibroids to remind us that huge tumours may also occasionally cause abdominal distension.

Fluid

The detection of free fluid (Fig. 6.25) in the abdomen by clinical examination is a rela-

Revision Panel 6.10

Causes of abdominal distension

Fluid (ascites).

Flatus (gaseous distension).

Fetus.

Fat.

Faeces (megacolon).

Fibroids (and other huge masses such as ovarian cysts, polycystic kidneys etc.

tively crude technique and at least 500-1000 ml are required to produce abnormal physical signs (Fig. 6.26). By contrast ultrasound can detect as little as 50 ml.

The diseases, which may be complicated by ascites (Fig. 6.25), are many and are listed in Revision Panel 6.11 but in practical terms there are three important common causes.

Cirrhosis Look for the stigmata of chronic liver disease and for hepatosplenomegaly.

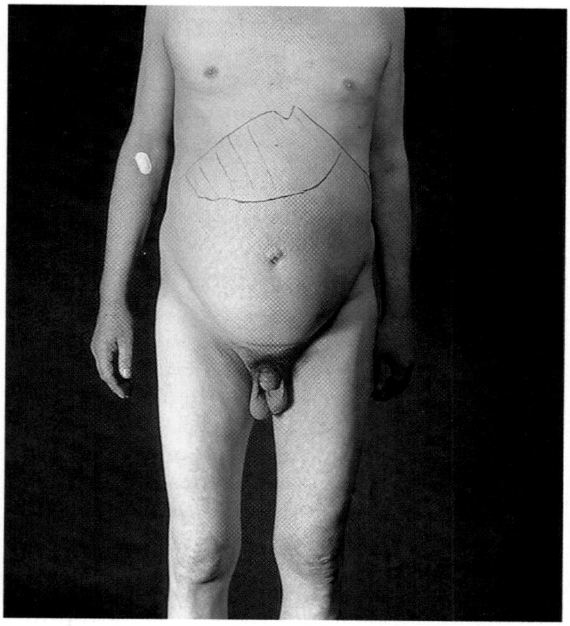

FIG. 6.25 Ascites due to cirrhosis of the liver. Note the hepatomegaly and the relative lack of body hair.

Revision Panel 6.11

Causes of ascites

Associated with chronic diseases	*Associated with acute abdomen*
Cirrhosis of the liver.[a]	Haemoperitoneum following trauma.
Heart failure.[a] Abdominal malignancy.[a] Liver disease without malignancy. Hepatic vein occlusion (Budd–Chiari syndrome). Constrictive pericarditis. Polyserositis (e.g. systemic lupus). Hypoproteinaemia (e.g. the nephrotic syndrome). Chronic peritonitis (e.g. tuberculosis). Lymphatic obstruction (chylous ascites).	Acute peritonitis. Acute pancreatitis.

[a]Mainly in older patients.

Congestive cardiac failure Examine carefully for other signs of heart failure such as raised jugular venous pressure, hepatomegaly and oedema.

Abdominal malignancy Examine the abdomen for masses. Do a pelvic examination to check for carcinoma of the ovary.

Flatus (gaseous distension)

In the early stages the distension is localized to that part of the abdomen containing the distended gut, such as in the right iliac fossa when the caecum is distended. As the distension progresses the whole abdomen becomes distended. The physical signs are those of hyperresonance but when there is also obstruction visible peristalsis will be seen.

Fetus

Many doctors have misinterpreted the physical signs of advanced pregnancy in obese

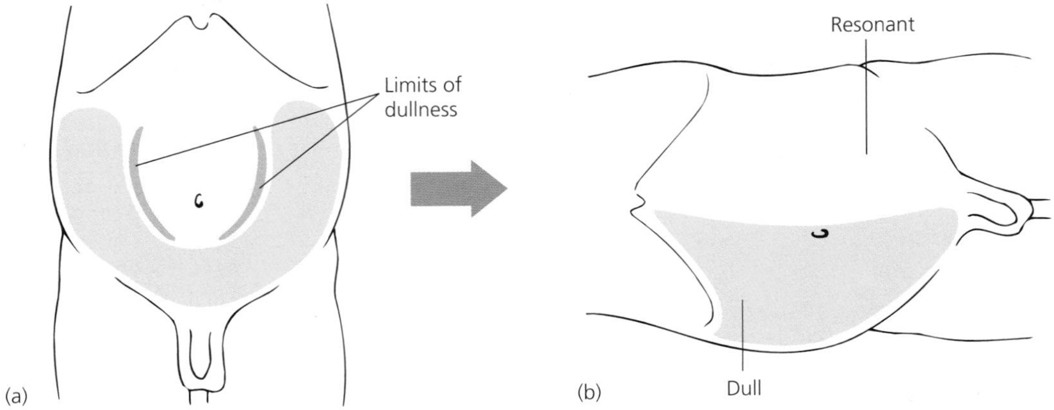

FIG. 6.26 Shifting dullness. (a) Patient lying on back – both flanks are dull. (b) Patient lying on side – fluid shifts so the upper flank only is resonant.

patients and indeed many will continue to do so in the future. It may seem a very basic point but this error will be avoided if pregnancy is considered in any woman with abdominal distension in the reproductive phase of life.

Fat

Obesity is not usually difficult to diagnose but sometimes fat is localized in the abdomen in a patient who is not unduly fat elsewhere. Fat accumulates in subcutaneous tissues and in the omentum but not necessarily to the same degree in each. The potbelly seen in beer drinking men is usually due to excessive deposits in the omentum. In women huge deposits in the abdominal wall may cause an apron of fat to hang down over the pubis.

> Revision Panel 6.12
>
> **Causes of marked distension of the abdomen due to solid or cystic lesions**
>
> Massive tumours which may actually distend the abdomen (e.g. hypernephroma).
>
> Hepatomegaly (particularly metastases).
>
> Massive splenomegaly.
>
> Polycystic kidneys (and liver).
>
> Lymphadenopathy (as with non-Hodgkin's lymphoma).
>
> Ganglioneuroma (in children).
>
> Nephroblastoma (in children).

Fibroids and other massive swellings in the abdomen

As part of the checklist it is useful to think of the last F (fibroids) to remind oneself of other solid masses, organs or cysts which may be so large as to actually distend the abdomen (Revision Panel 6.12).

THE ANUS AND RECTUM

The examination of the perineum, anus and rectum completes and is an integral part of the examination of the abdomen and gastrointestinal tract. Whilst it is unnecessary in children and young adults without relevant complaints it is essential in middle-aged and elderly adults. Without it the asymptomatic rectal carcinoma or rectal polyp will be missed. There are, of course, many conditions which present primarily as pain in the anorectal region or simply as a lump (see Revision Panel 6.13).

Revision Panel 6.13

Anal conditions presenting with pain

Pain alone	
Fissure	Pain with and after defaecation.
Proctalgia fugax	Attacks of severe cramping pain in the rectum. Usually at night lasting minutes to hours. Cause unknown.
Anorectal abscess	Pain usually localized.
Pain and lump	
Perianal haematoma	At all ages but common after childbirth.
Anorectal abscess	
Pain with lump and bleeding	
Prolapse of rectum	Almost always in women.
Prolapsed haemorrhoids	
Carcinoma of anus or anal canal	
Pain with bleeding	
Fissure	Stool streaked with blood.

For the patient this is the most embarrassing and unpleasant part of their physical examination.

- Be considerate, explain what you are doing and why.
- Be gentle.
- Place the patient in the left lateral position, with hips and knees flexed, and with buttocks on the edge of the bed.
- Put on gloves and inspect the anus and perineum by lifting the right buttock with the left hand.

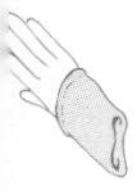

At this stage look for:

- Soiling of the perineum or underwear with faeces, discharge or blood.
- Prolapsed piles.
- Condylomata or anal warts (see also Chapter 19).
- Scarring and/or fistula formation (see Fig. 35.1).
- Ulcers or fissures.
- Rashes.

Then lubricate the right index finger and place the pulp on the anus. Ask the patient to push down as though having his bowels open and gentle pressure on the anus will allow the finger to slip into the anal canal and rectum. In performing the procedure press gently backwards; this will exert pressure on the sling of the puborectalis muscle which overcomes the tone in the anal sphincter (Figs. 6.27a, and b). Three important don'ts in performing rectal examinations:

- Don't insert the finger tip straight into the rectum.
- Don't attempt the examination if it appears to be too painful; there may be a fissure.
- Don't attempt to force the finger through a tight stricture.

Once the finger is inserted into the rectum sweep it round to assess the condition of the rectal mucosa, to feel for any abnormal lumps or ulcers and to define the normal structures. By placing the left hand on the abdomen in the suprapubic region you will be able to palpate pelvic structures bimanually. Note the presence and consistency of any faeces within the rectum. A hard mass of faeces in a frail elderly patient may indicate impaction.

In the male the most obvious landmark anteriorly is the prostate gland (Fig. 6.27c). It is firm, rubbery and is 2–3 cm in diameter. A shallow central groove may be palpable and nodu-

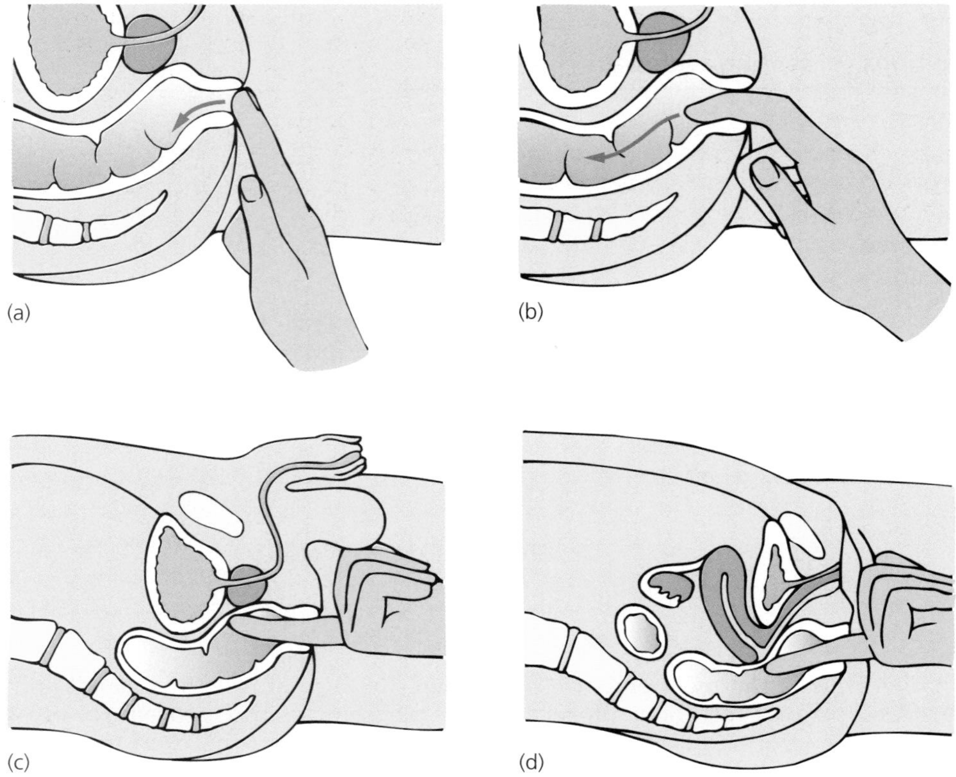

FIG. 6.27 (a, b) How to perform a rectal examination. (c) The position of the prostate gland. (d) The position of the cervix.

lar seminal vesicles may be palpable at the tip of the finger on either side. With advancing age the prostate hypertrophies with enlargement and progressive protrusion into the rectum, which is not necessarily symmetrical. The overlying rectal mucosa should be smooth and mobile. Carcinoma of the prostate starts as a hard nodule within the gland which is impossible to differentiate from an area of calcification. As the tumour enlarges it produces a hard asymmetrical irregular mass which invades the overlying mucosa. As the tumour extends laterally into the pelvis it produces 'winging' of the gland. In acute prostatitis the gland is extremely tender to palpation.

On either side of the rectum are the ischiorectal fossae which may be the site of abscess formation.

Posteriorly it is usually possible to feel the concavity of the coccyx.

In the female the corresponding landmark anteriorly is the cervix which, depending on its maturity feels like a firm mass, like the end of a nose (Fig. 6.27d). Using the bimanual technique it should be possible to define the size and shape of the uterus and to palpate any ovarian swellings.

In both sexes the rectal wall must be carefully examined for polyps or a rectal carcinoma. Up to 90% of rectal carcinomas can be felt digitally. Smaller tumours may be papilliferous or nodular but the extent of large ulcerating tumours can sometimes be difficult to define. As the tip of the examining finger explores over the edge of the mass it seems to enter a cavity; this is the necrotic ulcer base. When the rectal mucosa is inflamed, as with ulcerative colitis, it may have a velvety feel. However the state of the mucosa can only be accurately evaluated by direct vision through a proctoscope or sigmoidoscope and biopsy.

On withdrawing the finger examine the glove.

- Blood and/or mucus suggest an ulcerating tumour or chronic inflammatory bowel disease such as ulcerative colitis.
- Smelly, pale, sticky stools suggest malabsorption of fat or steatorrhoea.
- Pale stools suggest obstructive jaundice.
- Copious mucoid watery discharge suggests a villous adenoma.
- Mucus and watery discharge with a hard mass of faeces in the rectum suggest impaction.

7 Basic guide to diseases of the nervous system

POSSIBLE PROBLEMS

This chapter offers you a guide to examining the nervous system. You must start by learning how to do this comprehensively so that you can deal with any of a wide range of problems that may come your way. These may include:

- Sudden loss of consciousness.
- Strokes.
- Deteriorating intellectual functions.
- Problems with speech.
- Weakness.
- Difficulties with walking and of gait.
- Pain and other sensory disturbances.
- Involuntary movements.
- Headache (see Chapter 26).

Having said this, you will quickly learn that there is no such thing as a routine neurological examination. The examination of an unconscious elderly female with a catastrophic stroke will differ materially from that of young man with recurrent headaches. You have to match what you do with the needs of your patient. Only experience will tell you what must be emphasized and what can be left out. Let us start by considering how these common problems may present in the surgery, in the Accident and Emergency Department or in hospital.

SYMPTOMS

Loss of consciousness

Here much depends on the circumstances, the age and previous health of the patient, and the rapidity of recovery. The way in which you deal with the unconscious patient is reviewed in Chapter 15, but it is essential to:

- Ensure that witnesses, friends, or relatives do not disappear before being fully interrogated.
- Determine, in detail, the circumstances of the episode.
- Look for clues of present or past illnesses such as Medi-Alert badges and hospital outpatient appointment cards.
- Keep any tablets or bottles.
- Find out the name of the patient's doctor.

Revision Panel 7.1 lists some of the more common causes of loss of consciousness *with spontaneous recovery* and pointers to possible diagnoses.

Strokes

Most lay people understand what is meant by the term stroke – one of the most common causes of emergency admission to hospital. In all patients you must seek out possible aetiological factors.

Revision Panel 7.1

Sudden loss of consciousness with spontaneous recovery

	Type of attack	*Circumstances*	*What might be found on examination*
In the young	Syncope. Vasovagal.	Anxiety. Prolonged standing in hot, stuffy surroundings.	Pale, sweaty, slow pulse.
	Hypoglycaemia.	Known diabetic on insulin.	Pale, sweaty, recovery with glucose.
	Hyperventilation.	Excitement or anxiety.	Carpopedal spasm +/– tingling in extremities.
	Epilepsy.	At any time.	Dependent on type, but may be evidence of tongue biting or incontinence.
In middle-aged or elderly	As in young.		
	Postural hypotension.	Psychotrophic or hypotensive drugs, autonomic neuropathy.	Systolic BP falls > 20 mm on standing.
	Cough or micturition syncope in men.	Collapse after prolonged bout of coughing or in elderly men whilst standing and straining to pass water.	Nil.
	Rhythm disturbances, usually heart block.		May be back in normal rhythm when seen (see Chapter 4).
	Aortic stenosis.	With exertion.	Characteristic physical signs.

Basic questions must be asked about:

- Previous episodes and transient ischaemic attacks.
- History of hypertension.
- Family history.
- Smoking.
- Predisposing factors e.g. atrial fibrillation, valvular heart disease, vascular disease.

Deteriorating intellectual function

The family, concerned friends and employers are more likely to bring this to attention. The nature of your questions will depend on the degree of deterioration. Explain what you are doing and don't embarrass the more alert patients with offensively simple questions. You might start off some general questions such as:

- Do you think that your memory is getting worse?
- Do you have difficulty in always finding the right words in everyday conversation?
- Do you think your mood has altered?
- Have you got lost on familiar routes?
- Have you problems coping with your job?

We deal with the problems of dementia in Chapters 8 and 13.

Problems with speech

Here, history taking is closely woven into clinical examination. It will be apparent quickly whether your patient has problems of putting thoughts into words (expressive dysphasia) or understanding the spoken word (receptive dysphasia) or whether the problem is difficulty in articulation (dysarthria). How to do this will be dealt with in more detail later.

Weakness

Be careful to differentiate between true weakness and tiredness. Because of the difficulty that patients (and also doctors and students) have in making this distinction we have devoted two separate chapters to this in the problems based section of the book (see Chapter 28: Tiredness and Chapter 41: Limb Weakness).

It is essential to determine the time course and distribution of the weakness. Relentlessly increasing weakness in the limbs in a young boy may point to a muscular dystrophy; remitting attacks of weakness in a young woman may indicate a demyelinating disorder whereas quickly progressive weakness of the legs in an elderly man may indicate cord compression.

Problems with gait

Your patients are unlikely to complain of 'problems with gait'. They are more likely to say that their legs feel stiff, that they cannot get going or that they stagger and fall. You can assess the gait as your patient approaches. Questioning can then be more focussed. Some features of gait are summarized in Revision Panel 7.2.

Involuntary movements

Patients complain of movements that they cannot control in terms such as tremor, shakes, jerks or writhing.

THE EXAMINATION

After your general observations, assess intellectual function and speech and then move on to the cranial nerves, the motor and sensory systems. Most clinicians start at the top and move down.

First appearances

The examination and management of the drowsy or unconscious patient is dealt with in more detail in Chapter 15. In particular assess the level of consciousness, using the Glasgow scale if necessary, check the temperature, look for evidence of hemiplegia and consider metabolic causes for coma.

Practical Point

Always consider the possibility of meningitis, brain abscess or encephalitis in patients with fever and disturbed consciousness. It is all too easy to assume that the elderly patient, admitted with a presumed stroke, has fever due to an associated chest infection.

During history taking in the conscious patient you may be able to make a spot diagnosis from:

Revision Panel 7.2
Some features of gait

Type of gait	*Possible symptoms*	*Findings*
Spastic	Legs stiff and heavy, scrape toes of shoes.	In hemiplegia, arm flexed and adducted with leg extended. If both legs are spastic, thrusts of the trunk are used to assist in locomotion.
Sensory ataxic gait	Not sure where legs are, much worse in dark and with eyes closed.	Positive Rhomberg's sign (p.134). Posterior column loss.
Cerebellar ataxia	Unsteadiness. Staggering.	Broad-based gait.
Parkinsonian gait	Difficulty in getting going, whole body feels stiff. Can't turn quickly.	Tremor, no arm swing, leans forward and 'chases centre of gravity'.
Waddling gait	Difficulty in standing up or getting out of a chair.	Often due to proximal myopathy.
Foot drop	Frequent tripping, scuffs toe of shoe on affected side.	May be bilateral or unilateral. Often due to peripheral neuropathy.

- The facial appearances – depression, facial tics, neurofibromatosis (see Fig. 11.5), myopathy, tuberose sclerosis.
- Gait and posture – hemiplegia, Parkinson's disease, foot drop etc.
- General appearance and responses – dementia (Revision Panel 7.3) (remember that evidence of self-neglect may be concealed by an attentive family or carers smartening up the patient to see the doctor).
- Attitude and behaviour – hypomania, depression.

Mental functions

The assessment of the mental state will have begun with the patient entering the consulting room. The examination must be 'directed' towards making a working diagnosis and emphasis may vary between physician, neurologist, psychiatrist and geriatrician. Factors which are taken into account, but which may not necessarily need to be examined formally in every case, include:

- Appearance, behaviour, communication.
- Emotional state.
- Orientation in time and space.
- Possible delusions and hallucinations.
- Memory. When testing memory, try to differentiate between immediate recall, recent memory and remote memory. Immediate recall is memory for a few seconds or minutes and is tested by asking the patient to repeat for you a series of numbers and then another series in reverse order. Patients should be able to recall at least six numbers forwards and four backwards. Recent memory loss is conveniently tested by asking about orientation in time and space and quizzing your patient about the news or programmes seen recently on television. Long-term memory is often surprisingly well retained in spite of severe dementia.
- Intelligence.

Revision Panel 7.3

Clinical features of dementia

Frontal lobe features
Changed and dulled personality.
Impaired emotional control.
Poor judgement.
Loss of inhibitions.
Difficulty in generating speech.

Temporal lobe features
Can't remember recent events.
Impaired immediate recall.
Language disorder.

Parietal lobe features
Disturbed body image.
Left hemisphere concerned with speech, reading, calculation etc.
Right hemisphere concerned with spatial and construction skills i.e. dressing, laying the table.

Speech

Dysphasia is usually due to a combination of an expressive defect, i.e. problems in putting thoughts into words and receptive defect i.e. difficulty in understanding the spoken word. Test the receptive component by asking your patient to do a simple everyday task e.g. 'take off your glasses', 'take out your handkerchief' (Revision Panel 7.4). Test expressive speech by asking the patient to name objects such as a book, a pillow, or a plate.

Dysphasia indicates damage or disturbance of function of the dominant temporal lobe or

Revision Panel 7.4

Assessment of speech

Listen to spontaneous speech – articulation, content and fluency.

Ask patient to name simple objects – book, table and pen.

Check understanding of spoken and written instructions.

Ask to repeat words or phrases.

Ask to read aloud and to write a simple sentence.

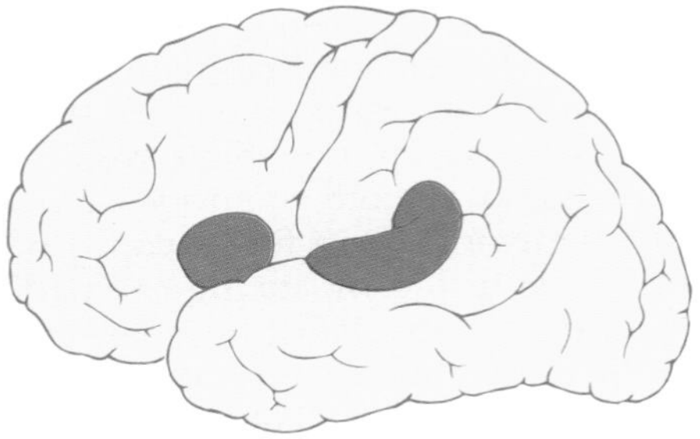

FIG. 7.1 Main anatomical sites where damage causes dysphasia (note this is the left hemisphere).

the dominant premotor cortex (Fig. 7.1). In right-handed people the dominant cortex is almost always the left; in left-handed people it is also on the left in 60%.

Dysarthria is simply a defect of articulation but may be due to a wide variety of causes including:

- Lesions of the brainstem as in the bulbar palsy of motor neuron disease.
- Bilateral pyramidal deficits after multiple small strokes, which may result in spastic speech (pseudobulbar palsy).
- Cerebellar dysarthria with slurred consonants and a staccato cadence of speech.
- Extrapyramidal disorders such as Parkinson's disease which gives a low and monotonous voice.

Primitive reflexes

These reflexes are of limited value in the specific localization and diagnosis of lesions but their features are summarized in Revision Panel 7.5.

The cranial nerves

The olfactory nerve

Examination of the function of the olfactory (I) nerve need not be performed routinely as it rarely contributes to the solution of a neurological problem. If you need to test the sense of smell use everyday substances such as coffee or perfume. Do not use a pungent substance such as ammonia vapour which has a direct effect on the nasal mucosa supplied by the Vth nerve.

Loss of the sense of smell (anosmia) is usually due to local nasal conditions such as rhinitis. When due to a neurological lesion it is usually the result of head injury but it may occasionally be due to structural lesions within the anterior cranial fossa. Anosmia

Revision Panel 7.5
Features of primitive reflexes

Reflex	*How to perform it*	*Significance*
Palmomental reflex	Scratch the palm of the hand with the sharp end of a tendon hammer.	Ipsilateral contraction of the mentalis muscle suggests a contralateral frontal lesion. (may be found normally in some individuals.)
Glabellar tap	Tap on the glabella[a] repetitively.	Normally blinking stops after 5–6 taps. Persistent blinking occurs in the dementias and in Parkinson's disease.
Grasp reflex	Firmly stroke the palm of the hand from radial to ulnar aspect.	Tight grasping on one side only may suggest a contralateral frontal lobe lesion.
Pout response	Tap the lips with the index finger.	Pouting suggests diffuse bilateral hemisphere disease.

[a]Glabella is the area of the forehead between the eyes.

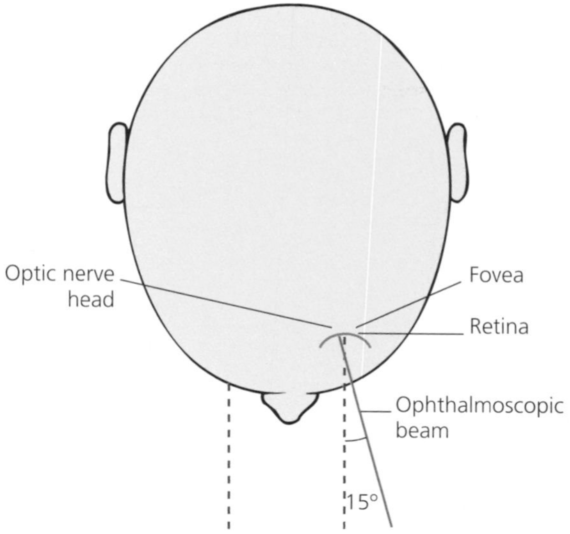

FIG. 7.2 Direct the ophthalmoscopic beam in a line 15 degrees to the axis of fixation. This should lead you directly to the optic disc.

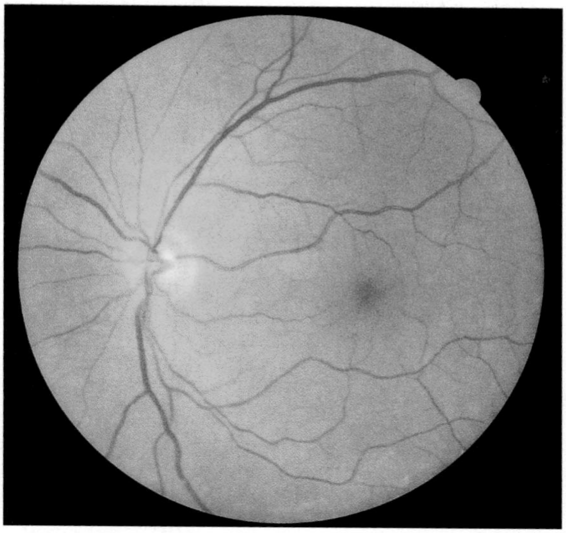

FIG. 7.3 The normal fundus. Note that the normal disc is pale pink and tends to be paler on the temporal side.

may be a very early sign of Parkinson's disease. Smell sensitivity declines with age in both sexes.

The optic nerve

Every student and doctor must learn to examine the optic (II) nerve efficiently and critically. This involves the proper use of the ophthalmoscope (see also Chapter 16). Take every opportunity to examine fundi, both normal and abnormal. Looking at the fundus with a beam of light from the ophthalmoscope through the pupil is rather like looking into a darkened room through the keyhole. To get the best from this examination:

- Put your patient into a darkened room so that the pupil will be dilated.
- Approach the pupil at about 15 degrees to the axis of fixation (Fig. 7.2). In this way the light will not shine directly on the macula, causing the pupil to constrict. You will be able to see the region of the optic disc immediately.
- If necessary dilute the pupil with a short-acting mydriatic such 1% tropicamide. Drugs of this kind can be safely used in the majority of patients though they are best avoided in those predisposed to narrow-angle glaucoma. Reverse the effects of the mydriatic at the end of the examination with 2% pilocarpine.

The normal optic disc (Fig. 7.3) is pale pink, the temporal side being usually paler than the nasal side. The central part is depressed – the physiological cup. The edge of the cup is normally well-defined and there is often a pigmented or stippled choroidal ring around the disc. Do not be confused by the presence of white areas radiating from the disc with feathered edges. These areas are due to medullated nerve fibres, which are a variant of normal, and of no clinical significance.

Papilloedema is passive swelling of the optic nerve head secondary to raised intracranial pressure. In the early stages of papilloedema there is increased pinkness of the disc with blurring of the edges. The physiological cup fills in and the veins become distended.

As papilloedema progresses the disc becomes more swollen and protrudes forwards. You can measure the degree of protrusion by focusing first on the centre of the disc

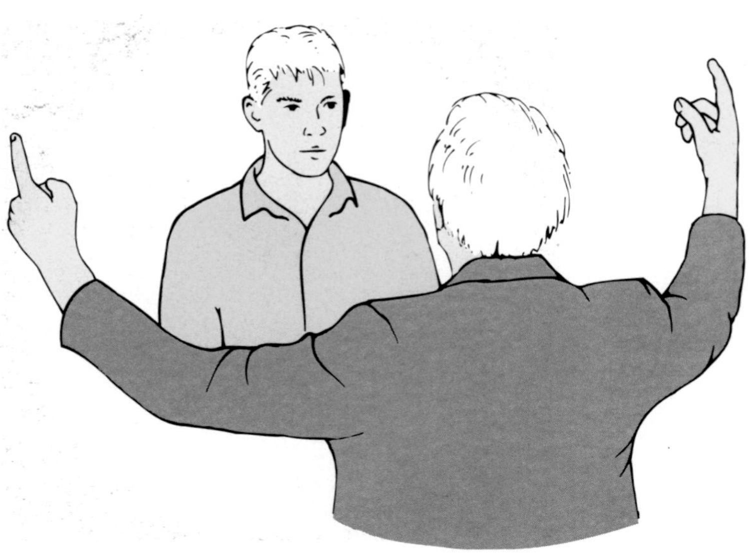

FIG. 7.4 Testing the visual fields by confrontation. To compare the patient's visual fields with your own, ensure that your object fingers are equidistant from yourself and the patient.

and then on the retina nearby. Three dioptres is equivalent to 1 mm of swelling. If papilloedema develops rapidly the veins engorge and haemorrhages and exudates develop in cartwheel fashion around the disc. The retinal vessels can often be seen climbing up over the edge of the disc. The causes of papilloedema are listed in Revision Panel 16.4.

> **Practical Point**
>
> Early papilloedema is difficult to assess. If in doubt ask for a more experienced opinion.

Optic neuritis is caused by inflammatory, demyelinating or vascular disease of the optic nerve. It causes loss of vision and pain on moving the eye. The pupil is often dilated and reacts slowly to light. When optic neuritis affects the nerve head (papillitis) and can therefore be seen with the ophthalmoscope, it produces an appearance similar to papilloedema with redness and swelling of the disc. However, it differs from papilloedema in that:

- There is severe visual disturbance.
- The swelling of the disc is less.
- The veins are less distended.

Optic atrophy (See Fig. 16.13) frequently follows optic neuritis but may be due to a wide range of conditions which are listed in Chapter 16. Because the nerve fibres become atrophic the disc becomes abnormally pale and its edges are sharply demarcated from the retina.

Vision and visual field testing

Non-specialists sometimes overlook these basic tests but they are of critical importance. They are dealt with in Chapter 16. Sometimes patients may be unaware of quite gross visual defects in one eye. Start by simple finger counting and then proceed to Snellen chart testing with and without spectacles.

Visual field testing is performed by confrontation. This depends on comparing the patient's visual field with your own. Seat yourself opposite the patient about one metre away. The testing is best performed in stages:

- Ask your patient to keep both eyes open and to look at the bridge of your nose.
- Then move your finger in each of the peripheral quadrants of the visual field, asking the patient if he can detect movement (Fig. 7.4). In this way a homonymous field defect may be detected (Fig. 7.5).

- Move the fingers in the right or left fields simultaneously. This may detect an 'inattention defect' even though the visual fields appear full at the first test stage.
- Test each eye separately. First ask the patient to cover the right eye with his right hand whilst you cover your left eye with your left hand. The visual field of the patient's left eye can be compared with your own right eye by moving your right

Practical Point

You may need to determine if a semiconscious patient has a homonymous hemianopia. To do this move your hand suddenly on one side of the face. Normally a patient will flinch; if there is a hemianopia to that side the stimulus will not be seen and there will be no response.

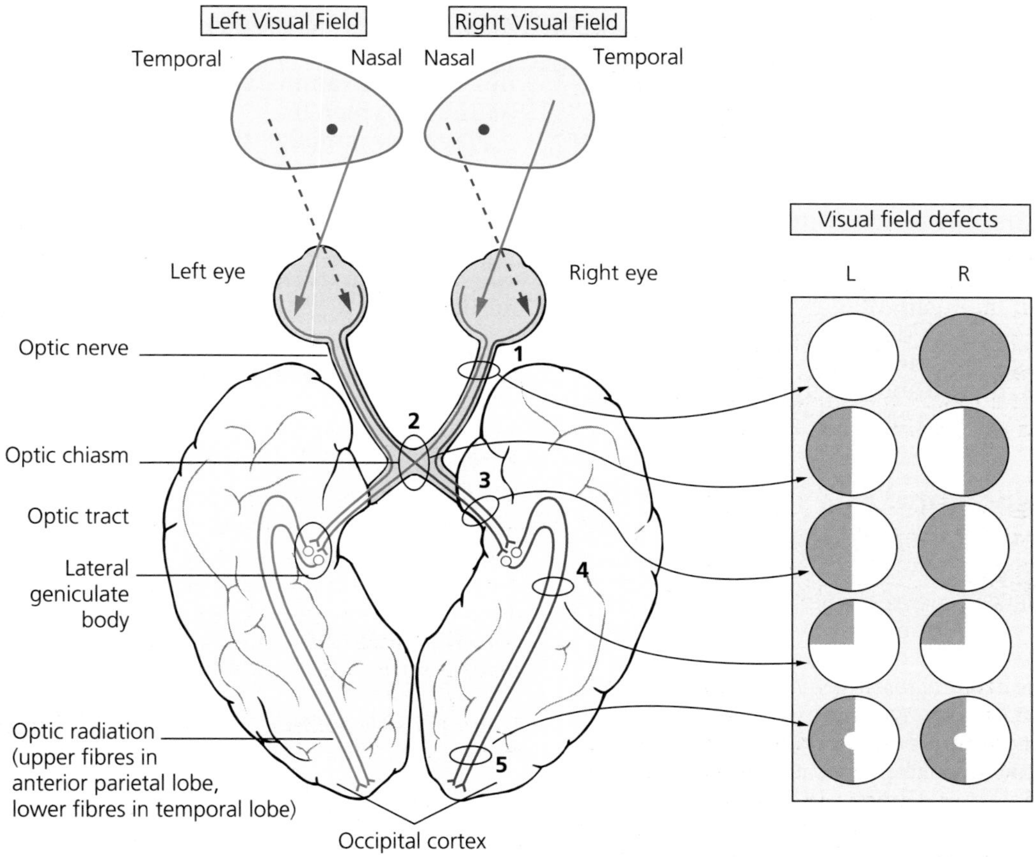

FIG. 7.5 Diagram of the visual pathways with visual field defects produced by lesions at specific sites. A lesion at (1) causes complete blindness in the right eye with loss of the direct light reflex in that eye. A lesion at (2), as with a pituitary tumour, produces a bitemporal hemianopia. In practice it is unusual to have a strictly symmetrical visual field defect. With lesions at (3), the optic tract, there will be a left homonymous hemianopia with macular (splitting) involvement. Lesions in the optic radiation will produce a left quadrantic hemianopia. With damage to the lower fibres of the optic radiation in the temporal lobe this will be an upper quadrantic hemianopia (4). Less commonly, with damage to the upper fibres of the optic radiation in the anterior part of the parietal lobe there will be a lower quadrantic hemianopia (not illustrated in the diagram). A lesion at (5) will produce a left homonymous hemianopia.

hand in from the periphery and asking when it is first seen. The procedure is then repeated for the other eye.

Visual testing by confrontation is a crude method of assessment and it cannot match the accuracy of formal perimetry using an instrument such as the Humphrey perimeter. Nevertheless, the patterns of visual field defects give useful localizing information for lesions of the visual pathway and retina. These are summarized in Fig. 7.5.

Subjective visual sensations

It is important to ask about visual sensations. Amongst the more common are:

- Zigzag lines, flashing lights or shimmering areas which may occur during the first few minutes of an attack of classical migraine.
- Floaters – these are little specks seen on looking at the sky or a white background; they are normal and of no significance.
- Visual hallucinations – as in the aura of epilepsy or in delirium tremens.
- Photopsias – tiny white flashes which may occur in retrobulbar neuritis and which may be precipitated by movement.

The oculomotor (III), trochlear (IV) and abducens (VI) nerves

These nerves are responsible individually or collectively for eye movements, pupillary responses and elevation of the eyelids. However, when testing eye movements, you may also detect nystagmus or defective conjugate eye movement which may indicate cerebellar, brainstem disease or a defect of the supranuclear pathways in the cerebral hemispheres. Similarly, when testing the pupillary responses and elevation of the upper lid you may also be checking for a defect of the sympathetic or parasympathetic nervous system. Fortunately it is not necessary to have a detailed knowledge of the complex neuroanatomical pathways to be able to reach a working diagnosis in the majority of clinical problems.

Practical Point

When testing the pupillary reaction to light, shine your torch at the pupil obliquely. If you shine the torch directly at the pupil the patient will automatically focus on the light source and accommodation will occur as well.

Start by examining the pupils The pupils (P), should be equal (E) and react (R) to light (L) and accommodation (A). It is probably acceptable to use the abbreviation PERLA in medical notes, but remember that doctors in other specialities may not understand what this means. Examination of the pupils is dealt with in Chapter 16.

Having examined the pupils move on to check *eye movements* by asking your patient to follow the your index finger, held one metre away, in all directions to the limits of binocular vision. If there is any defect test with each eye closed in turn. Whilst doing this note additionally:

- Drooping of the upper lid (ptosis).
- Squint, whether this is convergent or divergent.
- Double vision (diplopia) with normal forward gaze or with movement.
- Nystagmus.
- Defects of conjugate deviation.

Practical Point

Ocular muscle disorders, such as myasthenia gravis and thyrotoxicosis, may cause diplopia.

The actions of the individual eye muscles are complicated and depend on whether the eye is in abduction or adduction. However a simplified scheme of the action of the ocular muscles is shown in Fig. 7.6. From an examination of eye movements performed in the way described it should be possible to identify and localize the more important abnormalities (see Revision Panel 7.6).

Revision Panel 7.6

Abnormalities revealed by examination of eye movements

Abnormality of eye movement	*Site of lesion*	*Features*	*Disease*
Weakness of elevation and adduction i.e. eye looks down and out on forward gaze.	IIIrd nerve lesion.	Usually associated with ptosis and a dilated unreactive pupil (Fig. 7.7).	Trauma, diabetes, tumours, multiple sclerosis, aneurysms on or near Circle of Willis. Note that the parasympathetic fibres supplying the pupil are not always involved in vascular lesions such as diabetes.
Double vision and torsion of the globe on downward gaze.	IVth nerve lesion.	Rare as an isolated lesion.	As for IIIrd nerve.
Weakness on abducting eye.	VIth nerve lesion.	May occur in raised intracranial pressure as a false localizing sign.	Trauma, diabetes, multiple sclerosis, aneurysms.
Loss or impairment of conjugate vertical or horizontal gaze.	Above level of brainstem oculomotor nuclei.		Vascular or structural lesions, multiple sclerosis.
Weakness of adduction in one eye with nystagmus in the abducting eye on lateral gaze.	Median longitudinal bundle between IIIrd and VIth nerve nuclei (see Fig. 7.8).		Usually in multiple sclerosis.
Vertical nystagmus on upward gaze.	High in brainstem.		Vascular or structural lesions, multiple sclerosis.
Vertical nystagmus on downward gaze.	Low in brainstem.		Vascular or structural lesions, multiple sclerosis.

The trigeminal (V) nerve

The trigeminal nerve supplies sensation to the face and motor function to the muscles of mastication.

Figure 7.9 shows the distribution of the three sensory divisions. Important points are:

- Herpes zoster of the ophthalmic division of the Vth nerve is common (see Fig. 7.10).
- Trigeminal neuralgia (attacks of severe lancinating pain) may affect one or more divisions of the nerve but is usually unilateral.
- The ophthalmic division supplies sensation of the cornea. The corneal reflex tests corneal sensation and is elicited by touching the cornea with a wisp of cotton wool with the patient looking away. Loss of this reflex is abnormal but is also dependent on the integrity of the facial nerve for its motor component. The corneal reflex is the most delicate test of function of the ophthalmic division of the Vth nerve. Awareness of the sensory supply of the cornea is essential in the management of ophthalmic herpes.
- The maxillary division also supplies sensation to the upper teeth and hard palate on the same side.
- The mandibular division also supplies pain and touch sensation to the tongue and lower teeth on the same side.

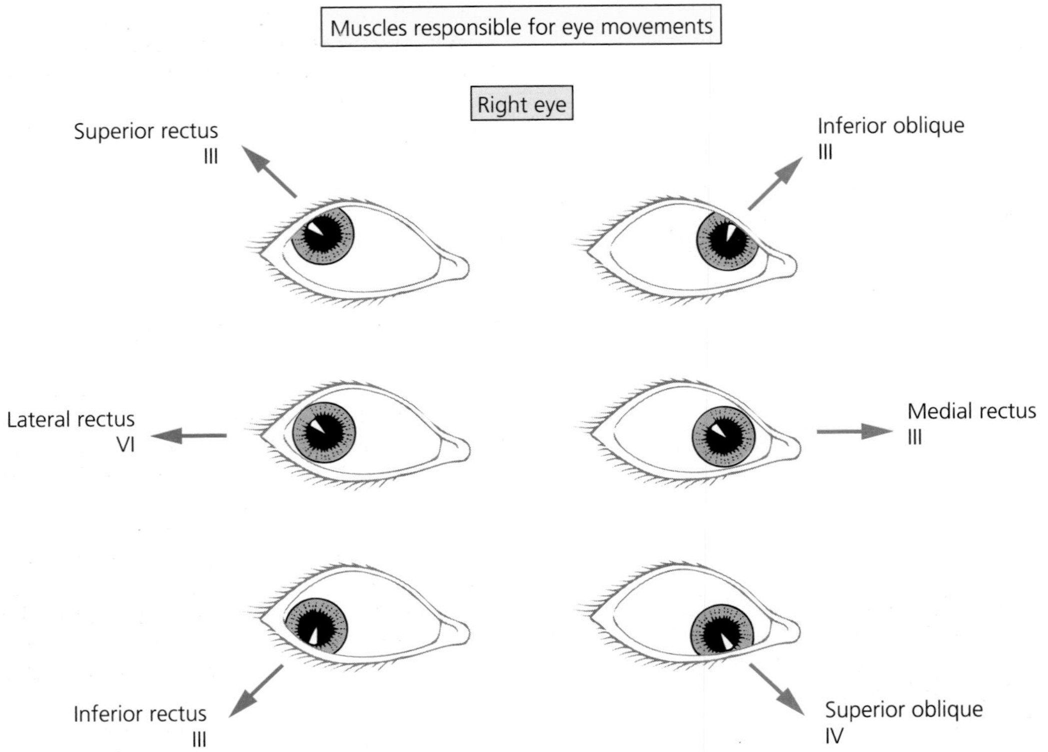

FIG. 7.6 A simplified scheme of the action of the IIIrd, IVth and VIth nerves and the individual muscles on eye movements.

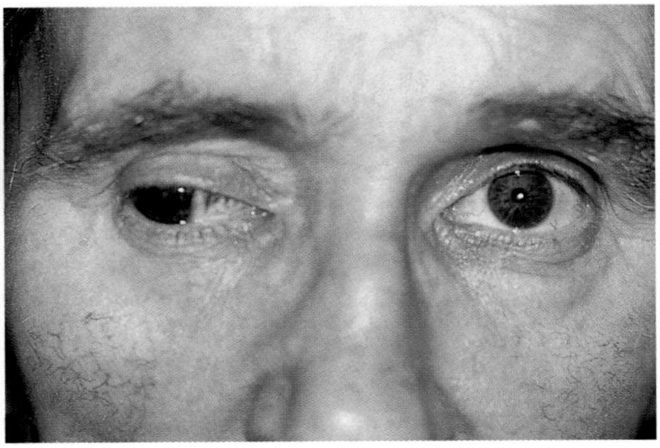

FIG. 7.7 Right IIIrd nerve lesion showing the eye deviated downwards and outwards, ptosis and a large (unreactive) right pupil.

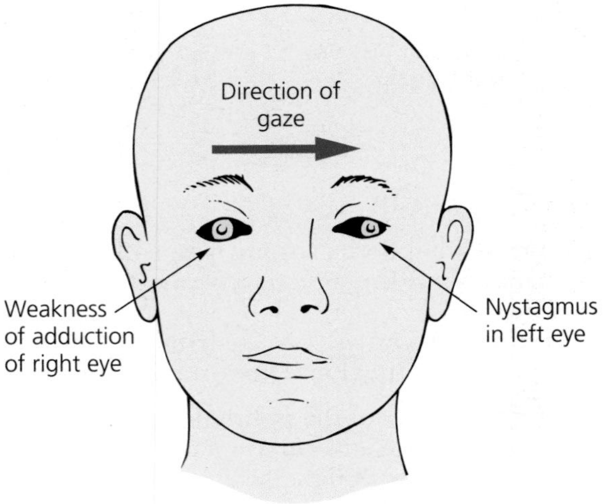

FIG. 7.8 Eye movements in a lesion of the median longitudinal bundle. On looking to the left the right eye fails to adduct, whereas the abducting left eye develops nystagmus.

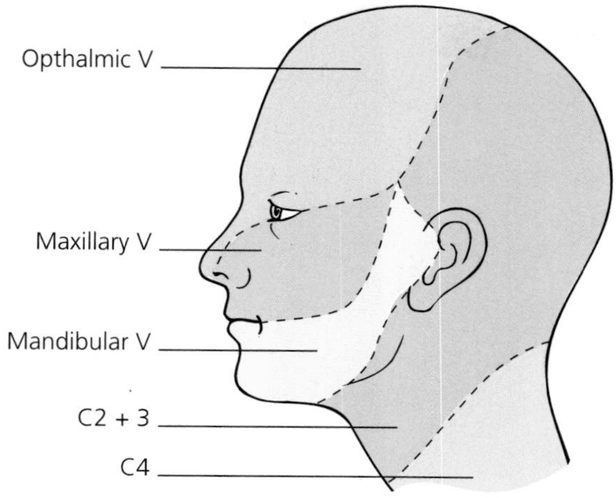

FIG. 7.9 The sensory distribution of the Vth nerve.

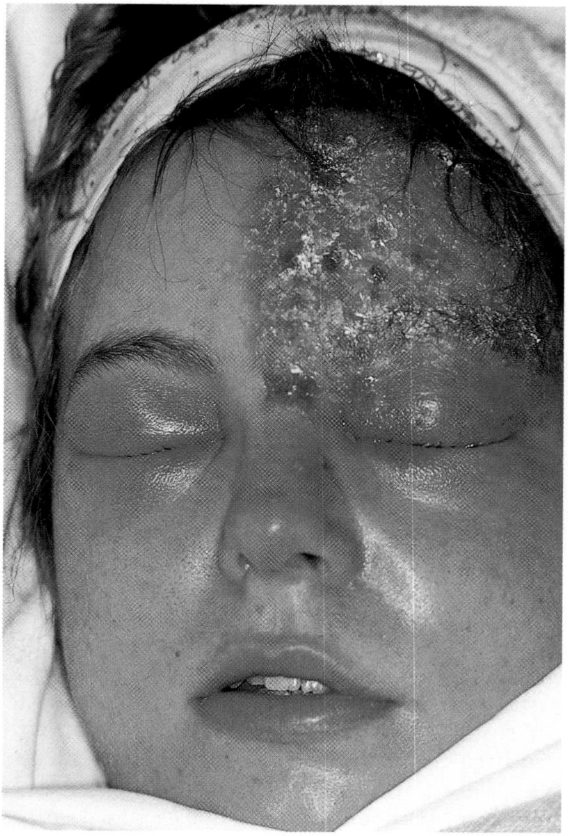

FIG. 7.10 Ophthalmic herpes.

The motor component of the trigeminal nerve supplies the temporalis muscles, the masseters and the lateral pterygoids. Simply placing fingers over the muscles in turn and asking the patient to bite can test the first two muscles.

The facial VII nerve

The facial nerve supplies the muscles of the face and scalp except the levator palpebrae superioris. During its course through the temporal bone it is joined by the chorda tympani nerve, which carries taste sensation from the anterior two-thirds of the tongue. The muscles of the upper part of the face are bilaterally innervated. Because of this, with a supranuclear paralysis, the upper and lower parts of the face will be equally affected. An exception to this rule is that the patient who has recently and suddenly sustained a stroke may have upper and lower face affected.

If the lesion of the facial nerve is within the facial canal the fibres of the chorda tympani will be involved and there will be loss of taste sensation over the anterior two-thirds of the tongue.

Practical Point

A glance at a patient with mild facial weakness will reveal smoothing out of the nasolabial fold and a droop at the angle of the mouth on the affected side.

When continuing testing of facial nerve function, formally start at the top and work down. Ask your patient to:

- 'Look up without moving your head': this normally causes wrinkling of the forehead and will clearly demonstrate if there is any weakness of the frontalis muscle. With an upper motor neuron lesion the brow will wrinkle on both sides.

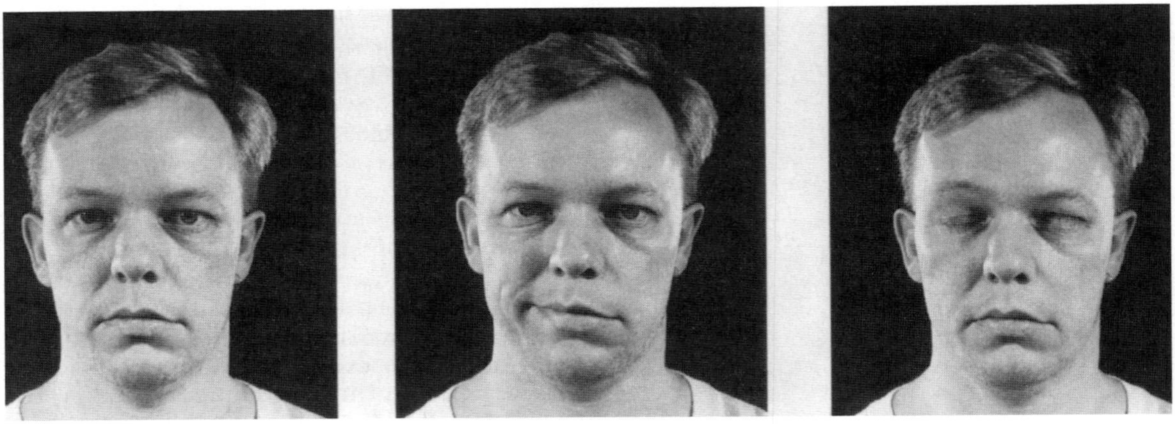

FIG. 7.11 Left Bell's palsy. (a) At rest the nasolabial fold is less prominent and the corner of the mouth droops. (b) On smiling. (c) On attempted closure of the eyes the left globe rolls upwards.

Revision Panel 7.7

Causes of a lower motor neuron facial weakness

Bell's palsy[a] – a benign condition characterized by pain in the region of the ear followed by unilateral weakness of the face.

Middle ear disease.[a]

Ramsey–Hunt syndrome – herpes of the geniculate ganglion.

Sarcoidosis – uveoparotid fever.

Carcinoma of the parotid gland.

Surgical damage to the nerve during ear or parotid gland surgery.

Leprosy – in tropics.

[a]Common causes

- 'Screw up your eyes': note if the eyelashes are buried equally. With a lower motor neuron facial palsy (Revision Panel 7.7) the eyeball rolls upwards, often to such a degree that the pupil disappears under the upper lid (Fig. 7.11).
- 'Show me your teeth': in unilateral facial paralysis the mouth is pulled away from the affected side.

The auditory and vestibular (VIII) nerves

Auditory nerve

The assessment of auditory nerve function is dealt with in Chapter 17.

Vestibular nerve

Vertigo is a sense of rotation either of the individual or of the environment. True vertigo is usually a result of disruption of either the labyrinthine system (termed peripheral vertigo) or the central connections of the vestibular nerve (termed central vertigo). There are no true bedside tests of vestibular function and the diagnosis of vertigo rests heavily of the history. Nevertheless in some cases the analysis of nystagmus (Revision Panel 7.8) (which is present in only a minority of patients with vertigo) may be of value.

Vestibular nystagmus typically has two components, a rapid phase and a slow phase, the direction of the rapid phase being used to define the direction of the nystagmus, i.e. rapid phase to the right equals nystagmus to the right. An irritative labyrinthine lesion will produce a nystagmus to the ipsilateral ear whereas a paralytic nystagmus will produce it to the opposite ear.

Rhomberg's test is sometimes used for the assessment of patients with vertigo but it is

Revision Panel 7.8
Causes of nystagmus

Congenital

Physiological
For example railway nystagmus or end-point nystagmus (taking the direction of gaze more than 60 degrees either side of the midline).

Pathological
Ocular.
Vestibular.
Of central nervous system origin.

non-specific. The patient is asked to stand with eyes closed and heels together. The test is regarded as being positive if the patient cannot maintain balance. This usually indicates defective joint position but vestibular impairment may also cause Rhombergism when position sense is normal. Don't attach too much significance to this sign.

The glossopharyngeal (IX) and vagus (X) nerves

The IXth and Xth cranial nerves are mixed nerves supplying tongue and pharynx, larynx and soft palate and sensory and motor fibres supplying the heart, lungs and abdominal viscera. There is no need to test these nerves routinely unless there are symptoms of dysarthria, dysphonia, or dysphagia or signs of brainstem damage.

Practical Point

Isolated lesions of the glossopharyngeal nerve are extremely rare but glossopharyngeal neuralgia (resembling trigeminal neuralgia) may cause lancinating pains at the back of the throat.

Depressing the tongue and touching each side of the posterior wall of the pharynx can test sensation in the pharynx (IX nerve). Reflex gagging to this stimulus causes elevation of the soft palate which should move centrally. The gag reflex has therefore as its afferent arm the glossopharyngeal nerve and as its efferent arm the vagus nerve which supplies the soft palate. Deviation of the uvula to one side indicates a Xth nerve lesion on the opposite side.

Isolated lesions of the vagus are rare. When unilateral lesions do occur at the base of the skull as the result of tumours or trauma, the adjacent IXth and XIth nerves are usually also implicated. However, damage to the left recurrent laryngeal branch due to bronchial carcinoma is common. The earliest sign of recurrent laryngeal palsy is an abductor palsy of the vocal cord causing hoarseness. Later the adductors are affected and the cord lies in mid position.

The accessory (XI) nerve

This is a purely motor nerve supplying the sternomastoid and trapezius muscles.

The sternomastoid muscle can be tested by getting the patient to turn the head to one side against pressure applied to the side of the chin. The muscle on the opposite side can be felt to contract. Asking the patient to push forward against pressure applied to the forehead allows you to compare the two muscles.

Asking the patient to shrug the shoulders can test the accessory muscle, which causes the trapezius muscle to contract.

The hypoglossal (XII) nerve

This is a purely motor nerve to the muscles of the tongue.

Bilateral upper motor neuron lesions of the tongue, usually due to multiple bilateral vascular lesions, produce what is termed pseudobulbar palsy with a spastic poorly moving tongue causing dysarthria, dysphagia and a brick jaw jerk.

Bilateral lower motor neuron lesions of the tongue cause wasting and fasciculation (continuous, rapid, irregular contractions of groups of muscle fibres). Examine for fasciculation with the tongue resting within the mouth; it is an extremely important physical sign and usually indicates motor neuron disease (Revision Panel 7.9).

If the hypoglossal nerve is paralysed the tongue protrudes towards the paralysed side.

Revision Panel 7.9
Involuntary movements of the tongue

Type of movement	*Usual cause*
Rapid protrusion and retraction (trombone tremor).	Parkinson's disease.
Choreiform movements.	Huntington's chorea.
Irregular, 'churning' movements of the tongue.	Drugs such as phenothiazines.
Fasciculation.	Motor neuron disease.

The motor system

Test the motor system bearing the following aspects in mind:

- Gait.
- Muscle bulk and/or wasting.
- Tone.
- Power.
- Coordination.
- Reflexes.
- Involuntary movements.

Gait

If your patient is mobile you will have noted this already as part of 'first impressions'. Almost unconsciously you will have recorded local problems such as a stiff back due to severe pain or a limp caused by osteoarthritis. Whilst you may not necessarily be able to make an accurate spot diagnosis at this stage it will direct the examination. (See Revision Panel 7.2 on gait at beginning of this chapter.)

Muscle bulk and/or wasting

With your patient suitably undressed you must look at muscle bulk and patterns of generalized or localized wasting (see Revision Panel 7.10). Atrophy of muscles is not always caused by neurological disorders – an injured knee can quickly cause quadriceps wasting. Look for pseudohypertrophy if you suspect a muscular dystrophy. If you are doubtful about degrees of muscle wasting, compare one side with the other; in the limbs the circumference can be measured with reference to a fixed bony point.

Tone

Correct assessment of tone requires much practice. Muscle tone may be increased (hypertonia) or decreased (hypotonia). Move the limb passively utilizing flexion/extension and pronation/supination at the elbow, and flexion/extension at the knee.

Hypertonia may be spastic (pyramidal) or rigid (extrapyramidal). In the spasticity of a pyramidal lesion the resistance to passive movement is greatest initially and then falls away – like a penknife opening. The rigid hypertonia of extrapyramidal disease is uniform throughout the movement though the tremor in Parkinson's disease often gives it a

Revision Panel 7.10
Muscle bulk and/or wasting

Causes of generalized muscle wasting	*Causes of localized muscle wasting*
Malignancy.	Disuse atrophy.
Malnutrition.	Peripheral neuropathy.
Other debilitating diseases.	Muscular dystrophy.
Prolonged immobility.	Poliomyelitis.
Malabsorption.	Cord lesions.
AIDS.	Motor neuron disease.
	Local nerve injury.

jerky 'cogwheel' effect. The hypotonic limb feels floppy on passive movement. If you are uncertain about the tone of the lower limbs try rolling the thigh, with the patient supine. Watch the foot; with the hypotonic limb the foot flops from side to the other as the limb is rolled whereas the hypertonic limb and foot roll like a log in one piece.

Measuring muscle power

Much information is gained from just watching your patient walk into the room, climb onto the examination couch, standing up from sitting and undertaking all those other movements which those who are fit do without thinking. If you need to evaluate muscle power systematically, ask your patient to undertake the following simple tasks, showing him what to do as you go along.

- Grip your fingers tightly.
- Spread out his fingers against resistance.
- Grip a piece of card firmly between finger and thumb.
- Flex and extend, in turn, the wrist and elbow against resistance.
- Flex and extend, abduct and adduct the shoulder against resistance.
- Sit up from the supine position on the couch without using the arms.
- Lift the leg off the couch with knee extended (checking hip flexion).
- Push the elevated leg downwards onto the couch (checking hip extension).
- Squeeze your fist between the knees (checking hip adduction).
- Push the knees apart (hip abduction)
- Flex and extend the knee in a sitting position.
- Plantarflex and dorsiflex the foot against resistance.

Any weakness should be graded and recorded so that serial assessments will show degrees of recovery or deterioration (see Revision Panel 7.11).

Revision Panel 7.11
Grading of muscle power

Grade 0: Total paralysis.

Grade 1: Trace of movement.

Grade 2: Able to move the limb only if supported against gravity.

Grade 3: Weak but just able to oppose gravity.

Grade 4: Weak but able to overcome gravity and resistance.

Grade 5: Normal power.

Practical Point

Check these points in assessing motor function

Gait.
Wasting.
Tone.
Power.
Coordination.
Reflexes.
Involuntary movements.

Coordination

Any weakness may be associated with a degree of clumsiness but incoordination is particularly prominent in sensory and cerebellar ataxia. Useful tests of coordination are:

- The finger–nose test. To perform this, ask your patient to hold each arm outstretched in turn and to touch the tip of their nose with the index finger tip. This test is then repeated with the eyes closed. The patient with a sensory ataxia will perform these tests smoothly whilst compensating with eyes open but will perform badly when the eyes are closed. The patient with cerebellar ataxia will have a marked intention tremor getting worse as the finger approaches its target with the eyes open and closed.
- The heel-shin test. Ask your patient to place a heel on the opposite shin and then slide the heel slowly up and down the shin. With a cerebellar ataxia the heel slithers off the shin from one side to the other.

- Disdiadochokinesis. This long word means impairment of rapid alternating movements which occurs in cerebellar disorders. Ask your patient to tap the back of one hand with first the palm, then the back of the other hand as quickly as possible. Bear in mind that some people are relatively clumsy with their non-dominant hand.

Reflexes

Eliciting the tendon reflexes is a skill only acquired after practice. Here are some points about the commonly used tendon reflexes, starting from the top down.

Biceps jerk C5 and 6 Place your thumb on the biceps tendon and strike with your thumb with the tendon hammer. This is a good reflex to test if you think your patient is myxoedematous and you want to demonstrate delayed relaxation.

Triceps jerk C6 and 7 Flex the elbow and allow the forearm to rest across the chest. Make sure that you tap the triceps tendon just above the olecranon and not the muscle belly itself.

> **Practical Point**
>
> *Tips about eliciting tendon jerks*
>
> Use a hammer with a firm rubber ring or head.
>
> Make sure that your patient is relaxed.
>
> Use a gentle free-fall swing – avoid sledgehammer blows or woodpecker taps.
>
> Use the same technique each time but try alternative positions of the patient if you have problems.

Supinator jerk C5 and 6 With the forearm in the semipronated position across the chest, strike the radial aspect of the forearm over the styloid process. This stretches the supinator and causes supination of the elbow. With lesions of C5/6 level the reflex may be lost to be replaced by finger flexion. This is known as inversion of the reflex.

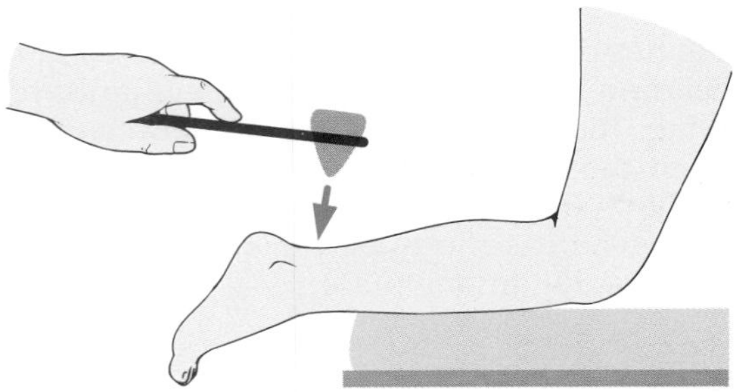

FIG. 7.12 Eliciting the ankle jerk in a kneeling patient (another reflex to use to assess myxoedema clinically).

Knee jerk L (2), 3 and 4 Support the flexed knee to 90 degrees with the left hand and strike the patellar tendon. Make sure that the knees are not touching. Note the contraction of the quadriceps. Some physicians elicit this reflex with their patient sitting on a chair.

Ankle jerk L5 and S1 (and 2) Flex the knee slightly and hold the foot in partial dorsiflexion. Strike the tendon and observe the contraction of gastrocnemius. If you have difficulty in obtaining the ankle jerk ask your patient to kneel on a padded chair facing away from you (Fig. 7.12).

Reinforcement When there is difficulty in obtaining a reflex, attempt to reinforce it by asking your patient to forcibly contract muscles remote from those being tested. For leg reflexes for example ask the patient to grip his hands together and to attempt to pull them apart whilst you test the reflex.

Clonus When reflexes are grossly exaggerated, as the result of an upper motor neuron lesion, clonus may be present. This is most easily elicited at the ankle by flexing the knee slightly, sharply dorsiflexing the foot and then maintaining the stretch on the calf muscles. A few rhythmic beats of contraction and relaxation may occur normally but sustained clonus is always abnormal (see Revision Panel 7.12).

Revision Panel 7.12
Grading of reflexes

In the notes reflexes may be graded or recorded as follows:

Grade 0: Absent, even with reinforcement.

Grade 1: Present.

Grade 2: Brisk but normal (as in nervousness).

Grade 3: Very brisk.

Grade 4: With clonus.

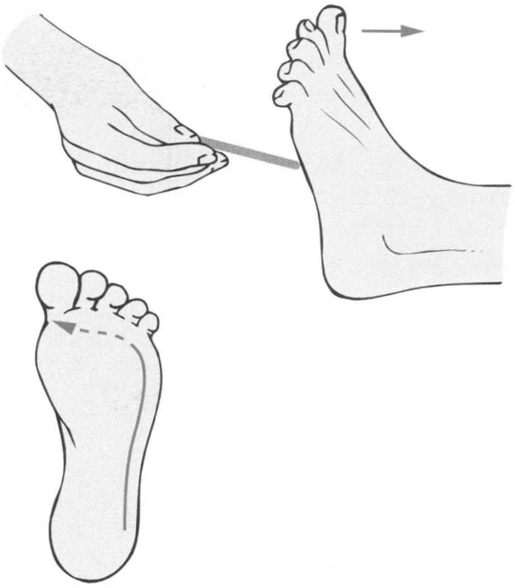

FIG. 7.13 The plantar reflex. Note the direction of the stimulus on the sole. An extensor response is shown.

The plantar reflex This is undoubtedly the most important reflex in the whole clinical examination of the nervous system. Learn how to do it properly. With your patient relaxed stroke the outer edge of the sole with a stick or key and draw it across medially under the metatarsal arch (Fig. 7.13). The normal response is flexion of the great toe and clawing of the other toes (a flexor plantar response). In lesions of the corticospinal tract an *extensor* plantar response replaces the normal *flexor* response. Here the first movement is extension of the great toe followed by fanning of the other toes. Babinski described these reflexes but it is better to describe them as simply flexor or extensor responses rather than positive or negative Babinski signs, which can be rather confusing.

The abdominal reflexes These are elicited by stroking each quadrant of the relaxed abdominal wall in turn. Each stroke produces a contraction of the underlying muscle, pulling the umbilicus in the direction of the stimulus. The abdominal reflex is absent in upper motor neuron lesions above the level of the reflex arc (Revision Panel 7.13).

Involuntary movements

You will have noted these whilst taking the history and examining your patient formally.

Revision Panel 7.13
Upper and lower motor neuron lesions

Features of an upper motor neuron lesion	*Features of a lower motor neuron lesion*
Muscle weakness.	Muscle weakness.
Increased tendon reflexes.	Decreased or absent tendon reflexes.
Depressed or absent abdominal reflexes.	Fasciculation (marked when cranial nerve motor nuclei or anterior horn cells are affected).
Extensor plantar response.	Wasting.
Spasticity.	Flaccidity.

Revision Panel 7.14

Causes of tremor

Anxiety.

Essential (familial) tremor – Absent at rest, appears with volitional activity, affects face and neck as well as upper limbs.

Thyrotoxicosis – Obvious with outstretched hands.

Parkinson's disease – Present at rest, partly abolished by activity.

β-Agonist overdosage.

Hypercapnia.

Hepatic coma – Flapping or twitching in type.

Chronic alcohol abuse.

Terms which are used to describe them are:

- Tremor – regular rhythmic repetitive movements at a joint (see Revision Panel 7.14).
- Chorea – jerky random repetitive movements. Patients seem fidgety. Seen in Sydenham's chorea, Huntington's chorea and L-dopa overdosage.
- Athetoid dystonia – writhing, slow movements which are non-repetitive and associated with disturbance of posture.
- Tics – repetitive (but often complex) jerking movements which may be suppressed voluntarily but only temporally. Usually in the young.
- Myoclonus – jerky repetitive movements (irregular or rhythmic), which are outside voluntary control.
- Fasciculation – diffuse irregular muscle twitching. Note that coarse involuntary twitching may occur around the shoulders in health.
- Myokymia – repetitive irregular muscle twitches localized to one part of a muscle. Common, usually as fine twitching of the eyelid.
- Asterixis – brief lapses of sustained posture. Seen in hepatic and renal failure.

The sensory system

How much of the sensory system has to be examined depends entirely on the circumstances; in many routine medical examinations it may be superfluous. For the localization of a cord lesion it has to be meticulous and may be time-consuming. When examining sensation think in terms of the possible anatomical lesion. If testing for a sensory level, as in a cord lesion, start at the feet and work up. Where the lesion is peripheral all modalities, i.e. touch, pain and temperature, will be affected. Where the lesion affects the central nervous system and the sensory pathways are separated anatomically, sensory loss will be disassociated. This is demonstrated in hemitransection of the cord in the Brown–Sequard syndrome (see Fig. 7.25).

Test the sensory modalities as follows:

Light touch Using a wisp of cotton wool, ask the patient to close his eyes and to tell you when contact is made after a single touch. Remember that the distal parts of limbs are more sensitive than proximal.

Proprioception Use a peripheral joint such as the first metatarsophalangeal joint. Hold the sides of the toe near its tip whilst moving it up and down. A normal patient should be able to detect a 5 mm movement. Rhomberg's test can be used to assess the quality of proprioceptive information coming from the limbs. Ask your patient to stand with feet together. Where there is proprioceptive loss there will be instability on closing the eyes.

Vibration loss Use a 128 Hz tuning fork. Start over the bony prominences of the malleoli and if sensation is absent there move up to the tibial tubercle and the iliac crest if necessary. Vibration sense may be diminished or lost in the fit elderly.

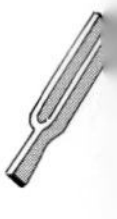

Pain Use a disposable pin and take care not to puncture the skin. Even if the skin is not punctured standard 'sharps' procedure applies.

Temperature Use tubes containing cold and hot water.

Revision Panel 7.15

Root and peripheral nerve supply of certain muscles

Joint	*Muscle*	*Action*	*Root supply*	*Peripheral nerve*	*Relevant clinical conditions*
Shoulder	*Deltoid.*	Abduction	C5,6	Circumflex	Stroke, neuralgic amyotrophy.
	Infraspinatus.	External rotation	C5,6	Suprascapular	
Elbow	Biceps.	Flexion	C5,6	Musculocutaneous	
	Triceps.	Extension	C7,8	Radial	
Wrist	*Extensor carpi radialis longus.*	Extension	C6,7	Radial	
	Extensor digitorum.		C7,8		
Fingers	Flexor digitorum profundus and sublimus.		C8	Median	
	Thenar muscles.		T1	Median	Injury to nerve at wrist. Carpal tunnel syndrome.
	Other intrinsic hand muscles.		T1	Ulnar	Injury to nerve at wrist.

The muscles in italics are those which tend to be weak in a mild pyramidal defect.

Shape recognition This is heavily dependent on cortical function. With eyes closed ask your patient to identify a simple object such as a coin or a biro.

Points about examining the upper limb

You must commit to memory the root and peripheral nerve supply of certain muscles in order to understand the common clinical conditions that are likely to be encountered in everyday practice. These are shown in Revision Panel 7.15.

After a stroke the arm will be spastic with adduction at the shoulder, flexion at the elbow and flexion at the wrist. Movement at the shoulder may be further limited by a frozen shoulder, which may develop after any period of prolonged immobility of the upper limb.

In advanced multiple sclerosis examination of the arm usually reveals a combination of an upper motor lesion and cerebellar signs. The limb is spastic with increased reflexes and a marked intention tremor.

In Parkinson's disease the combination of tremor and rigid spasticity produces a jerky or cogwheel resistance when the arm is taken passively through its range of movement. This, in combination with the resting tremor abolished by volitional movement, points to the diagnosis. An early sign is the fine pill-rolling tremor of the fingers at rest,

Ulnar nerve lesions (Revision Panel 7.16) are characterized by sensory loss over the ulnar side of the ring finger and both sides of the little finger. There may be a sensation of deadness in the hand (Fig. 7.14). On the motor side there is paralysis of the interossei, the 3rd and 4th lumbricals (which cannot be tested clinically), the hypothenar muscles and adductor

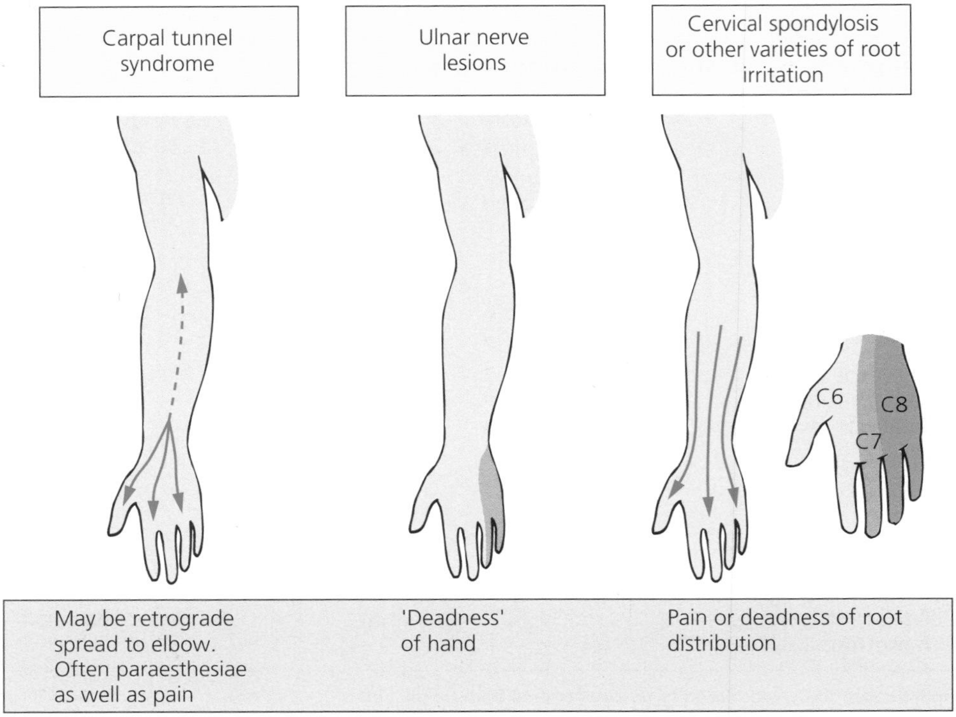

FIG. 7.14 Some common sensory conditions affecting the arm. (a) Carpal tunnel syndrome. Although it is the medial nerve which is compressed at the wrist, patients often complain of pain and paraesthesia in the whole of the hand. (b) Ulnar nerve lesions. (c) Nerve root pain.

pollicis (Fig. 7.15). Learn to test motor function by assessing the strength of the first interosseous muscle (Fig. 7.16).

Median nerve lesions (Revision Panel 7.16) are characterized by sensory loss over the palm of the hand, the palmar surfaces of the thumb, index and middle fingers, together with the radial side of the ring finger. On the motor side the median nerve supplies abductor pollicis brevis, opponens in 80% of patients and the 1st and 2nd lumbricals which again cannot be tested. The median nerve always supplies abductor pollicis brevis and this muscle provides a good test of median nerve function (Fig. 7.17).

Revision Panel 7.16
Wasting of the small muscles of the hand

Predominantly bilateral

Old age and frailty.
Rheumatoid arthritis.
Motor neuron disease.
Cervical myelopathy and spondylosis.
Peripheral neuropathy.
Syringomyelia.

Predominantly unilateral

Ulnar nerve lesions.
Median nerve lesions.
Lower brachial plexus damage e.g. trauma (Fig. 7.18) or secondary to carcinoma at apex of lung.
Thoracic outlet syndromes e.g. cervical rib.

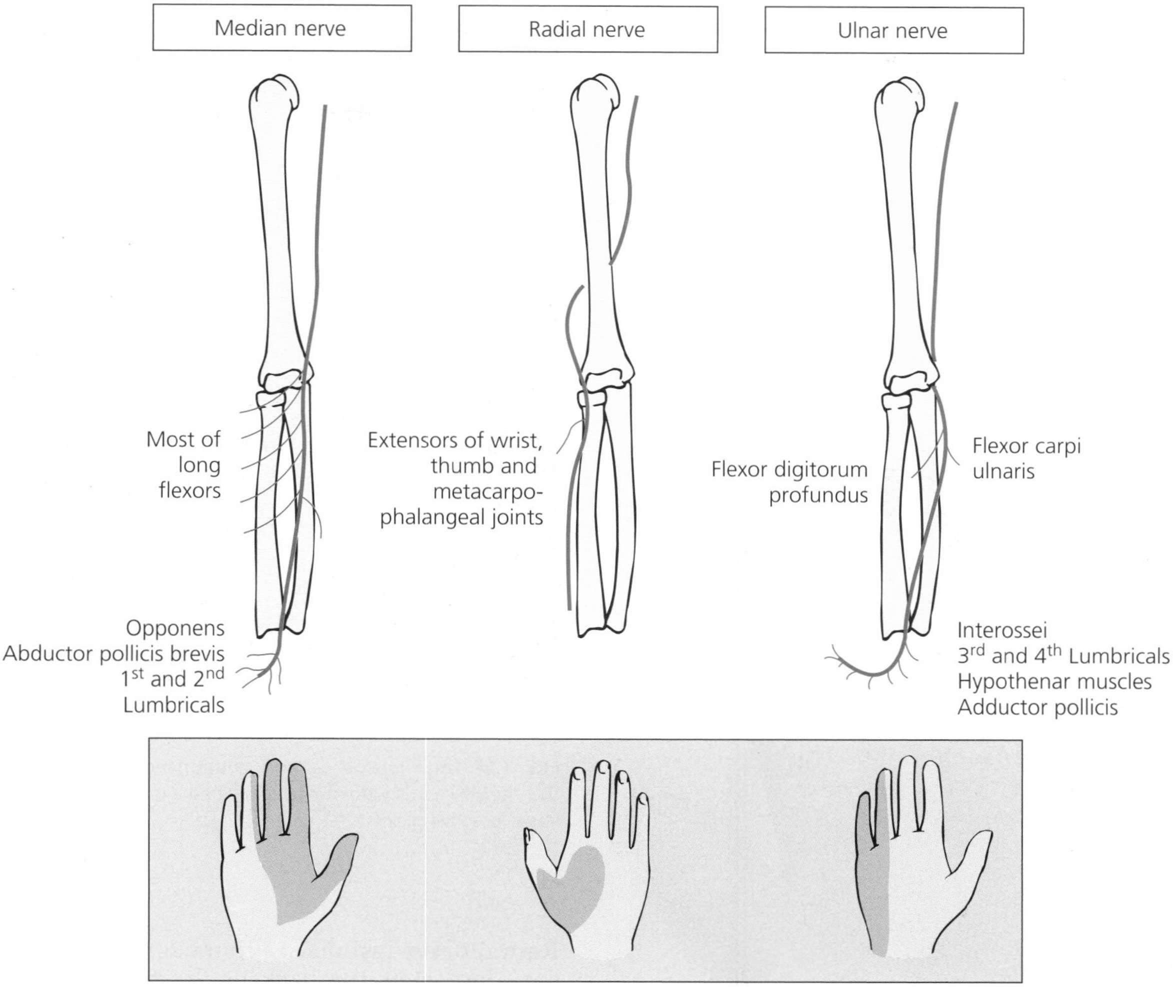

FIG. 7.15 The motor and sensory supply to the arm.

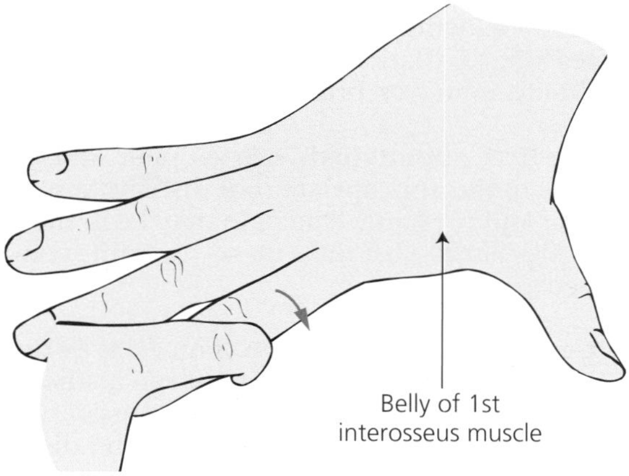

FIG. 7.16 Testing for weakness of the 1st interosseous muscle (ulnar nerve). Ask your patient to abduct the index finger against resistance as in the figure and then feel for contraction of the first interosseous (arrowed) with your finger tip on the belly of the muscle.

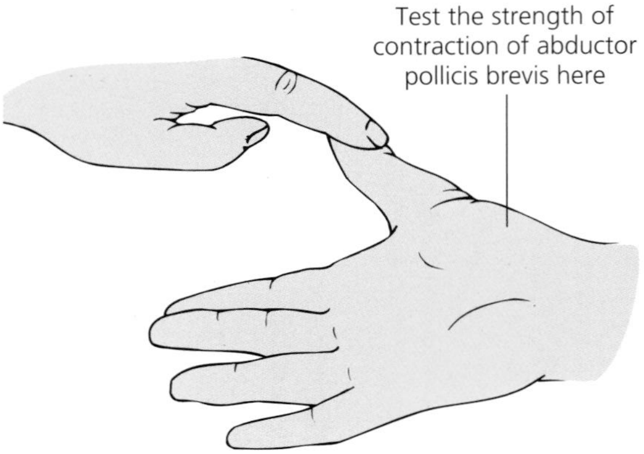

(a)

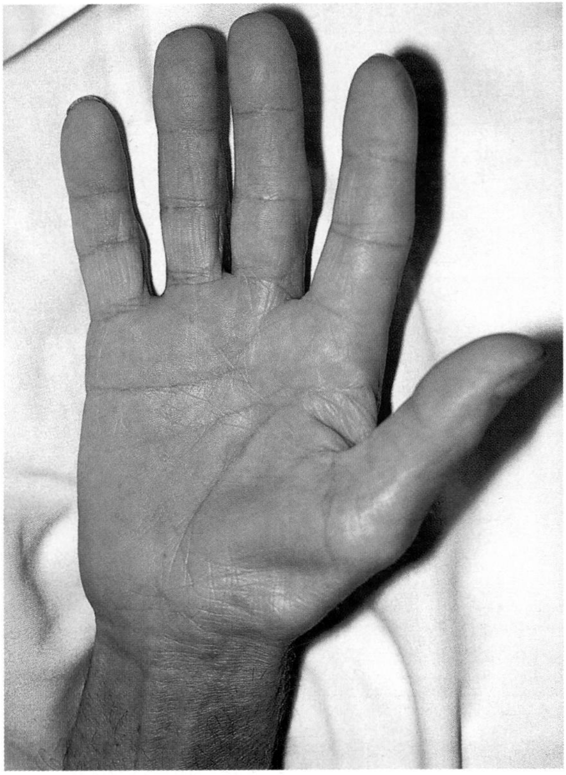

(b)

FIG. 7.17 (a) Testing for weakness of abductor pollicis brevis (median nerve). Ask the patient to place the hand on the table palm uppermost with the thumb nail vertical. The patient then tries to lift the thumb upward against resistance. The strength of the muscle can then be assessed with a fingertip on the muscle itself. (b) Wasting of abductor pollicis brevis in a patient with carpal tunnel syndrome.

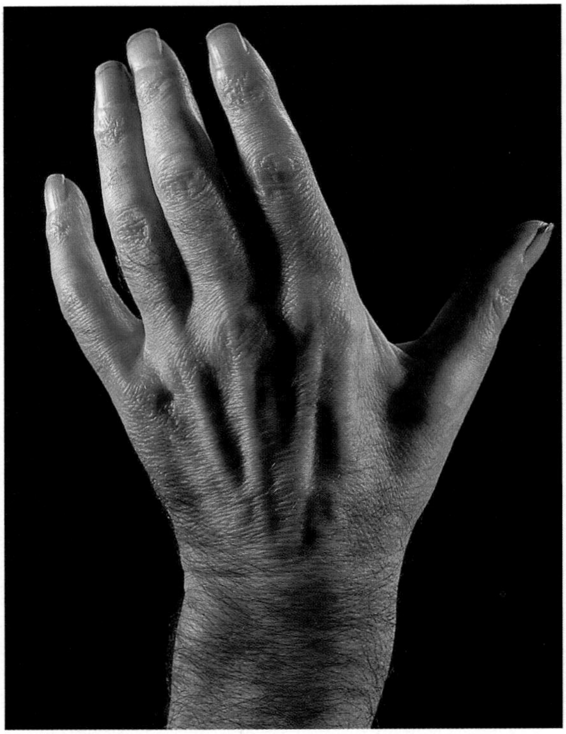

FIG. 7.18 Small muscle wasting in the hand, particularly of the interossei, in a patient who sustained a bullet injury to the lower brachial plexus.

Radial nerve lesions are characterized by sensory loss over the back of the hand mainly over the web of the thumb. On the motor side the nerve supplies the extensors of the wrist, thumb and metacarpophalangeal joints. Test motor function by extending the wrist against resistance. Radial nerve damage is usually due to injury or pressure in the upper arm.

Cervical spondylosis causes pain and deadness in the appropriate root distribution in the arm and/or hand. The pain may be in the back of the hand with little or no discomfort in the neck.

Carpal tunnel syndrome (Fig. 7.14) is due to compression of the medial nerve at the wrist within the carpal tunnel. It causes painful 'pins and needles' at night over the distribution of the median nerve, but often radiating elsewhere. These wake the patient but are relieved by changes in position or movement.

Points about examining the leg

As with the arm it is essential to be aware of the root supply of the more important muscles of the leg (see Revision Panel 7.17).

After a stroke the leg will be spastic and extended with the foot plantarflexed. In walking the leg swings forward and round to avoid the foot tripping.

In a spastic paraparesis the legs are in extension with the feet plantar flexed. The reflexes are very brisk, usually with clonus, with bilateral extensor plantar responses. Note that the immobility of the spastic paresis is often associated with leg oedema. With a complete cord lesion there will be sensory loss.

Practical Point

In *severe and chronic spastic paralysis* there is often so much oedema of the legs that it may be impossible to elicit knee and ankle jerks.

In advanced multiple sclerosis there is usually a combination of cerebellar and pyramidal signs. The legs are spastic with increased

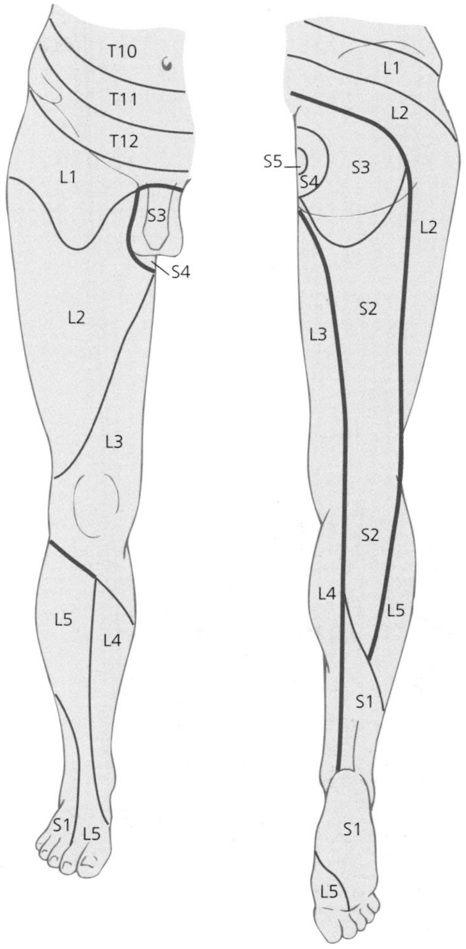

FIG. 7.19 The sensory dermatomes of the lower limb.

Revision Panel 7.17
Root supply of muscles of the leg

Hip	*Ilio-psoas*	Flexion	L1,2,3	Femoral nerve.
	Adductors	Adduction	L2,3,4	Obturator nerve.
	Gluteus maximus	Extension	L5,S1	Inferior gluteal nerve.
Knee	*Quadriceps*	Extension	L3,4	Femoral nerve.
	Hamstrings	Flexion	L5 S1	Sciatic nerve.
Ankle	Tibialis anterior	Dorsiflexion	L4,5	Anterior tibial nerve.
	Gastrocnemius/soleus	Plantar flexion	S1,2	Medial popliteal nerve.
Foot	*Extensor digitorum brevis*	Hallux dorsiflexion	S1	Anterior tibial nerve.

The muscles *in italics* are those which are mainly affected in a mild pyramidal lesion.

reflexes, bilateral clonus and extensor plantar responses; additionally, if it is possible to move the limbs volitionally, there will be gross ataxia obvious by the heel-shin test.

In the elderly there is often flexion at the hip and knee on standing. The ankle jerks may be absent and vibration sense impaired in apparently normal people.

Lumbar spondylosis commonly affects L5 and S1 roots. With the former, pain radiates into the top of the foot and there is weakness of extensor hallucis longus with sensory changes over the medial side (Fig. 7.19). With S1 root syndromes the pain is more lateral with weakness of plantar flexion of the foot and a depressed or absent ankle jerk.

Putting it all together

The last section of this chapter shows, in diagrammatic form, five common neurological syndromes and indicates some of the physical signs which are often, but not always, associated with them. The fifth figure, which shows the effects of hemitransection of the cord (the Brown–Sequard syndrome), illustrates the important principles of dissociated sensory loss (Figs 17.20–17.25).

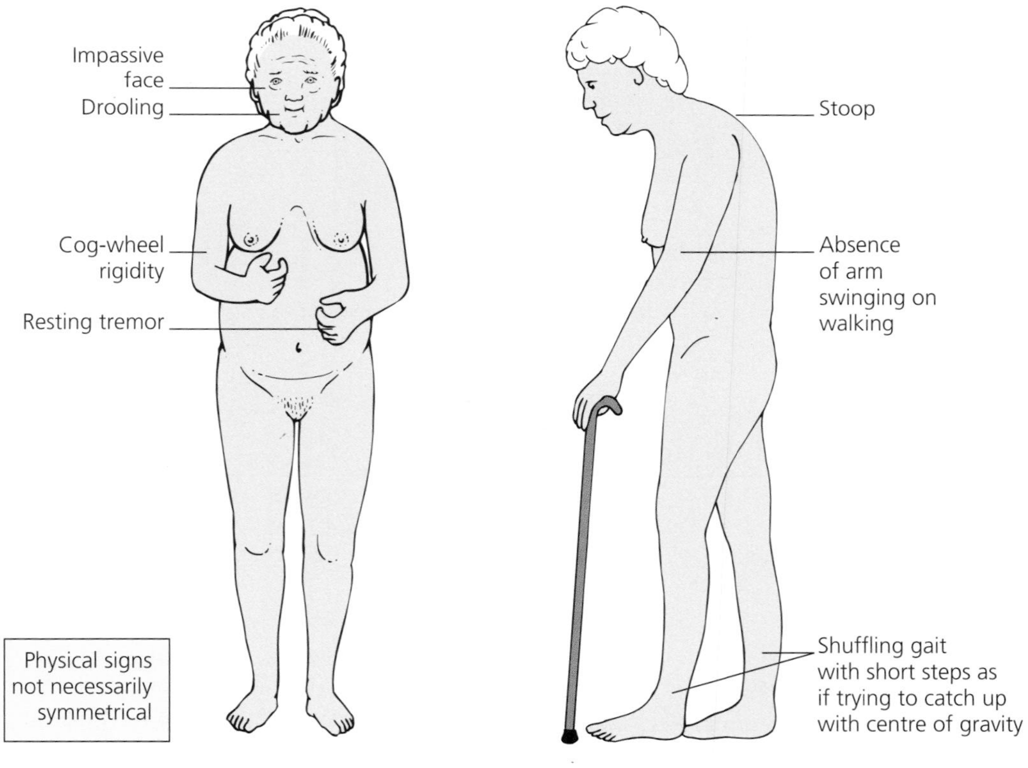

FIG. 7.20 A diagrammatic representation of the features of advanced Parkinson's disease.

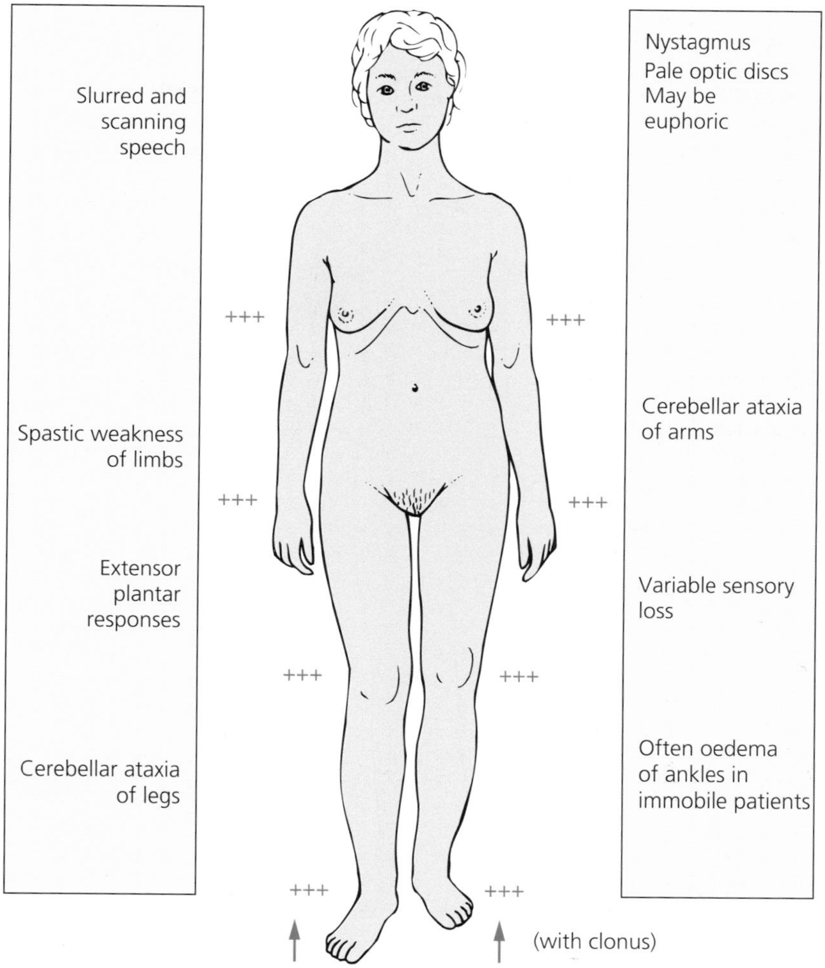

FIG. 7.21 A diagrammatic representation of abnormal physical signs that may be seen in advanced multiple sclerosis. +++: Very brisk reflexes. ↑: Plantar response extensor.

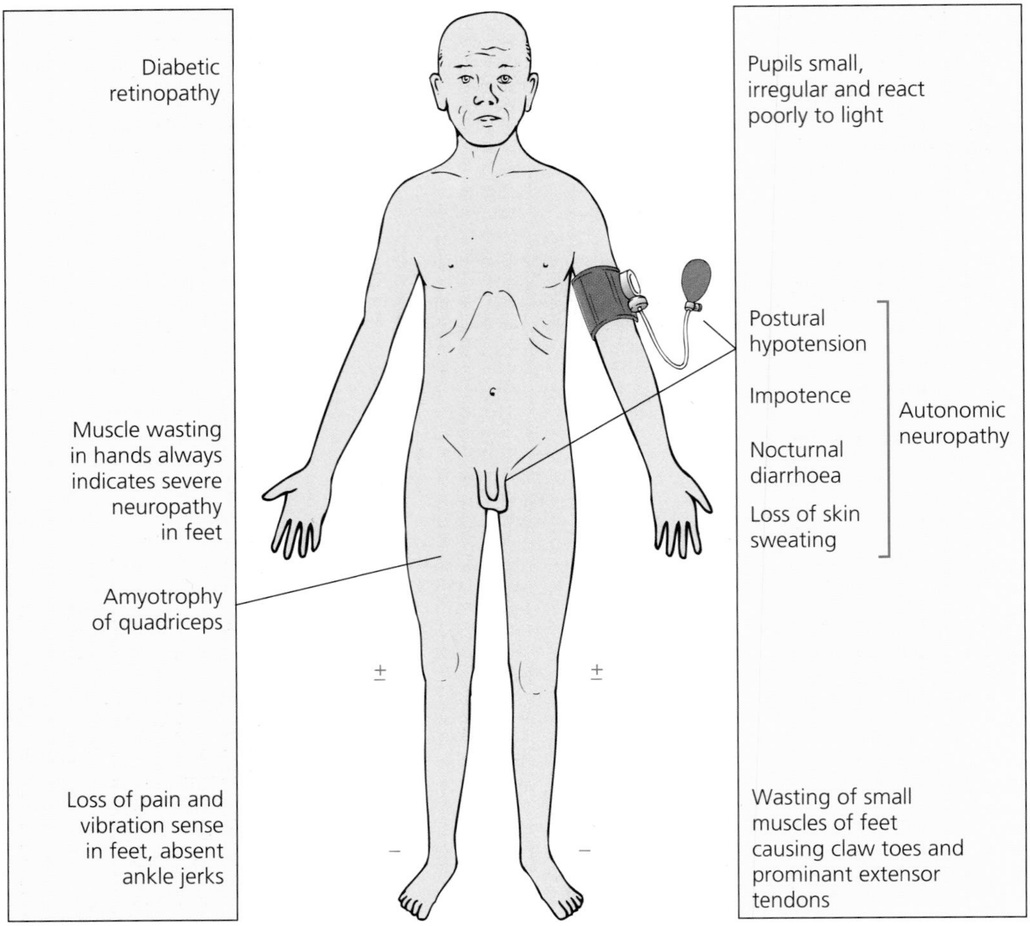

FIG. 7.22 A diagrammatic representation of the features of a mixed polyneuropathy as exemplified by diabetes mellitus. ±: Reflexes may be present or absent. –: Reflexes absent.

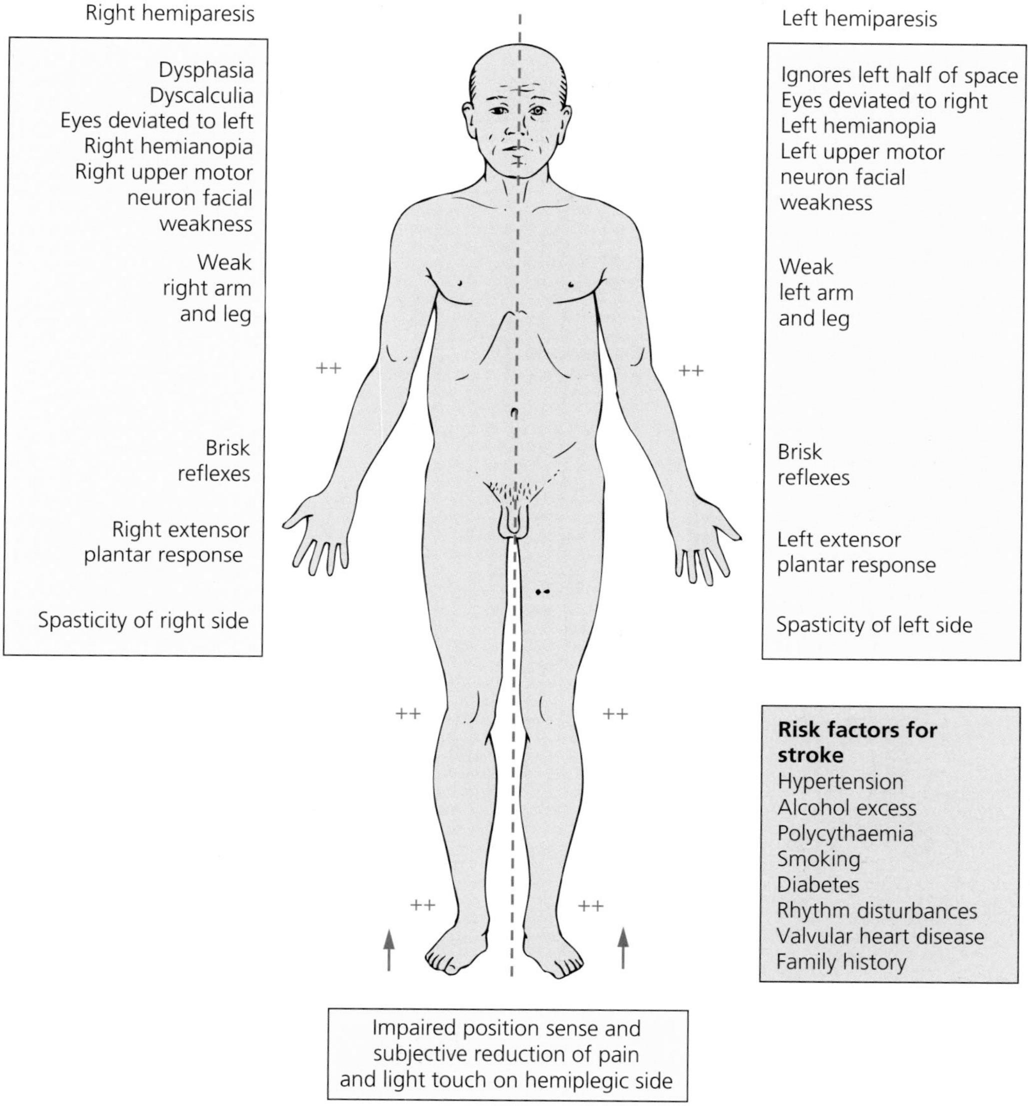

FIG. 7.23 A diagrammatic representation of the effects of right and left strokes in a right-handed person. ++: Brisk reflexes. ↑: Plantar response extensor.

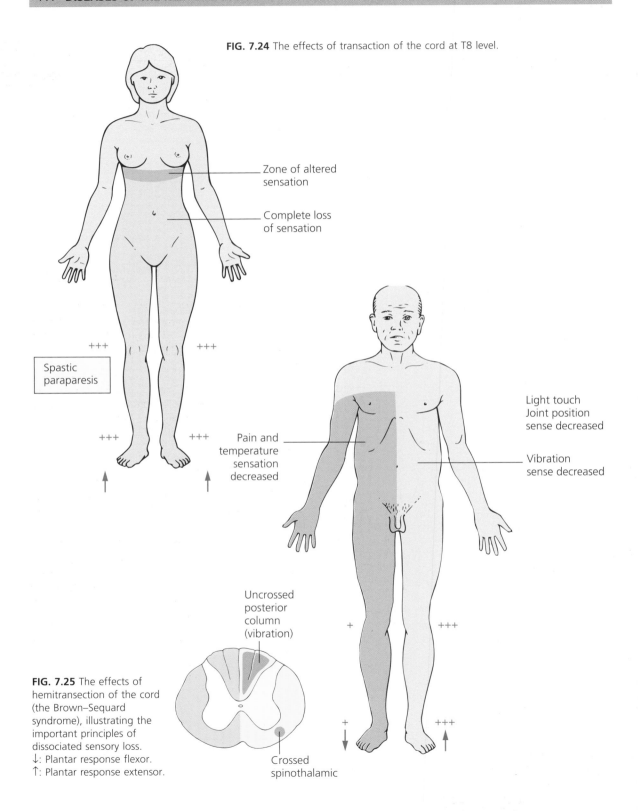

FIG. 7.24 The effects of transaction of the cord at T8 level.

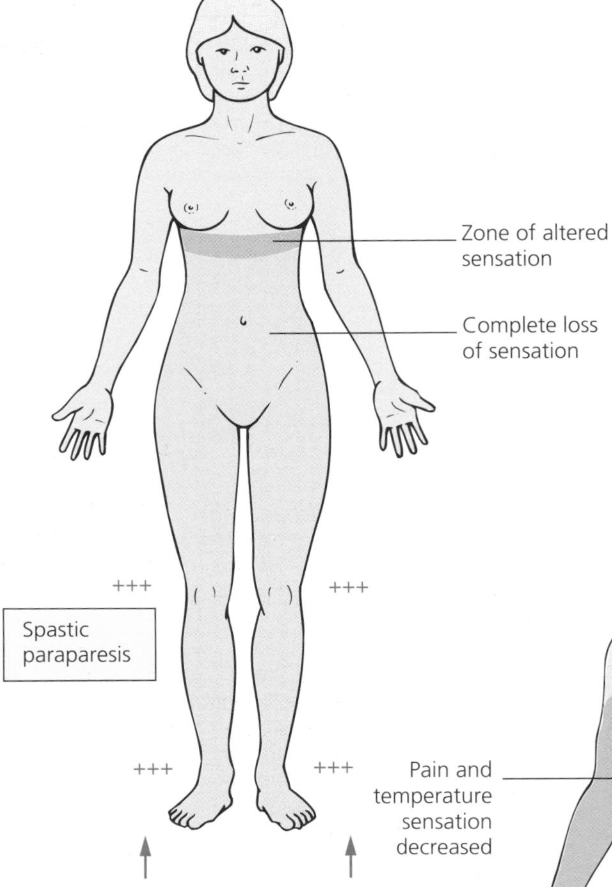

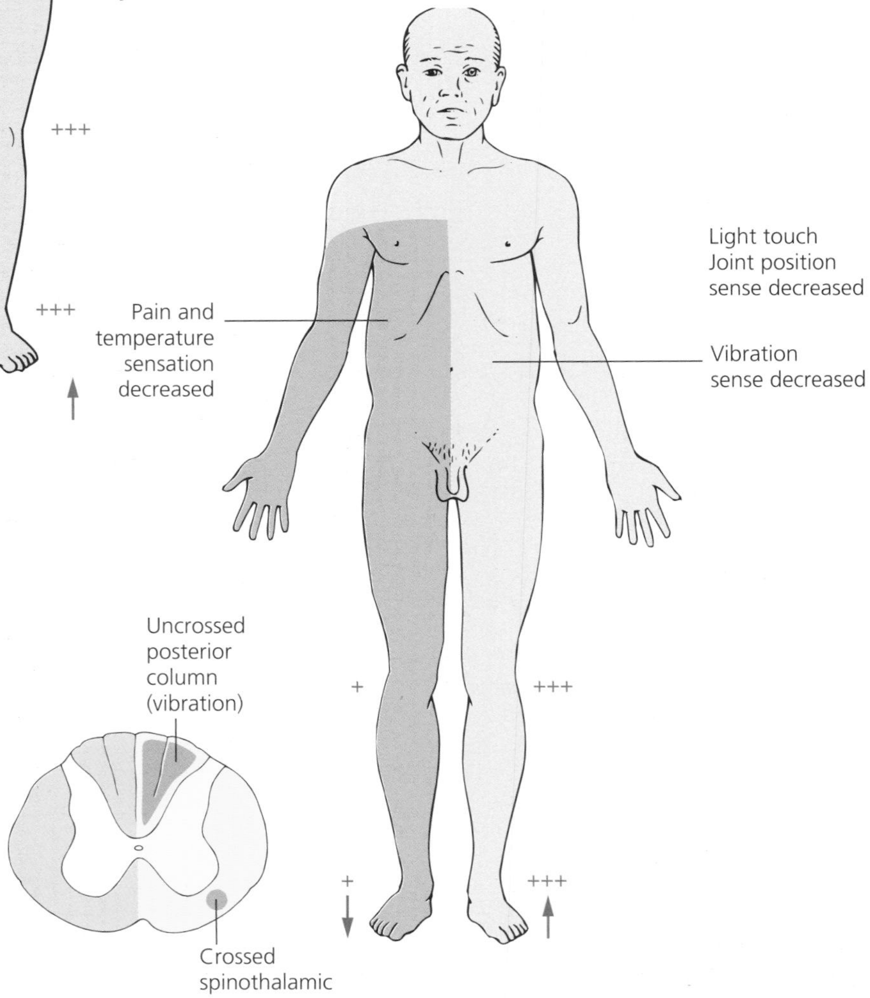

FIG. 7.25 The effects of hemitransection of the cord (the Brown–Sequard syndrome), illustrating the important principles of dissociated sensory loss.
↓: Plantar response flexor.
↑: Plantar response extensor.

Psychiatric disorders and how to spot them

8

In order to spot psychiatric disorders and arrive at the correct differential diagnosis, you will need to apply a systematic approach to taking a psychiatric history and carrying out a mental state examination.

INTERVIEWING THE PATIENT

Interviewing patients with general medical and surgical problems is covered in Section A (Chapters 1–3), but you will need to learn some additional points when carrying out a psychiatric interview.

First, you should try to make the patient feel at ease and encourage him or her to talk openly about their problems. It is better, particularly when starting the interview, to use open questions, such as: *'How are you in your spirits?'* rather than closed questions (such as *'Do you feel depressed?'*) that do not give the patient a chance to elaborate. Do encourage the patient to talk without interruption for the first five minutes about his or her presenting problems.

When first taking a psychiatric history or carrying out a mental state examination, you may feel uncomfortable about enquiring about the psychosexual history or asking about suicidal thoughts. In practice you will soon find that patients will not be surprised by this. In particular, don't worry that you will introduce the idea of committing suicide to them simply by asking a patient about suicidal thoughts – there is no evidence that this happens.

If your patient is deaf, but understands sign language, get the assistance of a professional signer. Similarly, if your patient does not speak English, you will need a professional translator.

Patients with psychiatric disorders do not always readily admit to their problems. Indeed, sometimes they may be mute, so it is useful to obtain information from other sources including:

- Relatives.
- The patient's GP.
- Other professionals involved in the case, such as social workers, community psychiatric nurses, psychologists and hostel nursing staff.
- Past psychiatric and medical case-notes.

Finally, do bear in mind issues of safety, as sometimes a patient may suddenly become violent, for example in response to hearing voices (auditory hallucinations). The following points are of particular importance:

- Always sit nearer the door than your patient.
- Always ensure that someone else knows where you are and whom you are interviewing.
- Always make sure you know where safety features such as alarms and panic buttons are located and how they operate.
- Remember that you cannot always calm down a violent patient by talking.

PSYCHIATRIC HISTORY

The following details should be obtained in the psychiatric history:

Reason for referral How and why the patient was referred.

Complaints In the patient's own words and including how long each complaint has lasted.

History of presenting illness For each symptom, give the chronology of its development, any precipitating factors and the effects on other aspects of the patient's life such as their social functioning.

Family history Details of parents and siblings.

Family psychiatric history Details of any family history of psychiatric disorders (including suicide) or neurological disorders.

Personal history Include details of childhood (date and place of birth), problems before or at birth or during pregnancy especially leading to premature delivery, early developmental milestones, childhood health, any history of 'nervous problems' and early emotional stresses such as bereavments:

- include details of schooling, relationship with peers and teachers, history of any difficulties at school such as truancy, qualifications and higher education,
- occupational history, including promotions or demotions,
- psychosexual history and, in the case of women, age of menarche, menstrual abnormalities, history of pregnancies and age of menopause, if relevant; sexual orientation, history of sexual/physical abuse, sexual and marital history,
- details of any children,
- current social situation and whom the patient lives with, marital status, occupation and financial status, nature and suitability of accommodation, hobbies and social interests.

Past medical history.

Past psychiatric history Nature and duration of the illnesses, hospitals and outpatient departments attended, treatment received and any current psychotropic medication and side-effects.

Psychoactive substance use

Alcohol:

- how much alcohol is currently drunk,
- any history of withdrawal symptoms,
- the score on the CAGE Questionnaire (see Revision Panel 8.1), which can be carried out routinely,
- any history of physical illnesses, injuries (e.g. road traffic accidents), legal problems (e.g. driving offences) or employment difficulties (e.g. being late regularly for work resulting in being sacked), that might result from excess alcohol.

Others:

- the type and number of nicotine-containing product(s) smoked and any previous history of smoking,
- any use of illicit drugs presently and in the past, including the types of drugs, the quantities taken, the methods of administration and the consequences.

Forensic history Any history of delinquency and criminal offences, including a history of any punishments received.

Premorbid personality – the patient's personality before the onset of psychiatric illness:

- attitudes to others in social, family and sexual relationships,
- attitude to self and character,
- moral and religious beliefs and standards,
- predominant mood,
- leisure activities and interests,
- fantasy life,
- reaction pattern to stress.

Revision Panel 8.1

The CAGE Questionnaire

Positive answers to two or more of the following four CAGE questions are indicative of problem drinking:

C Have you ever felt you should **C**ut down on your drinking?
A Have people **A**nnoyed you by criticizing your drinking?
G Have you ever felt **G**uilty about your drinking?
E Have you ever had a drink first thing in the morning (an **E**ye-opener) to steady your nerves or get rid of a hangover?

MENTAL STATE EXAMINATION

This covers the psychiatric symptomatology ('signs' of illness) exhibited at the time of the interview. In addition, information obtained by others, such as the observations of nursing staff in the case of inpatients, should also be used as the patient may not always admit to psychopathology. For example, a patient who is observed by the nursing staff to be responding to auditory hallucinations may deny during a formal interview experiencing perceptual abnormalities. The following details should be obtained in the mental state examination:

Appearance and behaviour

- General appearance.
- Posture and movements.
- Level of eye contact.
- Level of activity.
- Social behaviour.
- Degree of rapport.

(After Puri BK, Laking PJ, Treasaden IH (1996): *Textbook of Psychiatry*. Edinburgh: Churchill Livingstone.)

Revision Panel 8.2

Disorders of the form of speech

Circumstantiality
Thinking appears slow with the incorporation of unnecessary trivial details. The goal of thought is finally reached, however.

Echolalia
This is the automatic imitation by the patient of another person's speech. It occurs even when the patient does not understand the speech.

Flight of ideas
The speech consists of a stream of accelerated thoughts with abrupt changes from topic to topic and no central direction. The connections between the thoughts may be based on:

- chance relationships,
- chance associations,
- distracting stimuli,
- verbal associations – e.g. alliteration and assonance.

Neologism
This is a new word constructed by the patient or an everyday word used in a special way by the patient.

Passing by the point
The answers to questions, although clearly incorrect, demonstrate that the questions are understood. For example, when asked '*What colour is grass?*', the patient may reply 'Blue'.

Perseveration
In perseveration (of both speech and movement) mental operations are continued beyond the point at which they are relevant. Particular types of perseveration of speech are:

- palilalia – the patient repeats a word with increasing frequency,
- logoclonia – the patient repeats the last syllable of the last word.

Thought blocking
There is a sudden interruption in the train of thought, before it is completed, leaving a 'blank'. After a period of silence, the patient cannot recall what he or she had been saying or had been thinking of saying.

Disorders (loosening) of association (formal thought disorder)
These occur particularly in schizophrenia.

Speech

- Rate.
- Quantity.
- Articulation.
- Form – the way in which the patient speaks. Examples of disorders of the form of speech are given in Revision Panel 8.2.
- Record any neologisms (see Revision Panel 8.2).
- If the speech is abnormal, make a written record of an informative sample.

Mood

- Objective assessment (based on the history, appearance, behaviour and posture).
- Subjective assessment. Ask the patient a question such as 'How do you feel in yourself?', or 'How do you feel in your spirits?'
- Anxiety.
- Affect (see Revision Panel 8.3).

Revision Panel 8.3
Disorders of affect

Affect is a pattern of observable behaviours which is the expression of a subjectively experienced feeling state (emotion) and is variable over time in response to changing emotional states.

Blunted affect
The externalized feeling tone is severely reduced.

Flat affect
There is a total or almost total absence of signs of expression of affect.

Inappropriate affect
An affect that is inappropriate to the thought or speech it accompanies.

Labile affect
A labile externalized feeling tone which is not related to environmental stimuli.

Thought content

- Preoccupations (including morbid thoughts and worries).

Revision Panel 8.4
Obsessions

Obsessional themes include:

Fear of causing harm.

Dirt and contamination.

Aggression.

Sexual.

Religious.

Revision Panel 8.5
Phobias

Acrophobia – fear of heights.

Agoraphobia – literally a fear of the market place. It is a syndrome with a generalized high anxiety level about, or avoidance of, places or situations from which escape might be difficult, or embarrassing, or in which help may not be available in the event of having a panic attack or panic-like symptoms. Objects of fear may include:

- crowds,
- open and closed spaces,
- shopping,
- social situations,
- travelling by public transport.

Algophobia – fear of pain.

Claustrophobia – fear of closed spaces.

Phobias of internal stimuli – these include obsessive phobias and illness phobias, which overlap with hypochondriasis.

Social phobia – fear of personal interactions in a public setting, such as:

- public speaking,
- eating in public,
- meeting people.

Specific (simple) phobia – fear of discrete objects (e.g. snakes) or situations.

Xenophobia – fear of strangers.

Zoophobia – fear of animals.

- Obsessions (repetitive senseless thoughts that the patient recognizes as being irrational and that are unsuccessfully resisted (see Revision Panel 8.4). The patient may be asked 'Do you keep having certain thoughts that don't make sense in spite of trying to avoid them?'
- Phobias such as those shown in Revision Panel 8.5. A phobia is a persistent irrational fear of an activity, object or situation leading to avoidance. The fear is out of proportion to the real danger and cannot be reasoned away, being out of voluntary control.
- Suicidal thoughts. Begin probing with a question such as 'Have you ever felt life wasn't worth living?'
- Homicidal thoughts. The patient may be asked 'Have you ever felt the wish to harm others?'

Abnormal beliefs and interpretations of events

- Record their content, onset and degree of intensity.

Revision Panel 8.6
Delusions

Type of delusion	*Delusional belief*
Persecutory (querulant delusion)	One is being persecuted.
Of poverty	One is in poverty.
Of reference	The behaviour of others, and objects and events such as television and radio broadcasts and newspaper reports, refer to oneself in particular; when similar thoughts are held with less than delusional intensity they are called *ideas of reference.*
Of self-accusation	One's guilt.
Erotomania	Another person is deeply in love with one (usually occurs in women with the object often being a man of much higher social status).
Of infidelity (pathological jealousy, delusional jealousy	One's spouse or lover is being unfaithful .
Of grandeur	Exaggerated belief of one's own power and importance.
Of doubles	A person known to the patient has been replaced by a double.
Fregoli syndrome	A familiar person has taken on different appearances and is recognized in other people.
Nihilistic	Others, oneself, or the world do not exist or are about to cease to exist.
Somatic	Delusional belief pertaining to the functioning of one's body.
Bizarre	Belief is totally implausible and bizarre.
Systematized	A group of delusions united by a single theme or a delusion with multiple elaborations.

(After Puri BK, Laking PJ, Treasaden IH (1996): *Textbook of Psychiatry.* Edinburgh: Churchill Livingstone.)

- Delusions such as those shown in Revision Panel 8.6. A delusion is a false personal belief based on incorrect inference about external reality and firmly sustained in spite of what almost everyone else believes and in spite of what constitutes incontrovertible and obvious proof or evidence to the contrary. The belief is not one ordinarily accepted by other members of the person's culture or subculture (i.e. it is not an article of religious faith).
- Overvalued ideas. An overvalued idea is an unreasonable and sustained intense preoccupation maintained with less than delusional intensity. The idea or belief held is demonstrably false and is not one that is normally held by others of the patient's subculture, and there is a marked associated emotional investment.
- Delusional perception. A new and delusional significance is attached to a familiar real perception without any logical reason.

Abnormal experiences

- Sensory distortions. Changes in intensity, quality (e.g. visual distortions), or spatial form.
- Illusions. An illusion is a false perception of a real external stimulus.
- Hallucinations. As shown in Revision Panel 8.7. An hallucination is a false sensory perception in the absence of a real external stimulus. It is perceived as being located in objective space and as having the same realistic qualities as normal perceptions and is not subject to conscious manipulation.
- Pseudohallucinations are a form of imagery arising in the subjective inner space of the mind that lack the substantiality of normal perceptions and are not subject to conscious manipulation.
- Disorders of self-awareness (ego disorders) including depersonalization, in which the patient feels that he or she is altered or not real in some way, and derealization, in which the surroundings do not seem real. Both depersonalization and derealization may occur in normal people, during tiredness for example.

Revision Panel 8.7
Hallucinations

Different sensory modalities

Auditory hallucinations – may occur in depression (particularly second person hallucinations of a derogative nature) and in schizophrenia (particularly third person hallucinations and running commentaries).

Tactile hallucinations – usually involve sensations on or just under the skin, e.g. the sensation of insects crawling under the skin (*formication*).

Visceral hallucinations – of deep sensations.

Visual hallucinations – often indicative of the presence of an acute organic cerebral reaction.

Other special types of hallucination

Hallucinosis – hallucinations (usually auditory) occur in clear consciousness, usually as a result of chronic alcohol abuse.

Reflex – a stimulus in one sensory field leads to an hallucination in another sensory field; e.g. a man with schizophrenia would feel a sharp pain in his legs every time a certain patient called his name and he believed that the patient's voice was the cause of this pain.

Functional – the stimulus causing the hallucination is experienced in addition to the hallucination itself; e.g. a woman with schizophrenia would hear voices commenting about her every time she flushed the lavatory.

Autoscopy (also called the *phantom mirror image*) – the patient sees himself or herself and knows that it is he or she.

Extracampine – the hallucination occurs outside the patient's sensory field; e.g. a young man with schizophrenia believed he could just see Adolf Hitler standing behind him out of the corner of his eye but every time he turned around Hitler disappeared.

Trailing phenomenon – moving objects are seen as a series of discrete discontinuous images, usually as a result of taking hallucinogens.

Hypnopompic – the hallucination (usually visual or auditory) occurs while waking from sleep; it can occur in normal people.

Hypnagogic – the hallucination (usually visual or auditory) occurs while falling asleep; it can occur in normal people.

(After Puri BK, Laking PJ, Treasaden IH (1996): *Textbook of Psychiatry*. Edinburgh: Churchill Livingstone.)

Cognitive state

- If disorientation is suspected, orientation in time, place and person should be assessed by asking the patient to give the time, date, the place where he or she currently is, and questions about his or her name and identity.
- Attention and concentration can be checked by asking the patient to carry out the serial sevens test, in which the patient is asked to subtract seven from 100 and repeatedly subtract seven from the remainder as fast as possible, giving the answer at each stage – the time taken to reach a remainder less than seven is noted. If this is too difficult, use the number three instead of seven (serial threes) or ask the patient to recite the names of the days of the week or months of the year backwards.
- As concentration is sustained attention, the serial sevens can be administered first and if performed adequately there is no need to check attention separately. Disorders of attention include distractibility in which the patient's attention is drawn too frequently to unimportant or irrelevant external stimuli.
- Memory (see also Chapter 7)
  - immediate recall can be assessed by asking the patient to repeat immediately a sequence of digits (the normal range is five to nine digits, with a mean of seven),
  - registration can be assessed by giving the patient a name and address and asking him or her to repeat them; record any mistakes,
  - short-term memory can be assessed by asking the patient to repeat the name and address (given in the test of registration) five minutes later; record any mistakes,
  - memory for recent events can be assessed by asking the patient to recall important news items from the previous two days,
  - long-term memory can be assessed more formally by asking the patient to recall his or her date and place of birth,
  - abnormalities of memory are shown in Revision Panel 8.8.
- General knowledge can be assessed by asking the patient to name prominent national figures, the colours of the national flag or five capital cities in a given continent.
- Whether the patient's intelligence lies within the normal range, clinically, can be judged from the answers to the general knowledge questions, from the responses to questions regarding the history and mental state examination thus far, and from the level of education achieved (from the history). Dementia is a global organic impairment of intellectual functioning without impairment of consciousness, while pseudodementia resembles dementia clinically, but is not organic in origin.
- Further tests of the cognitive state which need to be carried out in those suspected of having an organic cerebral disorder, such as dementia, are given in Chapters 7 and 13 of this book.

Revision Panel 8.8
Abnormalities of memory

Amnesia is the inability to recall past experiences.
Hyperamnesia is an exaggerated degree of retention and recall.
Paramnesia is a distorted recall leading to falsification of memory, for example:

- *confabulation* – gaps in memory are unconsciously filled with false memories, as in the amnesic (or Korsakov's) syndrome.
- *déjà vu* – the subject feels that the current situation has been seen or experienced before.
- *déjà entendu* – the illusion of auditory recognition.
- *déjà pensé* – the illusion of recognition of a new thought.
- *jamais vu* – the illusion of failure to recognize a familiar situation.
- *retrospective falsification* – false details are added to the recollection of an otherwise real memory.

(After Puri BK, Laking PJ, Treasaden IH (1996): *Textbook of Psychiatry*. Edinburgh: Churchill Livingstone.)

Insight

- If the patient has a psychiatric disorder, their degree of insight into this can be assessed by determining whether the patient recognizes that they are ill, whether they accept that they have a psychiatric illness, and whether they accept that psychiatric treatment is necessary.

SOME COMMON PSYCHIATRIC SYNDROMES

SCHIZOPHRENIA

Characteristic clinical features of schizophrenia include one or more of the following:

- Changes in thinking.
- Changes in perception.
- Blunted or inappropriate affect.
- A reduced level of social functioning.

Cognitive functions are usually intact in the early stages of the disorder.

Schneiderian first-rank symptoms

In the absence of organic cerebral pathology, the presence of any of Schneider's first-rank symptoms is indicative, but not pathognomonic, of schizophrenia.

Auditory hallucinations

These may be of the following types:

- The voices heard may repeat the patient's thoughts out loud as they are being thought, just after they have been thought, or in anticipation just before they have been thought.
- The voices may discuss the patient and talk about him or her in the third person.
- The voices may give a running commentary about the patient.

Thought alienation

The patient believes their thoughts are under the control of an external agency or that others are participating in their thinking. The following types of thought alienation are included as first-rank symptoms:

- The patient may believe that external (alien) thoughts are being inserted into his or her mind by an external agency (thought insertion).
- The patient may believe that his or her own thoughts are being withdrawn from the mind by an external agency (thought withdrawal).
- The patient may believe that his or her thoughts are being 'read' by others, as if they were being broadcast (thought broadcasting).

Made feelings, impulses or actions

The patient may experience the feeling that his or her free will has been removed and that an external agency is controlling his or her:

- Feelings (made feelings).
- Impulses (made impulses).
- Actions (made actions or made acts).

Somatic passivity

This is the feeling that one is the passive recipient of somatic or bodily sensations from an external agency.

Delusional perception

This involves a real perception which is followed by a delusional misinterpretation of that perception.

Other symptoms

Symptoms which are sometimes described as having special importance in diagnosing schizophrenia but which are not pathognomonic include:

Other persistent delusions such as religious or political identity, or superhuman powers and abilities.

Persistent hallucinations in any modality, when accompanied either by fleeting or half-formed delusions without clear affective content, or by persistent overvalued ideas, or when occurring every day for weeks on end. An *overvalued idea* is an unreasonable and sustained intense preoccupation maintained with less than delusional intensity; the idea or belief is demonstrably false and is not one normally held by others of the patient's subculture. There is a marked emotional investment associated with overvalued ideas.

Breaks or interpolations in the train of thought, which can result in **incoherence** or **irrelevant speech**. They can also cause **neologisms**, which refer to new words constructed by the patient or to everyday words used in a special way by the patient.

Catatonic behaviour. The symptoms include **stupor**, in which the patient is unresponsive, akinetic, mute and fully conscious, and **excitement**; the patient may change between these two states. Other symptoms seen as part of catatonic behaviour include: **posturing**, in which the patient adopts an inappropriate or bizarre bodily posture continuously for a substantial period of time; **waxy flexibility** (also known as **cerea flexibilitas**), in which the patient's limbs can be 'moulded' into a position and remain fixed for long periods of time; and **negativism**, in which motiveless resistance occurs to instructions and to attempts to be moved.

Negative symptoms which typically occur in chronic schizophrenia. They include marked apathy, poverty of speech, lack of drive, slowness and blunting or incongruity of affect. They usually result in social withdrawal and lowered social performance. In identifying the presence of negative symptoms other possible causes of such symptomatology, such as depression and neuroleptic medication, should first be excluded.

A significant and consistent change in the overall quality of some aspects of **personal behaviour**, manifest as loss of interest, aimlessness, idleness, a self-absorbed attitude and social withdrawal.

DEPRESSIVE EPISODE

There is depression of mood, loss of interest and enjoyment (anhedonia), reduced energy (leading to tiredness and reduced activity), reduced attention and concentration, ideas of guilt and worthlessness, and lowered self-esteem. In turn, these can cause hopelessness and a belief that life is not worth living, so that suicidal thoughts may result.

Biological symptoms

The following somatic or physiological changes frequently occur:

- Reduced appetite leading to weight loss.
- Constipation.
- Insomnia including waking in the morning at least two hours before the usual time (early morning wakening).
- Diurnal variation of mood. Patients often wake feeling very low, with the mood gradually lifting during the day until it reaches its best in the evening. This diurnal cycle may repeat itself daily.
- A markedly reduced libido.
- Amenorrhoea.

Mental state examination

Signs on mental state examination may include the following:

Appearance

Depressive facies typically include downturned eyes, sagging of the corners of the mouth and the presence of a vertical furrow between the eyebrows. There is usually poor eye contact with the interviewer. There may be direct evidence of weight loss, with the patient appearing emaciated and, perhaps, dehydrated. Indirect evidence of recent weight loss may be indicated by the clothing appearing to be too large. Evidence of poor self-care and general neglect may include an unkempt appearance, poor personal hygiene and dirty clothing.

Behaviour

Psychomotor retardation typically occurs.

Speech

This is slow with long delays before answering questions.

Mood

This is characteristically low and sad with feelings of hopelessness. Anxiety, irritability and agitation may also occur. The patient may complain of reduced energy and drive, and an inability to feel enjoyment (anhedonia). There is a loss of interest in normal activities and hobbies.

Thoughts

Pessimistic thoughts concerning the patient's past, present and future occur, as may delusions of poverty or illness. Suicidal thoughts may occur and should be checked for. Homicidal thoughts may also be present.

Perceptions

In severe cases mood-congruent auditory hallucinations may occur which are typically in the second person and derogatory in content.

Cognition

Poor concentration may cause the patient to believe mistakenly that memory impairment has also occurred. In elderly patients the presentation may be very similar to that of dementia (see Chapter 13).

DEGREE OF SUICIDAL INTENT FOLLOWING PARASUICIDE

Following an act of parasuicide (deliberate self-harm), i.e. a self-initiated act deliberately undertaken that mimics the act of suicide but that does not result in death, it is important to ascertain the degree of suicidal intent that existed at the time of the act. A number of questions should be asked in order to carry out this assessment properly:

- What is the explanation for the attempt in terms of the probable reason(s) and goal(s)?
- Does the patient intend to die now?
- What problems confront the patient?
- Is there a psychiatric disorder and, if so, how relevant is it to the attempt?
- What are the patient's coping resources and supports?
- What kind of help might be appropriate, and is the patient willing to accept such help?

Practical Point

A high degree of suicidal intent is indicated by the following:

The act was planned beforehand.
Precautions were taken to avoid discovery.
No attempt was made by the patient to seek help afterwards.
A dangerous method was used, such as:
- shooting,
- drowning,
- hanging,
- electrocution.

There was a final act, such as:
- making a will,
- leaving a suicide note.

There was extensive premeditation.
The patient admits suicidal intent.

MANIA

The mood is elevated, which may result in either euphoria or irritability and anger. Other clinical features include increased energy, overactivity, pressure of speech, reduced sleep, loss of normal social and sexual inhibitions, and poor attention and concentration. During a manic episode a patient may overspend, start unrealistic projects, be sexually promiscuous, and, if irritable or angry, be inappropriately aggressive. In severe mania, there may be severe and sustained physical activity and excitement that may result in aggression or violence. Neglect of eating, drinking and personal hygiene may result in dangerous states of dehydration and self-neglect.

Mental state examination

Signs on mental state examination may include the following:

Appearance

The patient may be flamboyantly dressed in unusually bright colours. In severe cases there may be signs of self-neglect such as appearing unkempt and dehydrated.

Behaviour

Overactivity is characteristic – it may be difficult to persuade the patient to sit still and be interviewed.

Speech

Pressure of speech is characteristic – the speech is increased in rate and amount and may be difficult to interrupt.

Mood

The patient may be euphoric or else irritable and angry.

Thoughts

The patient may have an inflated view of their importance and may hold expansive and grandiose ideas about the significance of their opinions and work. Flight of ideas is common in severe cases, with the stream of accelerated thoughts showing abrupt changes from topic to topic and no central direction. In severe mania grandiose ideas may develop into delusions, and irritability and suspiciousness into delusions of persecution.

Perceptions

The appreciation of colours may become especially vivid, there may be a preoccupation with fine details of surfaces or textures, and subjective increased sensitivity to sounds (hyperacusis) may occur. In severe cases hallucinations may occur; these may be auditory, for example confirming the patient's grandiose delusions ('You are the most important person in the world'), or visual (in which the patient may, for example, see himself or herself seated on a throne or in a scene laden with religious motifs).

Cognitions

Attention and concentration are poor.

Insight

Insight is absent in a manic episode. Following the acute episode, recovery of insight, and in particular the realization of their behaviour whilst high, may tip the patient into depression.

NEUROTIC, STRESS-RELATED AND SOMATOFORM DISORDERS

Agoraphobia

This consists of a cluster of anxiety-causing phobias (see Revision Panel 8.5), including a fear of:

- Leaving home.
- Crowds.
- Public places.
- Travelling alone using public transport.

As a result, the patient may be housebound.

Social phobia

The phobias are centred around a fear of scrutiny by others in relatively small groups. As a result, the patient may avoid social situations such as eating in public, public speaking and encounters with the opposite sex.

Specific (isolated) phobia

The phobias are restricted to highly specific situations, such as:

- Proximity to animals.
- Heights.

- Thunder.
- Darkness.
- Flying.
- Closed spaces.
- Eating certain foods.
- Dentistry.

In addition there may be a fear of exposure to specific diseases, such as:

- AIDS.
- Radiation sickness.

Panic disorder

There are recurrent attacks of severe anxiety (panic) which are not restricted to any particular situation and which are therefore unpredictable. Symptoms include:

- A sudden onset of palpitations.
- Chest pain.
- Choking.
- Dizziness.
- Sweating.
- Trembling.
- Depersonalization.
- Derealization.

There may be a secondary fear of dying or going mad. Typically an attack will last just a few minutes.

Generalized anxiety disorder

Generalized and persistent anxiety occurs that is not restricted to, or even strongly predominating in, any particular environmental situation – i.e. it is free floating. Typical symptoms include:

- A continuous feeling of nervousness.
- Trembling.
- Muscular tension.
- Sweating.
- Lightheadedness.
- Palpitations.
- Dizziness.
- Dry mouth.
- Epigastric discomfort.
- Increased frequency and urgency of micturition.
- Sleep disturbance.

Obsessive–compulsive disorder

There are recurrent obsessional thoughts and/or compulsive acts which are recognized by the patient as being their own and which are unsuccessfully resisted (although in long-standing cases the resistance may be minimal). The obsessional thoughts are usually distressing (see Revision Panel 8.4); for example they may involve thoughts that are:

- Violent.
- Obscene.
- Blasphemous.
- Senseless.

The patient may also be depressed.

Post-traumatic stress disorder

This arises as a delayed and/or protracted response to a stressful event or situation of an exceptionally threatening or catastrophic nature such as rape or torture. Episodes of repeated reliving of the trauma occur in flashbacks, or dreams may occur against a persisting background of a sense of numbness, emotional blunting, anhedonia, detachment from others, and avoidance of anything that reminds the patient of the trauma.

EATING DISORDERS

Anorexia nervosa

The characteristic feature is deliberate weight loss, induced and/or sustained by the patient. The weight loss is self-induced using various strategies, such as:

- Avoiding 'fattening' foods.
- Self-induced vomiting.
- Purging.
- Excessive exercise.
- Abuse of diuretics.
- Abuse of appetite suppressants.

Symptoms and signs include:

- Thin and emaciated appearance (with the body mass being maintained at least 15%

below that expected, or a body mass index ≤ 17.5 kg/m^{-2}).

- Body-image distortion with a dread of fatness.
- Amenorrhoea in women (although if taking the oral contraceptive pill breakthrough vaginal bleeding still occurs).
- Low libido and erectile dysfunction in men.
- Signs of dehydration.
- Salivary gland swelling.
- Dental caries.
- Lack of breast development in females with prepubertal onset.
- Lack of genital development in males with prepubertal onset.
- Lanugo hair (often on the face and back).
- Axillary hair and pubic hair are present (cf. they are absent or scanty in hypopituitarism).
- Poor peripheral circulation.

Psychiatric symptomatology that is commonly associated with anorexia nervosa includes:

- Obsessive–compulsive behaviour, such as compulsive handwashing and weight checking.
- Anxiety – particularly related to food and eating.
- Mood disorder – depressive episodes and labile mood.

Bulimia nervosa

The characteristic features are repeated bouts of overeating and an excessive preoccupation with the control of body weight, with a morbid fear of fatness, leading to the adoption of extreme measures aimed at mitigating the 'fattening' effects of food eaten, for example by means of self-induced vomiting, purgative abuse and the abuse of appetite suppressants, thyroid preparations or diuretics. Symptoms and signs include:

- Body mass in the normal range (cf. anorexia nervosa).
- Normal menstrual cycle in women (cf. anorexia nervosa).
- Salivary gland swelling.
- Intermittent facial or peripheral oedema.
- Dental caries.
- Symptoms and signs of electrolyte disturbances (e.g. muscular weakness, cardiac arrhythmias, renal impairment, epileptic seizures, urinary tract infections, and tetany).

ALCOHOL ABUSE

This is one of the most common psychiatric problems that the student or newly qualified doctor is likely to meet. The use of the CAGE questionnaire in assessing the seriousness of a patient's drinking has been discussed (page 147). Further features of alcohol dependence are shown in the Practical Point below.

Practical point

Some features of dependence on alcohol

Compulsion to drink (cravings).
Increasing tolerance (more and more needed to achieve the same effect).
Withdrawal symptoms (morning shakes and delirium tremens).

In the domestic setting the physical and psychological dependence on alcohol sets up a whole sequence of social, legal, emotional and family consequences. Superimposed on these are the numerous physical complications which are mentioned elsewhere in this book.

In the hospital setting there are two situations in which alcohol is likely to pose serious difficulties. The first is when the intoxicated, confused and wildly disturbed and unmanageable drunk may present in the Accident and Emergency Department with other serious complications such as head injury. The second is when a previously unknown alcoholic develops withdrawal symptoms such as shakes or sweats whilst suffering some other primary illness such as pneumonia. This progresses after two to four days to delirium tremens with confusion, disorientation and fits.

9 Medical problems in pregnancy

This chapter highlights the ways in which normal pregnancy produces symptoms and signs, which under other circumstances would be considered abnormal.

SYMPTOMS

Most healthy pregnant women will have at least one of the following symptoms:

Breathlessness

Three-quarters of pregnant women notice some shortness of breath. About half of them will be breathless on climbing more than one flight of stairs whilst the remainder are breathless on trivial exertion such as walking on the level.

The cause is uncertain; it is not simply due to the gravid uterus since some women become breathless before 20 weeks gestation and symptoms reach their peak around 30 weeks. Therefore, mild breathlessness, by itself, coming on progressively in a previously healthy woman does not require investigation.

In contrast, breathlessness in pregnancy becomes a matter for concern if:

- It comes on suddenly.
- It is associated with wheezing.
- It is associated with chest pain and/or haemoptysis.
- There is a history of lung or heart disease.
- The past medical history is unknown and there might be undiagnosed congenital or rheumatic heart disease.

Palpitations

The heart rate increases in pregnancy but the patient rarely notices this. Occasional ectopic atrial and ventricular beats are common but are of no significance. Sustained palpitations, which may be accompanied by faintness or syncope, are usually caused by supraventricular tachycardia. This is more common than in the non-pregnant woman and may recur in successive pregnancies.

Remember also that thyrotoxicosis is common in pregnancy.

Ankle swelling

Pitting oedema of the lower limbs, increasing with the duration of the gestation and towards the end of each day, is a normal finding. It occurs in up to 80% of women and is due to a combination of the gravid uterus obstructing venous return and a reduced colloid osmotic pressure (resulting from the falling albumin concentration).

Ankle swelling should raise concern if:

- There is a history of renal or cardiac disease.
- It is unilateral, suggesting venous thrombosis.

Indigestion

Most women suffer from indigestion and heartburn during pregnancy, particularly in the third trimester. Peptic ulceration in pregnancy is rare.

Nausea and vomiting

Morning sickness in a young woman is virtually diagnostic of pregnancy. During pregnancy 85% of women experience nausea and/or vomiting. Whilst for most the symptoms are confined to the first trimester about 20% are troubled throughout the whole of pregnancy. When the vomiting is very severe it is termed *hyperemesis gravidarum*.

Constipation

This is very common in pregnancy and may be sufficient to cause abdominal discomfort. Taking iron tablets may aggravate it.

Urinary frequency

Urgency, frequency and nocturia are common in pregnant women. In some cases these symptoms are caused by a urinary tract infection; the only way to find out is to culture the urine.

*Jaundice occurring in pregnancy

Jaundice must always be taken seriously and referral to a gastroenterologist is essential.

Most cases of jaundice in pregnancy are due to intercurrent disease such as viral hepatitis. This is usually hepatitis A but virological studies are necessary to define the type of hepatitis and to establish the risk to mother and baby.

Two disorders are peculiar to pregnancy:

- Recurrent cholestasis of pregnancy occurs in the last trimester and is characterized by pruritus alone or with jaundice, dark urine and pale stools; once the baby is delivered the symptoms regress and the prognosis is good.
- Acute fatty liver of pregnancy is very rare and affects young primiparas in the third trimester. Patients become rapidly ill with jaundice, vomiting and abdominal pain. The outlook for mother and baby is grave.

Practical Point

Do not forget that pregnant women may develop other coincidental diseases

Tachycardia – thyrotoxicosis.

Urinary frequency – diabetes (but note that renal glycosuria is common in pregnancy).

Abdominal pain – acute appendicitis.

Breathlessness – asthma.

Jaundice – viral hepatitis.

PHYSICAL EXAMINATION (Fig. 9.1)

Changes in the skin and the cardiovascular system in pregnancy may simulate serious organic disease.

The skin

During pregnancy the skin undergoes several changes, most notably hyperpigmentation, but two signs, in the absence of jaundice, may suggest liver disease:

- Spider naevi – These occur in over 50% of pregnant women, appearing between eight and twenty weeks; they are indistinguishable from those of chronic liver disease.
- Palmar erythema – This somewhat nonspecific physical sign develops in about 70% of pregnant women, often over the whole of the palms.

The cardiovascular system

The circulation becomes hyperdynamic in pregnancy and the heart is rotated around its

* This is, of course, not a 'usual' symptom of pregnancy.

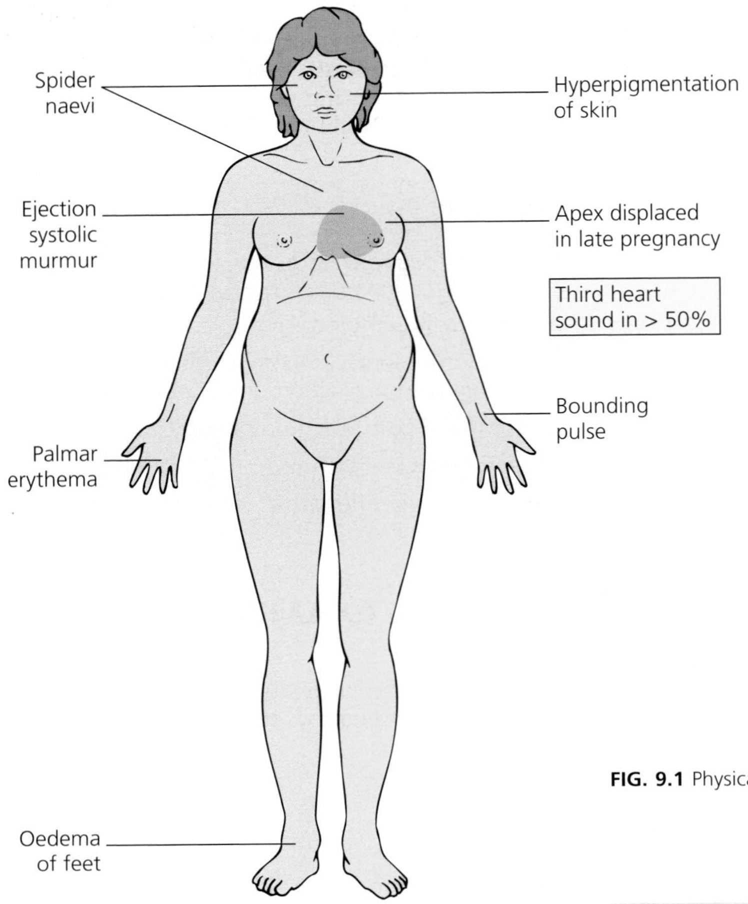

FIG. 9.1 Physical examination in pregnancy.

anteroposterior axis as the uterus enlarges. Several physical signs result from these changes:

- The peripheral pulse is of large volume and the heart rate is increased.
- The apex beat is progressively displaced and by the end of the third trimester may be up to 2 cm lateral to the mid-clavicular line in the 4th interspace.
- A third heart sound, resulting from rapid ventricular filling, may be audible in more than 50% of pregnant women.
- A systolic murmur, arising from either the pulmonary or tricuspid valve, can be heard in the majority of pregnant women; the murmur is never particularly loud but may be heard widely over the precordium.

Revision Panel 9.1
Symptoms and signs in pregnancy

Healthy pregnant women may suffer symptoms which in other circumstances would be considered abnormal:
Breathlessness.
Palpitations.
Ankle swelling.
Indigestion, nausea and vomiting.
Constipation.
Urinary frequency.

Physical signs in pregnancy include:
Palmar erythema.
Spider naevi.
Pigmentation of the skin.
Tachycardia with a full pulse.
Soft systolic murmurs.
A third heart sound.

- In addition to murmurs of valvular origin, systolic murmurs (probably due to increased flow in the mammary vessels) may be heard on each side of the sternum.

- In contrast, a murmur is likely to be important in pregnancy if it is loud and varies with respiration, and if it is pansystolic or late systolic.

10 Endocrine disorders

Diabetes mellitus and disorders of the thyroid gland are by far the most common endocrine disorders seen in clinical practice.

DIABETES MELLITUS

Diabetes mellitus affects 2–3% of the population of most Western countries. It is two to three times more common in Afrocaribbeans and people from the Indian subcontinent. In a patient with typical symptoms the diagnosis is confirmed if blood glucose is:

- Over 7.0 mmol/litre in a fasting patient.
- Over 11.1 mmol/litre on a random sample.

A glucose tolerance test is only needed if blood glucose is lower than these figures.

Hyperglycaemia in diabetes is due to a relative or absolute insulin deficiency and resistance to insulin action in peripheral tissues or both.

How diabetes presents

Typical presenting symptoms due to hyperglycaemia are:

- Thirst (see Revision Panel 10.1 for other causes).
- Polyuria caused by the osmotic diuresis induced by glycosuria.
- Weight loss (variable according to type of diabetes).
- Pruritis vulvae in women.
- Balanitis in men.

Revision Panel 10.1

Causes of thirst and polyuria

Diabetes mellitus.

Cranial diabetes insipidus – ADH deficiency.

Nephrogenic diabetes insipidus – ADH resistance.

Hypercalcaemia
- hyperparathyroidism,
- malignancy,
- sarcoidosis.

Hypokalaemia.

Drugs including diuretics.

Chronic renal failure.

Excess salt intake.

ADH: Antidiuretic hormone.

Classification (Revision Panel 10.2)

Most cases can be classified as:

- Type 1: Insulin-dependent diabetes with severe insulin deficiency.
- Type 2: Non-insulin-dependent diabetes with moderate insulin deficiency and insulin resistance.

Most newly diagnosed patients will admit to symptoms (see Revision Panel 10.3) but hyperglycaemia can be asymptomatic and may be detected on routine screening such as a *well person* clinic. An acute admission with diabetic ketoacidosis indicates severe insulin deficiency.

Revision Panel 10.2
Classification of diabetes

Type	*Suggestive clinical features*	*Type*	*Suggestive clinical features*
Type 1	Moderate or heavy ketonuria. Short history (few weeks). Severe symptoms. Rapid weight loss. First-degree relative taking insulin. Family history of autoimmune disease.	*Pancreatic*	
		Haemochromatosis	Pigmentation. Hepatomegaly. Hypogonadism.
		Chronic pancreatitis	Abdominal pain. Previous episodes of acute pancreatitis. Alcohol dependency.
Type 2 Obese	More than 120% ideal body weight in two-thirds of patients. Abdominal fat distribution (android). Insulin resistance greater than insulin deficiency.	Carcinoma	Abdominal pain. Disproportionate weight loss.
		Endocrine	
		Cushing's disease	
		Acromegaly	
		Hyperthyroidism	Typical clinical features.
		Phaeochromocytoma	
		Hyperaldosteronism	
Type 2 Non-obese	Less than 120% ideal body weight. Insulin deficiency greater than insulin resistance.	Glucagonoma	
		Drug-induced	
		Steroids	
		Beta-blockers	
		Thiazide diuretics	
Type 2 General features	No ketonuria. Longer history (months or years). Mild/moderate symptoms. Complications at diagnosis in 50%.	*Genetic syndromes*	
		MODY	Maturity onset diabetes of the young: autosomal dominant inheritance.
		DIDMOAD	Diabetes insipidus, diabetes mellitus, optic atrophy and deafness.

Patients are acutely unwell with dehydration, abdominal pain and acidotic (Kussmaul) respirations, metabolic acidosis, and ketones which give the breath a sweet peardrops-like smell, recognizable by most people.

Type 2 diabetes can present with hyperosmolar non-ketotic coma (HONK) in which progressive hyperglycaemia causes severe dehydration but insulin levels are sufficient to prevent ketoacidosis.

The history

Patients typically present with one of three main symptoms:

- Thirst.
- Polyuria.
- Weight loss.

Polyuria is caused by an osmotic diuresis induced by glycosuria, which causes the

Revision Panel 10.3
Presentation of diabetes

Routine screening
Health insurance/employment medical.

Symptoms
See text.

Hyperglycaemic emergencies
Diabetic ketoacidosis.
Hyperosmolar non-ketotic coma.

Complications at diagnosis
Type-2 diabetes only.

- Microvascular
  poor eyesight (retinopathy),
  foot ulcers (sensory neuropathy),
  renal failure (nephropathy).
- Macrovascular
  ischaemic heart disease,
  claudication.
- Cerebrovascular.

patient to feel thirsty. You should consider other causes of thirst and polyuria though these are much rarer (Revision Panel 10.1).

Checklist of other important points in the history

Diabetes can lead to other symptoms which the patient may not volunteer. You should enquire about:

- Pruritis vulvae in women and balanitis in men, the result of glycosuria and candida infection.
- Blurred vision due to glucose-related osmotic changes in the lens.
- Recurrent epigastric pain or continued weight loss due to pancreatic disease.
- 'Pins and needles' or 'burning' pains in the feet and calves or progressively insensitive feet without pain due to sensory nerve involvement.
- Clawing of the toes due to wasting of the intrinsic foot muscles, putting excess pressure on the metatarsal heads, the result of motor nerve involvement.
- Impotence and postural hypotension as autonomic neuropathy develops.
- Foot ulcers which develop as neuropathy masks awareness of abnormal pressure or trauma, for example from ill fitting shoes.
- Calf pain on walking (intermittent claudication); exertional chest pain due to coronary artery disease; and stroke due to cerebrovascular disease.
- Superficial tissues damaged by repeated injection of insulin into the same site (lipohypertrophy).

Some commonly used drugs are diabetogenic so remember to enquire specifically about steroids, beta-blockers and thiazide diuretics.

The physical examination

This varies to a certain extent according to how the patient presents. You should look for:

- Signs which suggest a possible cause for diabetes.
- Complications of diabetes particularly in patients with Type 2 diabetes where the pre-clinical phase lasts several years; half of these will have evidence of complications at diagnosis (Revision Panel 10.4).
- Any additional illnesses which may influence management.

Look first for possible causes such as:

- Striae and proximal weakness of Cushing's disease.
- Spade-like hands and lantern jaw which may suggest acromegaly.
- Prominent eyes, sweating and fast pulse of hyperthyroidism.
- Slate grey skin pigmentation and hepatomegaly which may suggest haemochromatosis.

Look for signs of weight loss and check previous hospital records for corroboration.

Specific signs you should look for are:

Retinopathy

Sight-threatening proliferative retinopathy is usually asymptomatic until a vitreous haemorrhage occurs when sight will be suddenly lost. This is more common in Type 1 diabetes. Dilate the pupil and examine the retina and macula of the eye carefully for:

'Dots and blots' – capillary microaneurysms and small retinal haemorrhages.

Hard exudates – small well-defined white plaques representing retinal lipid deposits.

Revision Panel 10.4
Complications at diagnosis

Complication	*Comment*
Retinopathy	
Visual acuity.	Snellen chart.
Cataracts.	Loss of red reflex. Dilate pupils with 1% tropicamide (retinal examination).
Nephropathy	
Blood pressure.	
Proteinuria.	Albustix.
Neuropathy	
Peripheral sensory.	Pin-prick. Vibration sense.
Motor.	Diabetic amyotrophy.
Autonomic.	Postural hypotension. Impotence.
Mononeuropathy.	IIIrd/VIth nerve palsy, foot drop.
Feet	
Callus.	Over pressure points.
Deformity.	Claw toes. Hallux valgus. Charcot arthropathy. Ulceration.
Vascular disease	
Peripheral.	Check pulses/bruits.
Coronary.	Check pulses/bruits.
Cerebrovascular.	
Skin	
Necrobiosis.	
Injection sites.	Lipohypertrophy.

Practical Point

You should always check a patient's urine for evidence of nephropathy – microalbuminuria and urinary protein each time you see the patient.

Retinal infarcts (Fig. 10.1) – also called 'cotton wool' spots.

New vessels (Fig. 10.2) – a key feature of proliferative retinopathy, arise from the optic disc or peripheral retina.

Venous irregularity and tortuosity

Maculopathy – more common in Type 2 diabetes, oedema or ischaemia develop in the macula region and cause gradual visual loss.

Neuropathy

Diabetic neuropathy has a 'glove and stocking' distribution so check the distal arms and legs for:

- Objective evidence of sensory loss.
- Objective evidence of muscle weakness.
- Neuropathic ulcers (Fig. 10.3) secondary to sensory loss and muscle weakness.

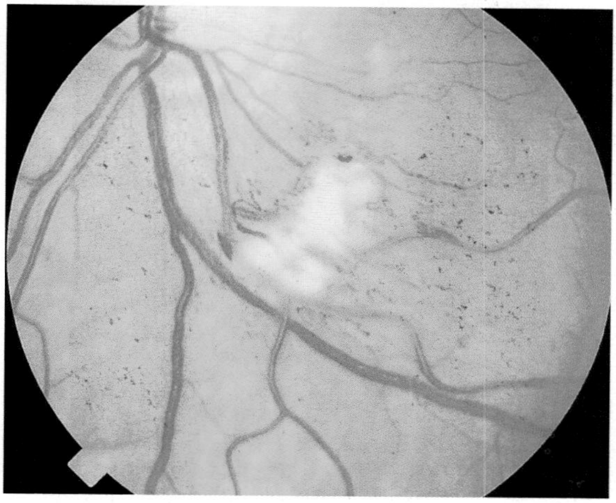

FIG. 10.1 A retinal infarct in diabetes. These appearances are non-specific and may be seen in other systemic diseases such as polyarteritis and subacute bacterial endocarditis. These appearances are sometimes described as 'cotton wool' spots.

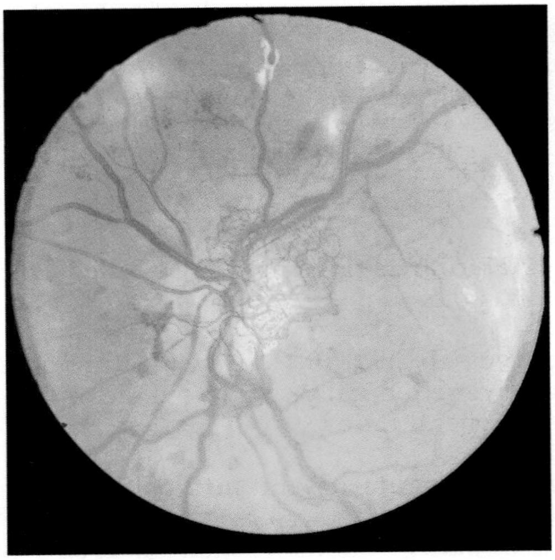

FIG. 10.2 Diabetic retinopathy. In this case the new vessels are seen on the optic disc. Other examples of diabetic retinopathy are seen in Figs 16.11a and b.

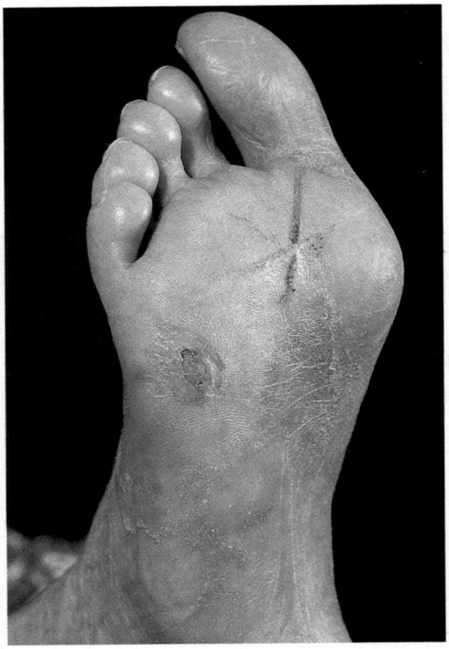

FIG. 10.3 A neuropathic ulcer in a diabetic foot. In diabetes there is a mixed neuropathy. The motor neuropathy leads to wasting of the intrinsic muscles of the foot with clawing of the toes and prominence of the heads of the metatarsals. Walking on the abnormally prominent but painless metatarsals causes ulceration under the heads of these bones.

Nephropathy

Microalbuminuria is the first sign of nephropathy. As urinary protein increases it becomes detectable with Albustix and this is usually associated with progressive hypertension and a rising creatinine. End-stage renal failure develops, on average, within 7-10 years.

Arterial damage

Always examine the major pulses. Vascular disease is common in patients with long-standing disease.

THYROID DISEASE

Disease of the thyroid gland may be present for some time before a patient complains of symptoms. This is particularly true of an underactive thyroid as vague symptoms of 'generally slowing down and putting on weight' may be attributed to simply getting older.

The history

Patients with a disorder affecting the thyroid gland complain of:

- Swelling of the neck, which is usually painless, due to enlargement of the thyroid (goitre) (Fig. 10.4a,b).
- Symptoms attributable to a change of thyroid function (hyper – or hypothyroidism).
- Swelling and symptoms of thyroid dysfunction.

Symptoms of hyperthyroidism or hypothyroidism are contrasted in Revision Panel 10.5.

The patient or a relative may notice a swelling in the neck and fear malignancy. You should ask whether the swelling is painful as this is an unusual feature of thyroid disease other than in de Quervain's thyroiditis or haemorrhage into a thyroid cyst. Swallowing may be affected by a large multinodular

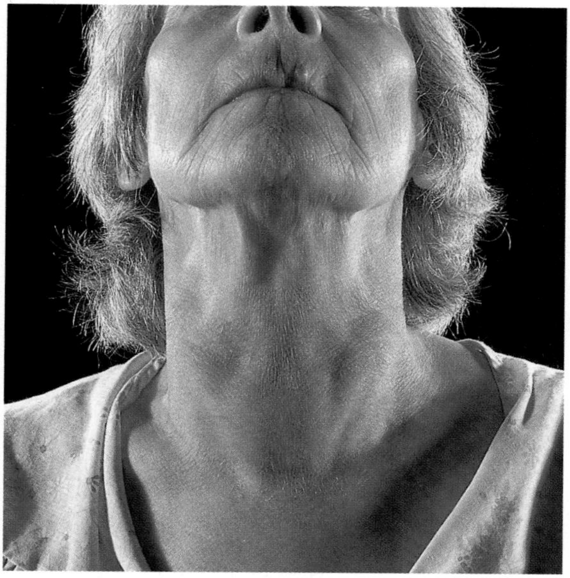

(a)

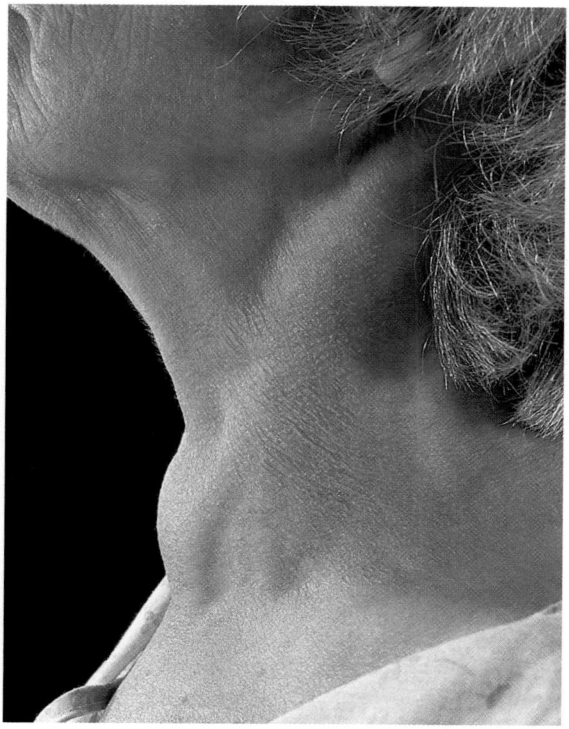

(b)

FIG. 10.4 Anterior (a) and lateral (b) views of a multinodular goitre with considerable enlargement of the isthmus.

Revision Panel 10.5
Symptoms of thyroid disease

Hyperthyroidism	*Hypothyroidism*
Weight loss.	Weight gain.
Heat intolerance.	Cold intolerance.
Diarrhoea.	Constipation.
Palpitations.	
Atrial fibrillation.	Bradycardia.
Oligomenorrhoea.	Menorrhagia.
Increased sweating.	Dry skin.
	Thinning hair.
Proximal myopathy.	Muscle pains.
Tiredness.	Tiredness.

goitre, which may (rarely) cause tracheal compression with stridor.

Examining the thyroid

Start by looking from the front to identify obvious swellings around the neck.

Next, stand behind the seated patient and palpate the central isthmus and the two lobes of the thyroid (Fig. 10.5), followed by a search for local lymph nodes, a common site of secondary spread of thyroid carcinoma.

Ask the patient to swallow a sip of water:

- Thyroid swellings usually move upwards on swallowing.
- A tethered immobile gland suggests malignancy.

Causes of an enlarged thyroid are shown in Revision Panel 10.6.

What to look for in suspected hyperthyroidism

First impressions are important. Visible clues to hyperthyroidism are:

- Appearing anxious and restless.
- A staring expression due to overactivity of the levator palpabrae superioris muscle.

Ask the patient to look up at your finger and follow your finger as you lower it from above

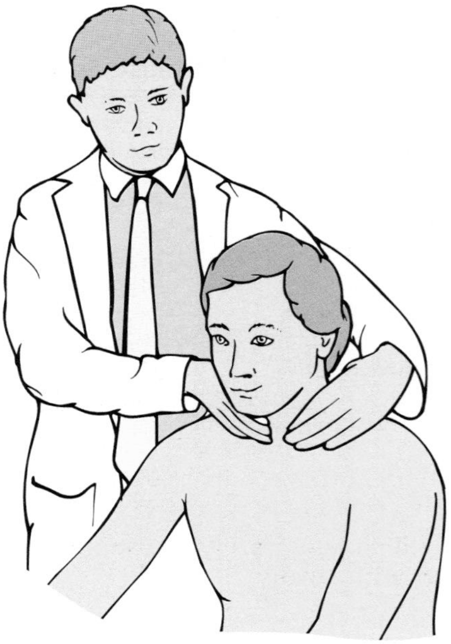

FIG. 10.5 Palpation of the thyroid gland. Stand behind or just to the side of the patient. During the examination ask the patient to take some water in the mouth and swallow it. The non-tethered gland moves upwards on swallowing.

the horizontal to below; a delay in descent of the upper lids is termed 'lid lag' and is frequently seen in hyperthyroidism. Notice that the hands are warm and sweaty and there will be a fine tremor of the outstretched arms. Feel the pulse – a resting tachycardia is common and atrial fibrillation occurs in 5–10% of cases. Systolic blood pressure may be increased with a wide pulse pressure. The thyroid may enlarge retrosternally but this is difficult to detect clinically.

Causes of hyperthyroidism are shown in Revision Panel 10.7.

Graves' disease is associated with other specific clinical signs.

Thyroid-associated ophthalmopathy usually co-exists with hyperthyroidism but may precede or follow disturbance of thyroid function by many years. Look specifically for:

Periorbital oedema affecting the eyelids and lachrymal glands, typically worse in the morning.

Revision Panel 10.6
Causes of goitre

Causes	*Clinical features*
Iodine deficiency	Endemic. Non-toxic.
Autoimmune	
▪ Graves' disease	Diffuse goitre. Systolic bruit. Hyperthyroidism. Ophthalmopathy.
▪ Hashimoto's thyroiditis	Diffuse goitre. Occasionally tender. Hypothyroidism.
Viral	Tender goitre. Transient hyperthyroidism.
Solitary nodules	Toxic adenoma. Simple cyst. Nodule in multinodular gland.
Enzyme deficiency	Rare.
Physiological	Puberty. Pregnancy.
Malignant	Usually carcinoma. Rarely lymphoma.

Revision Panel 10.7
Causes of hyperthyroidism

Common
Graves' disease (Fig. 10.6).
Multinodular goitre.
Toxic adenoma.

Less common
Quervain's thyroiditis.
Drugs – amiodarone.
Thyrotoxicosis fictitia.

Chemosis causing sore, gritty eyes, which may look red and infected.

Ophthalmoplegia which may cause diplopia, most commonly on upward gaze due to involvement of the inferior oblique muscle.

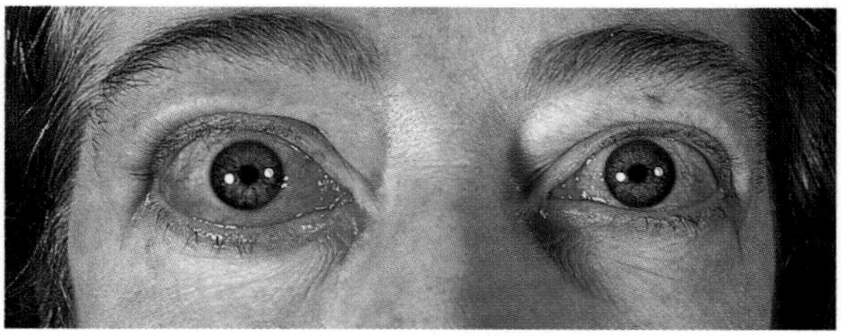

FIG. 10.6 Severe asymmetrical eye changes in Graves' disease. This woman has exophthalmos, oedema of the lower lids, and chemosis.

Exophthalmos produced by infiltration of inflammatory cells and swelling of the retro-orbital muscles. Increased pressure in the orbit pushes the globe forwards and the optic nerve may be compressed causing visual deterioration (Fig. 10.6).

Pre-tibial myxoedema is a raised purplish red thickening of the skin over the lower shins and feet in Graves' disease. The cause is unknown.

Thyroid acropachy resembles finger clubbing but also involves subperiosteal new bone formation seen on X-ray of the hands.

Myopathy particularly affecting the proximal muscles is common and, if severe, may prevent the patient from rising from a chair or climbing stairs.

What to look for in suspected hypothyroidism

(Fig. 10.7, see also Fig. 2.2)

Florid signs of hypothyroidism are rarely seen in developed countries because of the wide availability of thyroid function tests. Signs may be missed because they usually develop very slowly.

Gross hypothyroidism is characterized by:

- Dry scaly skin.
- Thinning hair and eyebrows.
- Puffiness of the face and hands.
- A slow low-pitched voice.

> **Revision Panel 10.8**
> **Common causes of hypothyroidism**
>
> Hashimoto's thyroiditis.
> Post-radioactive iodine.
> Post-thyroidectomy.
> Iodine deficiency (wordwide).

- Bradycardia.
- Slow relaxation of reflexes, best elicited at the ankle with the patient kneeling on a chair.

Common causes of hypothyroidism are shown in Revision Panel 10.8.

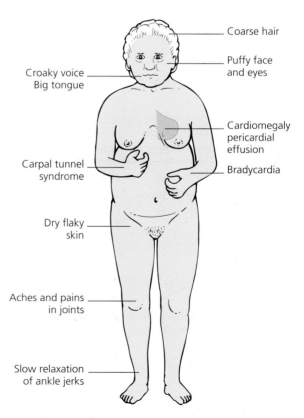

FIG. 10.7 Diagrammatic representation of the clinical features of hypothyroid myxoedema.

PITUITARY DISEASE

As with the thyroid the pituitary gland causes disease because of enlargement, changing function, or both. Pituitary adenomas under 1cm are termed microadenomas and those over 1cm are macroadenomas.

As a macroadenoma or parasellar tumour expands, it presses on surrounding structures such as the optic chiasm (Fig. 10.8). As a result, patients complain mainly of headache and visual disturbance.

Macroadenomas also damage normal pituitary tissue causing progressive hypopituitarism. The gonadotrophins and growth hormone are most susceptible, followed by thyroid stimulating hormone (TSH), then adrenocorticotropic hormone (ACTH) and rarely arginine vasopressin (AVP). The clinical consequences of pituitary failure are summarized in Revision Panel 10.9.

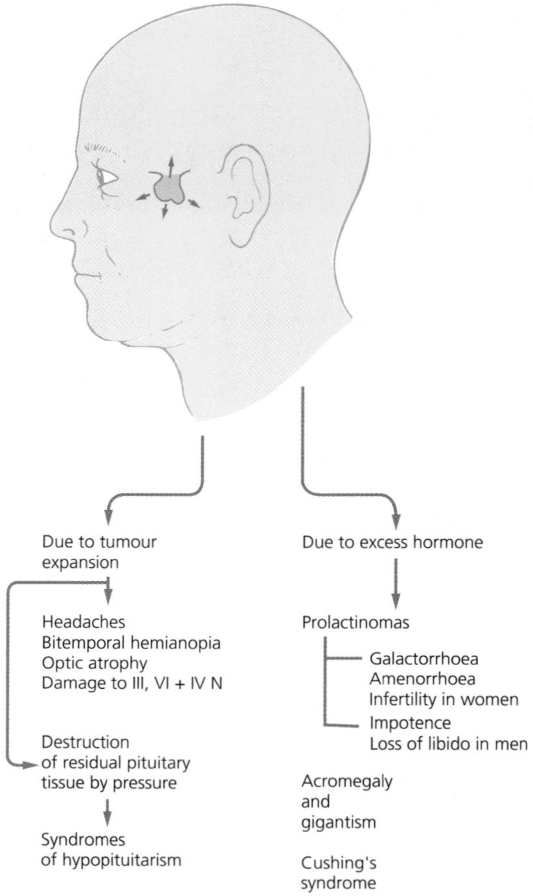

FIG. 10.8 The clinical presentation of pituitary tumours.

Revision Panel 10.9
Clinical consequences of pituitary failure

Deficiency	*Child*	*Adult*
LH	Pubertal delay	Amenorrhoea.
FSH		Infertility. Erectile failure. ↓Secondary sexual characteristics.
GH	Growth delay	↓Muscle strength. ↑Abdominal fat.
TSH	Hypothyroidism Growth delay	Hypothyroidism.
ACTH	Adrenal failure	Adrenal failure.
AVP	Diabetes insipidus	Diabetes insipidus.

LH: Luteinizing hormone. FSH: Follicle-stimulating hormone. GH: Growth hormone. TSH: Thyroid-stimulating hormone. ACTH: Adrenocorticotropic hormone. AVP: Arginine vasopressin.

Panhypopituitarism causes non-specific symptoms of lethargy, tiredness, anorexia and weight loss. Patients are usually pale with thin smooth skin. Secondary sexual characteristics are absent and, in the male the testes are small and soft while the breasts may be underdeveloped in women. There may be clinical signs of hypothyroidism.

Acute illness may precipitate a hypopituitary crisis characterized by coma, hypothermia, hypotension, hypoglycaemia and hyponatraemia.

Functioning tumours

Functioning tumours may produce excess hormone.

The most common is a prolactinoma. Excess prolactin causes galactorrhoea and amenorrhoea with infertility in women and impotence with loss of libido in men. Men usually present with larger tumours (macroprolactinomas) which cause local pressure symptoms.

A growth-hormone-secreting macroadenoma which occurs before puberty will cause accelerated growth and gigantisim. In adults, it causes acromegaly, with characteristic clinical features (Revision Panel 10.10). These occur so insidiously that only 50% of patients or their relatives notice them.

In the other 50% a doctor, nurse or medical student makes the diagnosis as an 'incidental observation'. Since growth-hormone secreting tumours are usually macroadenomas, patients may also have clinical features of hypopituitarism.

Revision Panel 10.10

Characteristic physical findings in acromegaly

Increased size of hands and feet.
Prominent supraorbital ridges.
Thickened lips and tongue.
Prominent nasolabial folds.
Mandibular growth (prognathism).
Overbite of lower teeth over upper teeth.
Enlarged tongue.
Sweaty and greasy skin.

Associated medical problems
Carpal tunnel syndrome.
Hypertension.
Diabetes mellitus.
Goitre.
Osteoarthritis.
Cardiomyopathy.

Cushing's syndrome

Although Cushing's syndrome is rare it produces clinical features including weight gain, hypertension and diabetes which are common. The syndrome results from prolonged exposure to excess glucocorticoid. There are four main ways this may occur:

Revision Panel 10.11

Comparison of clinical features of Cushing's syndrome and nutritional obesity

	Cushing's syndrome	*Obesity*
Fat distribution.	Abdominal. 'Moon face'. 'Buffalo hump'. Thin legs.	Generalized.
Skin.	Thin/fragile. Bruising ++. Purple striae on lower abdomen.	Normal/thickened. No bruising. White 'stretch marks'.
Muscle.	Proximal myopathy.	Normal.
Bone.	Osteoporosis.	Normal.
High blood pressure.	Yes.	Possible.
Diabetes.	Yes.	Possible.
Periods.	Oligomenorrhoea.	Usually normal.
Oedema.	++	±

- Exogenous steroid treatment.
- A benign or malignant adrenal tumour producing excess cortisol.
- Ectopic ACTH production from a non-pituitary tumour. The most common is an oat cell tumour of the lung.
- A pituitary adenoma secreting ACTH. Both adrenal glands are stimulated and are often enlarged.

Differentiating Cushing's syndrome from nutritional obesity is clinically important because of the high mortality of untreated Cushing's syndrome (see Revision Panel 10.11).

Patients with ectopic ACTH due to a malignant tumour do not usually survive long enough to develop classical features of Cushing's syndrome. They have very high ACTH levels and develop generalized pigmentation. High cortisol levels cause hypokalaemia, which makes the already severe myopathic symptoms worse.

Revision Panel 10.12

Summary: Endocrine disorders

In a patient with thirst, polyuria and weight loss, a random glucose of 11.1 mmol/litre or more confirms diabetes.

Most patients can be classified with Type 1 (absolute insulin deficiency) or Type 2 (relative insulin deficiency and insulin-resistance) diabetes.

Other causes of diabetes include pancreatic, endocrine, drug-induced and genetic syndromes.

At diagnosis, 50% of patients with Type 2 diabetes have complications.

Major microvascular complications are retinopathy, neuropathy and nephropathy.

Disease of the thyroid or pituitary gland present as a disturbance of size or function or both.

Hyperthyroidism in Graves' disease may coexist with thyroid-associated ophthalmopathy or may be separated by many years.

Non-functioning pituitary tumours cause hypopituitarism by damaging normal pituitary tissue.

ADRENAL DISEASE

Addison's disease

Autoimmune destruction of the adrenal cortex causes failure of both glucocorticoid and mineralocorticoid secretion. Symptoms include malaise, anorexia and weight loss with episodes of abdominal pain. On examination the patient is often thin and wasted with postural hypotension due to loss of salt and water because of aldosterone deficiency. Generalized skin pigmentation (see Fig. 2.7) is seen in about 50% of cases due to ACTH and related peptides from the anterior pituitary, the secretion of which is increased in response to low cortisol levels. Pigmentation is particularly noticable in the palmar creases (Fig. 10.9), in areas of pressure from clothing straps and in the buccal mucosa.

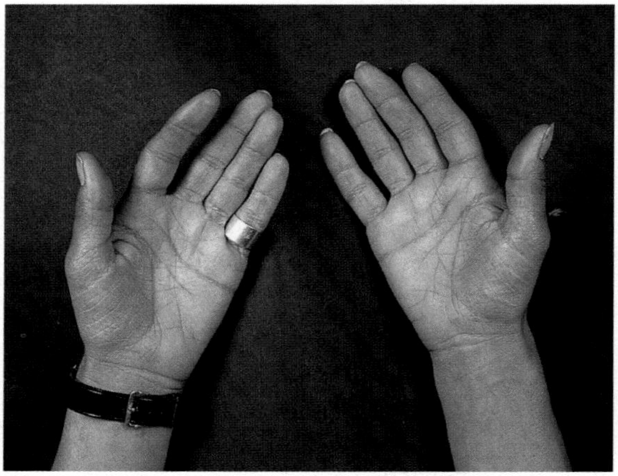

FIG. 10.9 Pigmentation of the palmar creases in Addison's disease.

Physical signs in skin disease

11

The skin is an organ with vital physiological functions. Because the skin is clearly visible, everyone wishes their own to be flawless. The multi-million pound cosmetics industry is based upon this understandable and inherent desire for perfection so it is easy to appreciate that skin disease causes a psychological strain out of proportion to disturbances in function which the pathology produces. Stigmatization frequently results in embarrassment and consequent avoidance of social and sexual contact.

The contribution that cutaneous physical signs make towards diagnoses which, at first, seem to be purely internal in their manifestations is often overlooked. For example the pallor of anaemia, the excessive sweating of phaeochromocytoma, the malar flush of mitral valve disease, the icterus of biliary obstruction or, quite simply, the age and sex of the patient are all conveyed at a glance by visible cutaneous signs. In addition there are specific reactions in the skin which may indicate an internal disorder, some of which are given in Revision Panel 11.1.

The purpose of this chapter is not to describe individual dermatological diseases in detail but to draw attention to the patterns of cutaneous reaction and outline the steps whereby a sensible approach to diagnosis can be made.

Revision Panel 11.1

Skin reactions which may indicate an internal disorder

Eruption	*Usual cause or association*
Acanthosis nigricans	Malignancy (usually stomach).
Dermatomyositis	Malignancy (ovary, bronchus).
Erythema nodosum	See Fig. 11.1 and Revision Panel 11.11.
Ichthyosis (acquired)	Malignancy.
Nailfold telangiectasia	Connective tissue diseases.
Necrobiosis lipoidica	Diabetes mellitus (Fig 11.2).
Nodules	Rheumatoid disease (Fig 11.3). Gout (see Fig. 17.1).
Pretibial myxoedema	Thyrotoxicosis (Fig 11.4).
Pyoderma gangrenosa	Ulcerative colitis (Fig. 11.4).
Livedo reticularis	Polyarteritis nodosa.
Xanthelasma	Hypercholesterolaemia.

THE HISTORY

When taking a history:

- Start by *just listening*.
- Be prepared to fit together the pieces of the patient's story like a jigsaw.
- Don't be tempted to skip the history in order to have a quick look at the skin and reach a speedy, if inadequate, diagnosis.
- Never pre-judge what a patient is going to tell you – a teenager with prominent facial acne may actually have come about his athlete's foot or an elderly woman with a visible rodent ulcer may want to discuss her

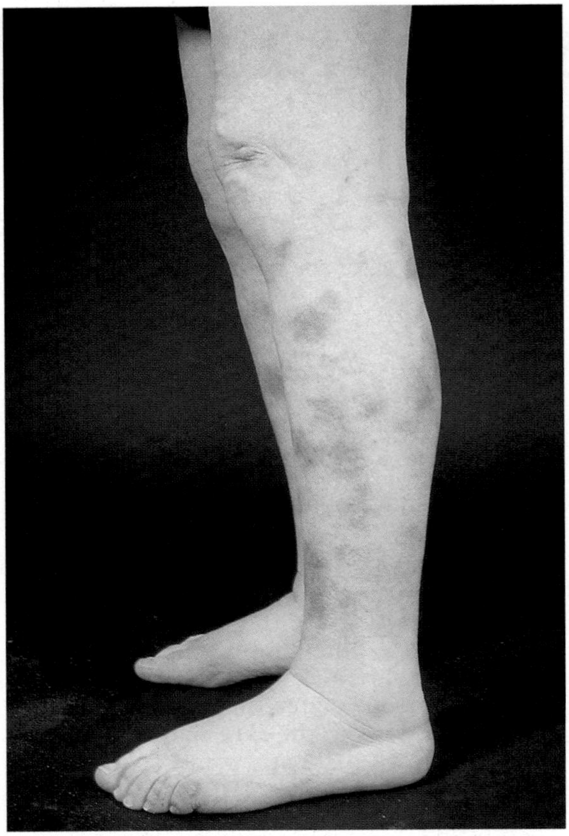

FIG. 11.1 Erythema nodosum. This shows the characteristic distribution of hot, tender nodules over the front of the shins.

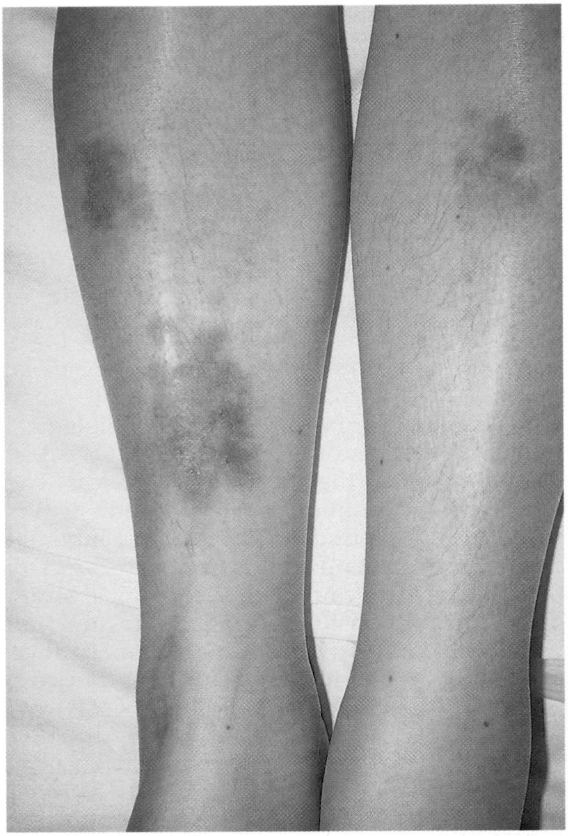

FIG. 11.2 Necrobiosis lipoidica. The site of this relatively uncommon complication of diabetes is typical.

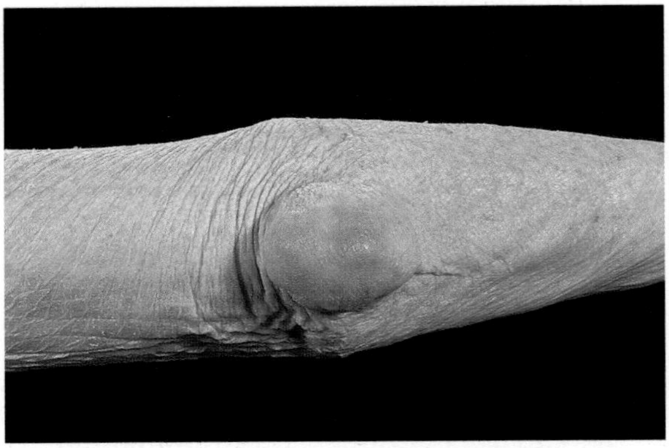

FIG. 11.3 A large rheumatoid nodule at the elbow. This lesion ulcerated at a later date.

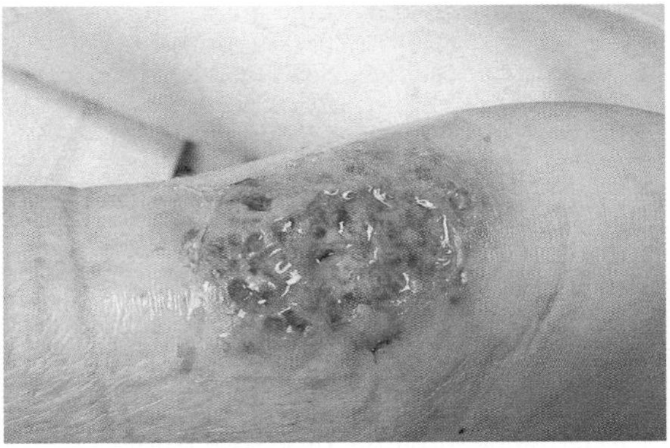

FIG. 11.4 Pyoderma gangrenosa of the knee in a woman with ulcerative colitis. This rare lesion healed three weeks after a total proctocolectomy.

intertrigo. Questioning about any additional abnormalities you have noticed can come later.

Generally, skin problems can be divided into two broad groups:

Skin tumours – both benign and malignant, together with localized blemishes and abnormalities which, although minor, may loom very large in the patient's mind (Fig. 11.5).

More generalized eruptions – and also problems with the skin appendages such as sweat glands, hair (Revision Panel 11.2) or nails (Revision Panel 11.3).

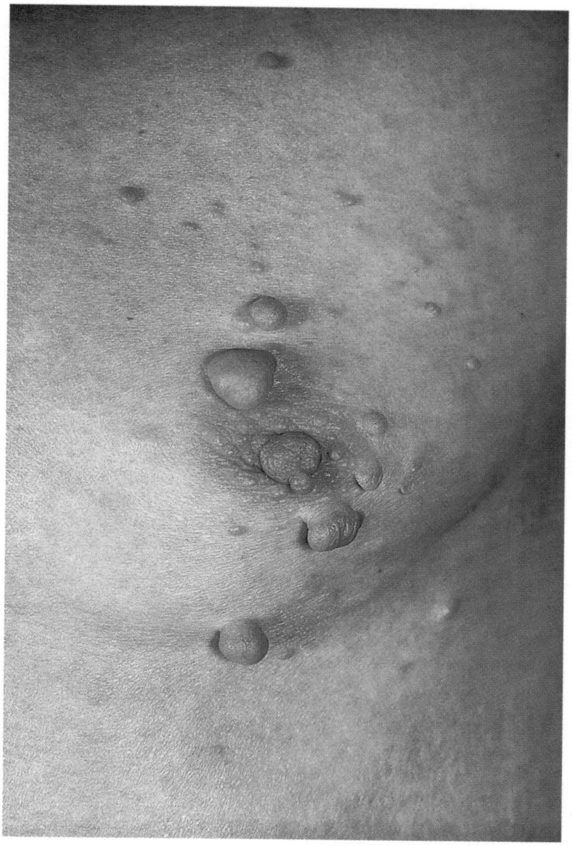

FIG. 11.5 Lesions of the chest wall in a patient with neurofibromatosis. Fortunately this patient's skin tumours were relatively minimal on the face and caused little distress.

Revision Panel 11.2

Abnormalities of hair

HAIR LOSS	
Generalized	
Severe illness	
Hypothyroidism	
Hypopituitarism	
Iron deficiency	
Drugs	Especially cytotoxics.
Localized	
Male pattern baldness	Characteristic distribution.
Alopecia areata	Normal scalp surface.
Scarring	Loss of follicles.
Infection	Bacterial and fungal.
Traumatic	Habit, hair style.
Lichen planus	Keratin plugged follicles.
Lupus erythematosus	Keratin plugged follicles.
INCREASED HAIR (HYPERTRICHOSIS)	
Generalized	
Racial	Indian subcontinent.
Familial	
Polycystic ovaries	Sometimes sole symptom.
Anorexia nervosa	Vellus or lanugo hair.
Drugs	e.g. Cyclosporin.
Androgens	Adrenal tumour.
Congenital adrenal hyperplasia	
Localized	
Naevoid	
Inflammatory skin disease	
Occlusion	e.g. Plaster of Paris.

The presenting complaint

What caused the patient to seek advice? Was it just the appearance of the rash or were symptoms present as well? Did symptoms such as itching or soreness develop before there was anything to be seen? What did the original lesion look like? Subsequent change and treatment, both appropriate and inappropriate, might have greatly altered the appearances. If the problem is widespread, where on the body surface did it start? Did a longstanding blemish suddenly change?

Revision Panel 11.3
Nail abnormalities

Abnormality	*Common cause*
Onycholysis (lifting free margin)	Psoriasis. Fungal infection.
Koilonychia (spoon shape)	Iron deficiency (see Fig. 40.1)
Pitting	Psoriasis (Fig. 11.6).
Longitudinal ridging	Age.
Transverse ridging (Beau's lines)	Systemic illness (Fig. 11.7).
Onychogryphosis (thickening and twisting)	Trauma ageing (see Fig. 14.2).
White streaks	Fungal infection.
Yellow nails	Slow growth.
Clubbing	Respiratory disease.

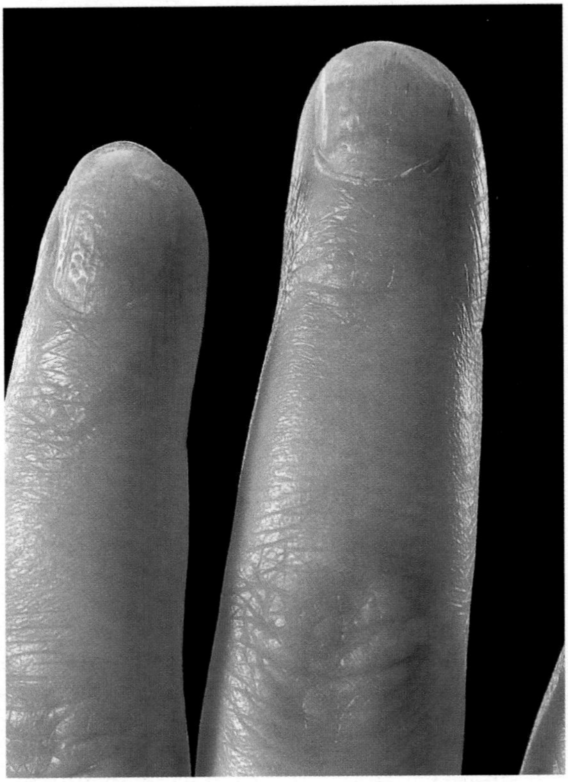

FIG. 11.6 Nail disease in psoriasis. Onycholysis of the nail of the middle finger and pitting of the nail of the ring finger.

Lesions which are out of sight, behind an ear or on the back may be noticed first by others if they are asymptomatic. Is there a fear of skin cancer?

Practical Point

The general rules of examination apply irrespective of lesion size. These rules will enable you to distinguish a harmless mole from a malignant melanoma or an innocuous dermatofibroma from a Kaposi's sarcoma.

Duration

It can be surprisingly difficult to get an accurate idea of the duration of skin conditions. This is particularly true of skin tumours and other readily visible conditions. As a general rule, patients tend to underestimate the time such lesions have been present, probably because of embarrassment and the expectation of a hostile reaction if they appear to have delayed seeking advice.

Subsequent change

What has happened to the lesions since they started? Have the original ones disappeared and been replaced by others or has there been relentless spread? Did the condition spread rapidly? Does the affected area fluctuate, sometimes returning to normal or is it persistent? Do the lesions occur in crops? Is there a pattern to their spread? Have they spread from the trunk to the extremities or vice versa?

The presence of scaling, blistering, weeping, bleeding, pain and, above all, itching should be noted. If present, the periodicity of the itching and exacerbating and relieving factors noted. The major causes of generalized pruritus and some illustrative examples of local pruritus are given in Revision Panel 11.4. Eruptions which start as, for example, a blister, may later produce an erosion or ulcer.

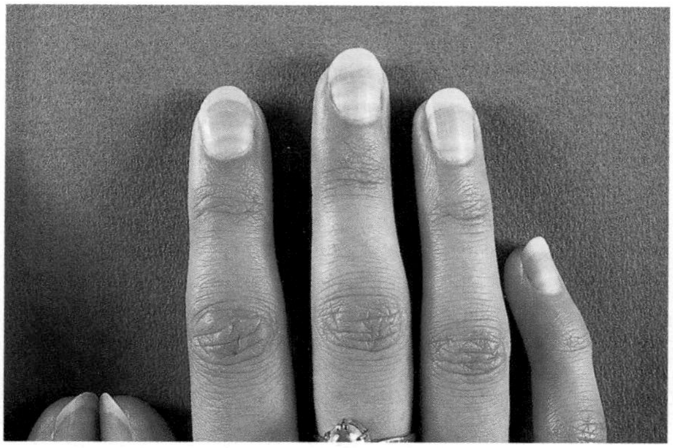

FIG. 11.7 White bands on the nails in a patient who had been having courses of chemotherapy for acute lymphoblastic leukaemia. Beau's lines are transverse depressions on the nails due to defective growth during severe illness.

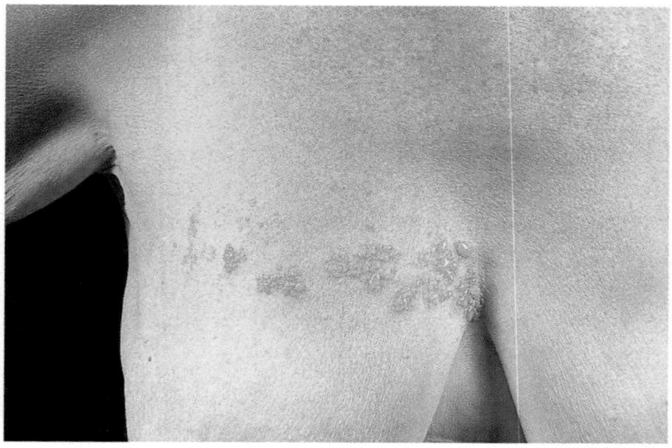

FIG. 11.8 Herpes zoster of the chest wall in a woman undergoing treatment for lymphoma.

Topical applications

Irrespective of what may have been prescribed, it is rare for a patient to have applied *nothing* to a rash before seeking medical advice. Often protestations of denial are belied by the odour of proprietary medicines. What is visible at the time of consultation might be the result of self-medication or inappropriate therapy, the original condition having been greatly modified.

Additional features of the history

Previous skin disease

The history should go right back to birth. Certain ichthyoses may present severely in the neonate as a so-called 'collodion baby' but subsequently improve considerably in later childhood. Others such as atopic eczema may settle in a year or two but problems recur in adult life.

Other illnesses

Both past and present illnesses and the medication prescribed might be important (Fig. 11.8). Some disorders recognizably due to internal diseases are listed in Revision Panel 11.1 and some distinctive drug eruptions are shown in Revision Panel 11.5.

Family and social history

Enquiries about other affected family members will reveal information not only about genetic disorders but more mundane contagious conditions such as impetigo, tinea or scabies which might spread between family and friends.

Geographical factors

Great Britain is a multiracial society and travel abroad is easy. Unusual tropical infections, including human immunodeficiency virus

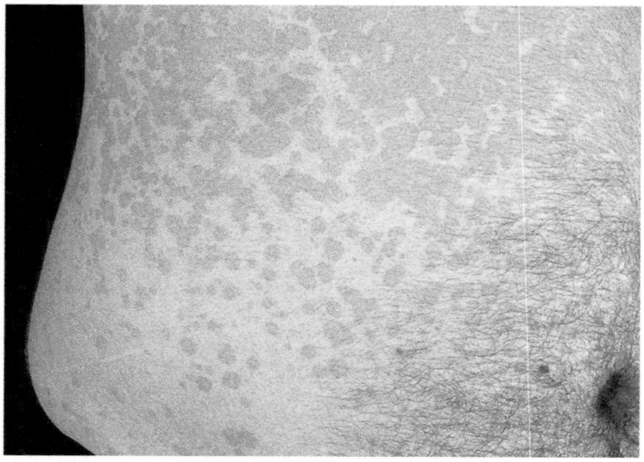

FIG. 11.9 Tinea versicolor. A common eruption in those working in hot environments. Note the variation in size of the lesions.

(HIV), can be acquired from even the shortest of stays in endemic areas. For those with fair skins, living for long periods in hot, humid climates can bring its own problems (Fig. 11.9). Many of the skin changes attributed to ageing (Revision Panel 11.6) are in fact brought about by solar damage, although this is not a popular gospel to preach on Mediterranean beaches. The effects are cumulative and it is believed that exposure in childhood might be more damaging than in adult life.

Revision Panel 11.4
Causes of pruritus

GENERALIZED

Due to skin disease	*Examples*
Infections/infestations	Tinea, scabies, pediculosis, insect bites.
Eczema of all types	
Miscellaneous	Lichen planus (Fig. 11.10), urticaria, prickly heat (milaria), dermatitis herpetiformis, pityriasis rosea.
Idiopathic	Senile pruritus.

Due to internal disorders
Cholestasis
Renal failure
Polycythaemia
Iron deficiency
Lymphoma

LOCALIZED

Eyelids	Allergic eczema due to make-up.
Perianal region	Idiopathic, haemorrhoids.
Legs	Asteatotic eczema.
Vulva	Candidiasis.
Scalp (in children)	Pediculosis.
Limbs	Insect bites.

Occupation

Skin disease is one of the major reasons for claiming industrial injury benefit. Many industrial chemicals can irritate the skin or give rise to an allergy, so precise details of work and working conditions are well worth determining. Anyone interested in skin problems

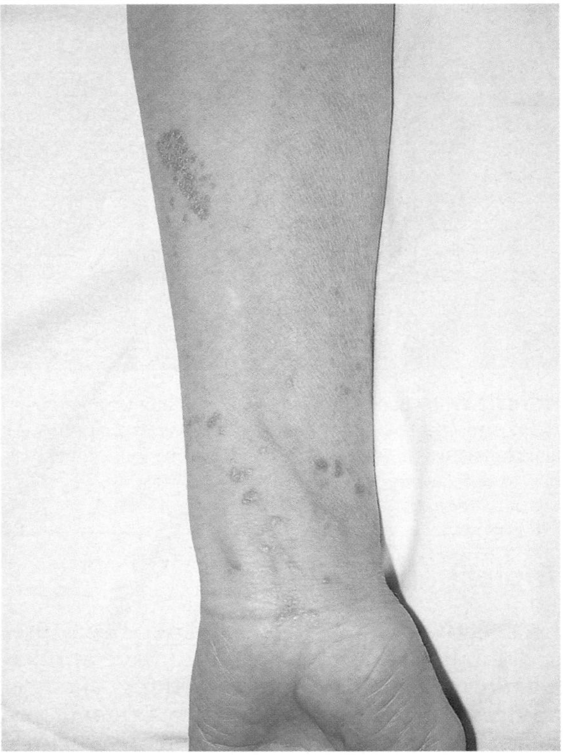

FIG. 11.10 Lichen planus. An itchy eruption commonly seen on the flexor surfaces of the wrist. The lesions may be polygonal in shape.

Revision Panel 11.5
Distinctive drug eruptions

Type of eruption	*Common cause*
Acneiform	Anabolic steroids.
Alopecia	Cyclophosphamide, other cytotoxics.
Erythema multiforme	Non-steroidal antiflammatory, sulphonamides.
Fixed drug eruptions	Phenolphthalein, sulphonamides.
Lichenoid	Gold, antimalarials.
Photosensitivity	Tetracyclines, phenothiazines.
Urticaria	Penicillin.

Revision Panel 11.6

Effects of age on the skin

General reduction in	
Epidermal thickness	
Scalp hair density	
Pigmentation	Especially hair.
Sweat gland function	Irreversible.
Sebaceous gland activity	
Elastic tissue	Especially sun-exposed areas.
General non-specific changes	
Dry skin	
Pruritus	
Eczema of the lower legs (Fig. 11.11).	
Gravitational diseases	
Local lesions	
Purpura	On minor trauma.
Telangiectasia	On light-exposed areas.
Benign tumours	
Campbell de Morgan spots	After age of 20 years.
Seborrhoeic keratoses	
Lentigines	On light-exposed skin.
Premalignant tumours	
Solar keratoses	Particularly tropical sun.
Lentigo maligna	Very slow growing.
Malignant tumours	
Basal cell carcinomata	On light-exposed areas.
Squamous cell carcinomata	On light-exposed areas.

should never miss an opportunity to visit local factories to see at first hand what is happening; knowledge of working practices and colloquial terms can also greatly aid rapport.

Hobbies

These, not work, may be the source of trouble.

THE EXAMINATION

Whilst inspection must have pride of place, palpation is also important not only to aid

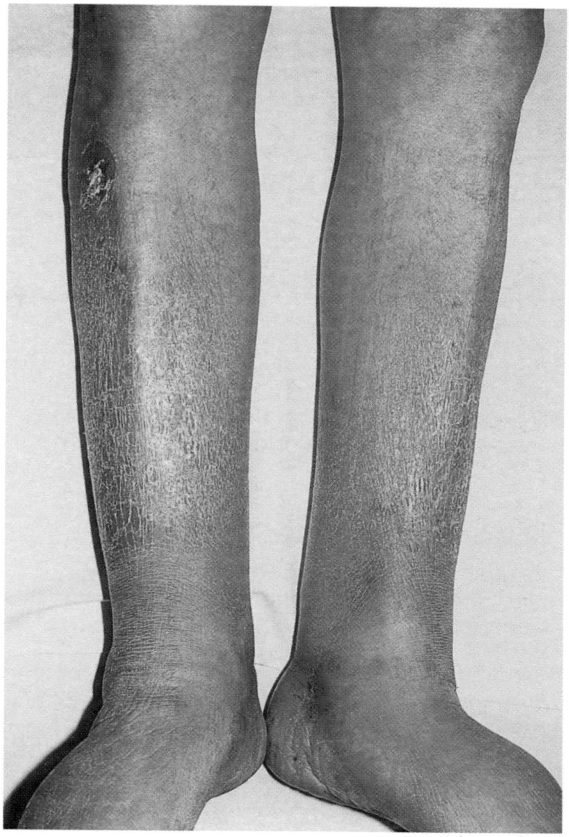

FIG. 11.11 Chronic changes in the skin of an elderly man who had been immobile.

diagnosis but also to reassure the patient that their skin disease is nothing to be afraid of.

Inspection

Distribution of lesions

Always carry out a proper examination of the skin with the patient fully undressed and seen in good natural light. Obviously common sense must prevail about how much to expose but do not be put off by a declaration that 'it only affects my hands and lower legs'. This usually indicates a disinclination to undress. Vital diagnostic clues might be concealed.

Inspection of the skin really starts with general observations:

Revision Panel 11.7
Causes of hypopigmentation

Generalized	
Albinism	Complete.
Hypopituitarism	Relative.
Vitiligo	With end-stage confluent disease.
Localized	
Piebaldism	Congenital.
Tuberose sclerosis	Congenital.
Vitiligo	Acquired.
Post-traumatic	Scarring, any cause.
Leprosy	With local anaesthesia
Morphoea	+ thickening (localized scleroderma).

Revision Panel 11.8
Causes of hyperpigmentation

Generalized	
Racial	
Tanning	
Pregnancy	
Addison's disease	Generally pigmented especially exposed areas (see Fig. 2.7) with brown patches on buccal mucosa.
Renal failure	
Cachexia	
Haemochromatosis	
Drug induced	e.g. Busulphan.
Localized	
Freckles	On light-exposed areas.
Lentigines	In elderly.
Chloasma	Pregnancy and the contraceptive pill.
Café-au-lait patches	Consider neurofibromatosis if more than six patches.
Peutz-Jeghers	Perioral.
Post-inflammatory	A common cause.
Acanthosis nigricans	Hyperkeratosis in axilla/other flexures.

- What is the general skin colour? Is it normal, hypopigmented (Revision Panel 11.7) or hyperpigmented (Revision Panel 11.8) or generally red or erythrodermic (Revision Panel 11.9).

Revision Panel 11.9
Causes of erythroderma

Psoriasis	Commonest.
Eczema	All types.
Toxic erythema	e.g. Viral infections.
Drug allergy	
Lymphoma	Rare.
Chronic lymphatic leukaemia	Rare.
Unknown	Seen occasionally in elderly men.

- What is the pattern of the lesions on the skin surface? Is it symmetrical? Is it more on flexor or extensor aspects of joints? Is it limited to exposed areas suggestive of photosensitivity (Revision Panel 11.10) or reaction such as in contact dermatitis to other external factors?

Examine the whole of the skin including the nails and nailfolds, hair and scalp, ears and external auditory meati and the mouth (see Chapter 6). Look at all the flexures including the axillae, umbilicus, inframammary folds, and genital and perianal areas. Finally, however reluctant the patient is, remove the socks and look at the feet and in between the toes.

Morphology

Having determined the overall pattern of the lesions it is necessary to inspect them individually. A nomenclature has been developed in order to simplify description:

- A lesion which is easily seen but impalpable (like a freckle) is described as a *macule*.
- A lesion which is easily seen and is palpable is described as a *papule*.
- A lesion which is easily seen and is palpable and extensive is a *plaque*.
- A lesion which is easily seen and is palpable, extensive and deep is a *nodule*.
- Oedema with no overlying epidermal change produces a *weal*.

Revision Panel 11.10
Causes of photosensitivity

Genetic	
Albinism	Total lack of melanin.
Metabolic and nutritional	
The porphyrias	Except acute intermittent.
Disorders of trytophan metabolism	e.g. Pellagra.
Drug-induced	
Phenothiazines	
Tetracyclines and derivatives	
Thiazide diuretics	
Piroxicam and other NSAIDs	
Chlorpropramide	
Idiopathic	
Polymorphic light eruption	Especially young women.
Solar urticaria	
Actinic reticuloid	Elderly men.
Topical photosensitization	
Chemical	e.g. Perfumes.
Conditions worsened by light	
SLE	
Discoid SLE	
Psoriasis	In acutely active phase.

NSAIDs: Non-steroidal anti-inflammatory drugs.
SLE: systemic lupus erythematosus.

Fluid-filled *blisters* on the skin are arbitrarily divided on the basis of size into smaller vesicles and larger bullae. Blistering is an important physical sign, occurring in a number of conditions such as:

- Pemphigoid which always blisters.
- Erythema multiforme which blisters occasionally.
- Pustules which contain debris, leukocytes and microorganisms as well as fluid but this does not automatically indicate infection; the pustules of psoriasis for example are sterile.
- An erosion which is due to loss of epidermis and the consequent oozing of serous fluid which then dries produces crusts. Erosions will heal without damage to the skin but ulcers produced by penetration into the dermis will scar.
- Scaling which is due to accumulation of keratin, either normal or abnormal, on the skin surface. It may be the only visible change, as in some ichthyoses or accompanied by inflammation as in psoriasis.
- Desquamation which is due to shedding of the horny layer and can follow an inflammatory disorder such as an exanthem, drug reaction or underlying cellulitis.

Outline

The margin of the individual lesions should be carefully examined. Some disorders give rise to lesions with a clearcut division between normal and abnormal skin whereas in others the abnormal blends into the normal.

- A convex border indicates the direction of spread.
- Where multiple small lesions have coalesced to produce larger patches the margin will appear scalloped.
- Lichen planus (Fig 11.10) is characteristically limited by fine skin creases producing polygonal lesions.

Practical Point

Blistering is an important physical sign.
Blisters occur in:
Pemphigoid: always.
Erythema multiforme: occasionally.
Psoriasis: never simple blisters but sterile pustules.

Practical Point

Beware of patients who talk of 'blisters' in the skin; the term is often used by lay people to mean a weal not a fluid-filled lesion so always clarify the point.

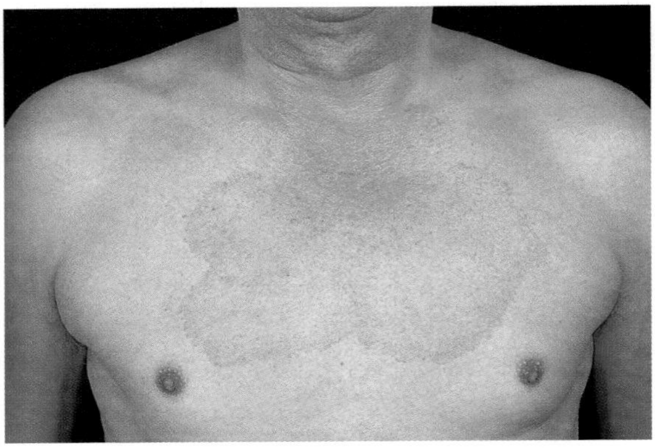

FIG. 11.12 Ringworm. Note the characteristic spreading edge.

- If the skin in the centre of a lesion returns to normal as it spreads it takes on an annular appearance. Whilst typical of ringworm (Fig. 11.12) it is not pathognomonic.
- Linearity may imply either an underlying structural defect or a response to external factors such as occurs in the Koebner phenomenon where non-specific injury, such as a scratch, turns into a specific skin disease. This occurs most commonly in psoriasis.
- Extensive chronic changes in the lower legs may be due to immobility (Fig. 11.11).

Colour

The subtle differences in erythema in different diseases can be very helpful diagnostically but to become expert requires practice. The same applies in interpreting colour changes in dark skins where redness may not be so obvious. As a general rule:

- Bright red erythema indicates an active disorder – as activity declines the lesions become paler and the redness may be replaced by post-inflammatory pigmentation which can last for many months.
- Erythema occurring beneath a thickened epidermis will tend to take on a slightly violaceous hue.
- Telangiectasia can be distinguished from purpura and petechiae by blanching on diascopy, that is looking through a glass slide pressed against the skin.

Practical Point

Active disease is usually indicated by bright red erythema and a convex border indicates the direction of spread.

Texture

If it is difficult to determine whether the surface of a lesion is scaling or not, removal of surface grease using a little ether is helpful. Conversely if scaling is present, obscuring the base of the lesion, a little oil can be applied to the surface. Characteristic scaling which turns silvery on scratching is seen in the lesions of psoriasis.

Palpation

This should never be omitted. It is reassuring for a patient to know you are not afraid to touch their skin. An extensive rash is as unpleasant to the patient as it would be to any of us. Patients with skin disease are not a special subgroup of humanity. Relatives and friends may keep a discrete distance and sexual activity may be non-existent, so the last thing a medical advisor should do is to confirm their untouchability.

Palpation is also informative. The skin may be thickened, in which case it should be possible to identify whether it is dermal or epidermal. The lesion might spread much further than is evident visually, be calcified or cystic, cooler or warmer than the surrounding skin, as in erythema nodosum (Revision Panel 11.11 and Fig. 11.1) or atrophic with loss of dermal collagen.

Crusts, when present, should be removed from a sample area so that the underlying surface can be inspected. As crusts are not firmly adherent to the surface, the simplicity of their removal will also help to distinguish them from keratin, which is an integral part of the lesion and can rarely be removed with ease.

Revision Panel 11.11

Some causes of erythema nodosum

Infection	
Streptococcus	Sometimes recurrent.
Primary tuberculosis	Early only, severe.
Deep mycoses	
Cattle ringworm	
Sarcoidosis	
Crohn's disease	
Ulcerative colitis	
Sulphonamides	
Malignancies	After radiotherapy.
Unknown	May be persistent.

Revision Panel 11.12

Summary

Learn the basic nomenclature used to describe skin lesions. Psychological problems due to skin disease should not be underestimated.

Be sure to take a full history.

Family, social and occupational history may provide vital information.

Examine the whole of the skin surface.

Look at the distribution of the lesions on the skin surface.

Examine closely the morphology of skin lesions.

Palpation is an important part of the examination.

INVESTIGATIONS

If it is not possible to make a diagnosis on clinical grounds alone, further investigations may be indicated. Simple tests should be seen as extensions of the clinical examination. These include:

- Isolating an acarus in scabies.
- Finding fungal hyphae in suspected ringworm.
- Using Wood's light to detect fluorescence or areas of hypopigmentation.
- Checking for allergy with prick or patch tests.
- Biopsy of the skin biopsy for light microscopy and immunofluorescence.
- Requesting clinicopathological investigations in microbiology, haematology, immunology or biochemistry may also be necessary.

12 What to look for in the acutely ill patient

The patient who becomes acutely and perhaps desperately ill over a few minutes or hours, or who is admitted having been found in such a state, taxes the diagnostic skills of every doctor. There is no time to waste, often not enough time to take a comprehensive history – indeed there may not be one available – or to examine the patient fully. Your course of action is dictated by the circumstances, in particular the age of the patient and the speed of onset of the illness.

Start by identifying the clinical syndrome which is dominating the illness. Is it:

- Shock?
- Fever?
- Hypothermia?
- Respiratory failure?
- Poisoning?
- Disturbed consciousness? (see Chapter 15).

SHOCK

The shocked patient will:

- Be cold with a clammy skin.
- Be restless and agitated.
- Have a fast thready pulse.
- Be hypotensive
- Have an impaired peripheral circulation.

The recognition of shock means that your patient is critically ill and you must move on rapidly to ask directed questions and to look for relevant signs (Revision Panel 12.1).

Cardiogenic shock

In a middle-aged or elderly patient the most likely cause will be some form of pump failure such as myocardial infarction,cardiac tamponade or aortic dissection. Pain may not necessarily be a feature of myocardial infarction, particularly in the elderly.

Hypovolaemic shock

Massive loss of blood due to gastrointestinal haemorrhage is usually easily recognized by the intense pallor, hypotension and tachycardia. It is not necessary for there to be accompanying haematemesis or melaena (Fig. 12.1). A large bleed from a duodenal ulcer may take time to pass through the gastrointestinal tract before appearing as frank melaena.

Hypovolaemic shock may also be due to salt and water loss in a wide range of clinical disorders including gastroenteritis, cholera, intestinal obstruction, heat exhaustion and Addisonian crisis. Here the loss of skin turgor and dryness of the tongue dominate the clinical signs.

Septic shock

In the early stages of septic shock the appearance of the patient is quite different from the other types of shock. The patient may not look

Revision Panel 12.1

Common causes of shock

Mechanism	*Possible diagnoses*	*What to ask about*	*Signs to look for*
Cardiogenic shock	Myocardial infarction.	Previous heart problems, particularly angina. Smoking. Diabetes. Hypertension.	Low output state. Left ventricular failure. Tachycardia. Rhythm disturbances.
	Dissecting or ruptured aneurysms.	As above but think of aneurysm when there is much back pain.	Absent or variable peripheral pulses. Much lower blood pressure in one arm.
Hypovolaemic shock			
■ Blood	Bleeding from gastointestinal tract.	History of dyspepsia or ulcers.	Melaena.
		Alcohol habits. Liver problems.	Stigmata of CLD. Hepatosplenomegaly.
■ Water and electrolytes	Gastroenteritis. Diarrhoea. Vomiting.	Possible sites of fluid loss.	Lax skin. Dry tongue. Soft eyeballs.
Septic shock	Gram-negative septicaemia.	Usually associated with recent surgery on gastrointestinal tract.	Flushed skin. Bright eyed. Warm peripheries. Bounding pulse.
Anaphylactic shock	Injections, insect stings.	Details of incident. Previous similar episodes.	Bronchospasm. Vasodilatation. Urticaria.
Surgical shock	Rupture of viscus. Pancreatitis.	(See also Chapter 27.)	Rigid abdomen. Release pain. Absent bowel sounds.

CLD: Chronic liver disease.

desperately ill, as indeed he or she is, and appears bright-eyed, with warm skin and a full bounding pulse. This pattern of illness is usually seen in Gram-negative infections following gastrointestinal or genitourinary surgery.

Anaphylactic shock

The causal factor, such as an injection or insect sting, is usually obvious. The clinical syndrome is due to massive release of histamine and other compounds which cause vasodilatation. The blood volume is unchanged but there is functional hypovolaemia with poor peripheral perfusion.

Surgical shock

Under these circumstances the clinical syndrome is dominated by the primary condition – e.g. perforation of a duodenal ulcer.

FEVER

This is usually the presenting feature in the acutely ill patient suffering from microbial infection. The majority of these infections have an onset over hours or a day or two but some, such as cryptogenic liver abscess, subacute bacterial endocarditis and tuberculosis, may have a more gradual onset.

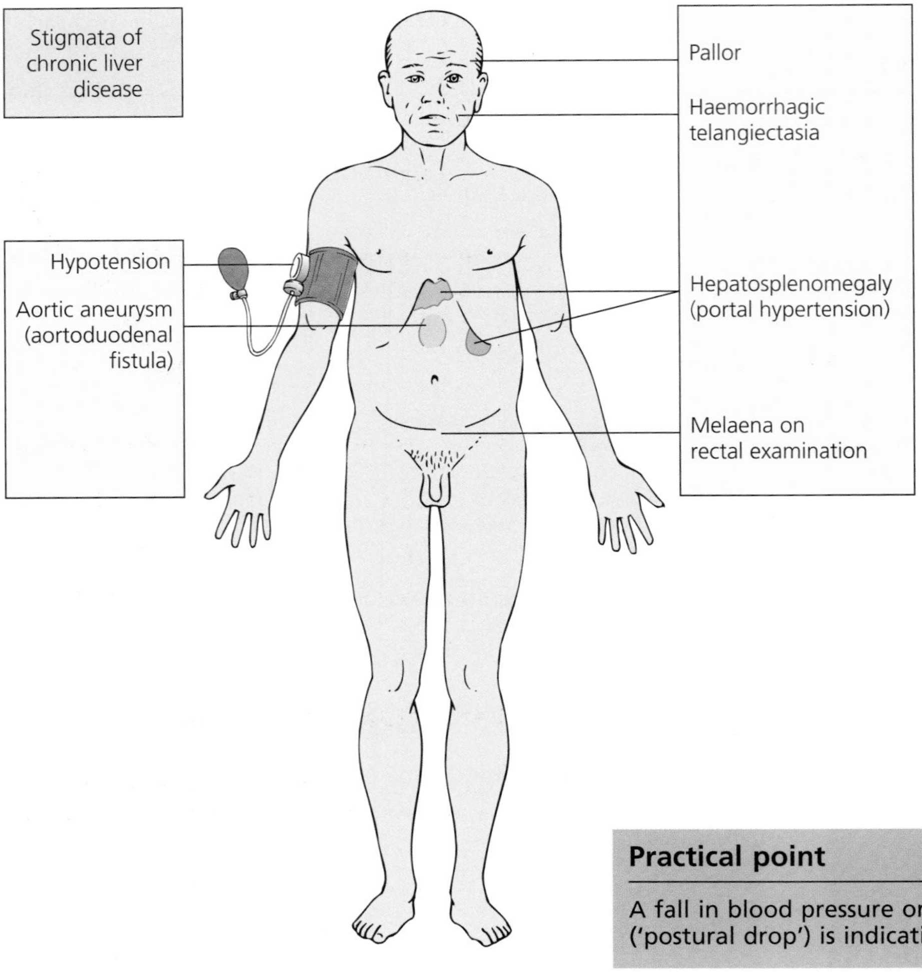

FIG. 12.1 Some signs to look for in a patient with shock due to massive gastrointestinal bleeding.

> **Practical point**
>
> A fall in blood pressure on sitting up ('postural drop') is indicative of hypovolaemia.

Some general points about the acutely ill febrile patient are worth remembering (Revision Panel 12.2):

- Rigors, or shivering attacks, commonly occur at the onset of bacterial infections of the biliary tract (cholangitis), of the urinary tract or with pneumonia.
- Rigors occurring in the tropics, or in a recently returned traveller, are due to malaria until proved otherwise.
- Some fevers have characteristic patterns, which may help with the diagnosis. For example in brucellosis the fever may be remitting in type and in dengue fever the fever may have a biphasic pattern.
- In untreated lobar pneumonia the fever may fall quickly with corresponding clinical recovery.
- Drenching night sweats may be due to tuberculosis or non-infective disease such as lymphoma.
- Meningococcal septicaemia may have a fulminant course progressing to death within 24 hours, in spite of prompt and appropriate therapy.
- Think of the possibility of associated human immunodeficiency virus (HIV) infection in any young person with an unusual febrile illness.
- Febrile responses to infection in the elderly may be less dramatic.

> **Revision Panel 12.2**
> **Physical signs of fever**
>
> Facial flushing.
>
> Sweating, particularly at night.
>
> Drenching nocturnal sweats in some fevers such as tuberculosis.
>
> Tachycardia (but bradycardia in some fevers such as typhoid).
>
> Herpes labialis.
>
> Delirium with high fevers (> 39°C in children and > 40°C in adults).
>
> Core temperatures of > 42°C may cause rhabdomyolysis, coma and death.

Remember that not every patient with fever has a microbial infection. Whilst most non-infective causes of fever have a gradual onset some, such as malignant lymphoma and polyarteritis, may occasionally have a surprisingly sharp onset.

HYPOTHERMIA

Whilst the majority of cases of hypothermia are due to obvious causes, such as exposure to extremely cold weather or immersion in cold water, hypothermia may be an important contributory factor in the acutely ill patient, particularly the elderly. It is essential to measure core temperature using a low-reading rectal or aural thermometer. Hypothermia may complicate:

- Myxoedema.
- Hypoglycaemia and hypopituitarism.
- Severe malnutrition.
- Any severe illness – e.g. stroke, diabetic ketoacidosis, septicaemia.
- Drug overdosage – e.g. alcohol, phenothiazines, narcotics.
- Injury, either accidental or surgical.

The signs of hypothermia are illustrated in Fig. 12.2.

RESPIRATORY FAILURE

In the acutely ill patient respiratory failure may be the primary cause of the illness or just one

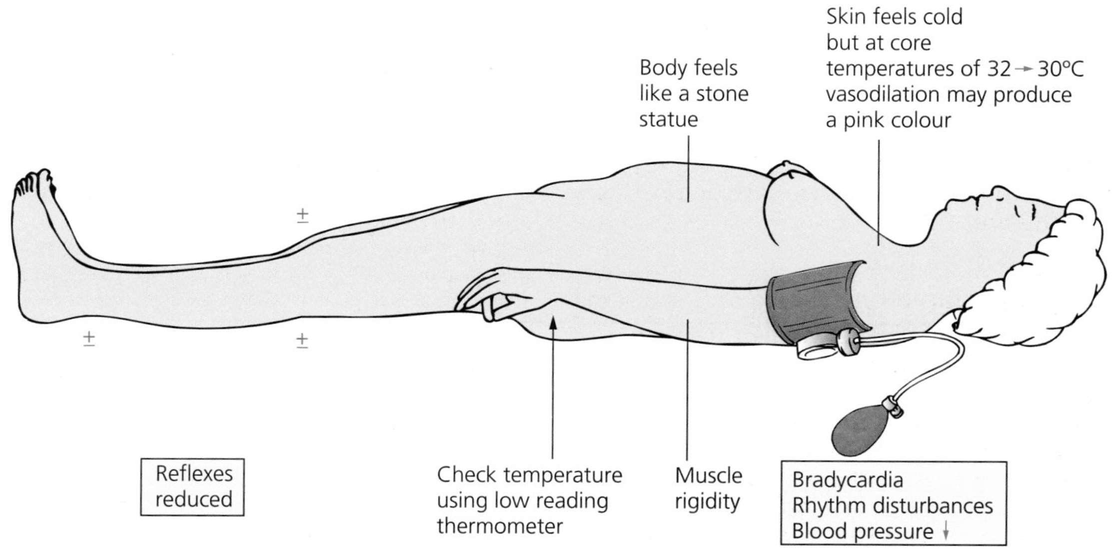

FIG. 12.2 Signs of hypothermia.

factor interacting with many others contributing to the parlous state of the patient. Whilst pulmonary disease of one sort or another accounts for the majority of cases of respiratory failure it may be encountered in a wide variety of other clinical settings including:

- Cardiac arrest.
- Left ventricular failure.
- Renal failure.
- Hepatic coma.
- Chest trauma.
- Poisoning.
- Serious neurological illness.

> **Practical Point**
>
> Respiratory failure is often part of many complex life-threatening illnesses.

The syndrome of respiratory failure is defined as the presence of hypoxaemia and/or hypercapnia due to respiratory disease at rest. Although hypoxaemia and hypercapnia commonly present together they may occur independently (See Revision Panel 12.3). Blood gas analysis is essential for correct management.

Clinical features

Hypoxaemia The presence and degree of hypoxaemia can only be assessed accurately by blood gas measurement and the clinical features, whilst critically important, are non-specific. The various components include:

- Neurological features such as restlessness, fatigue, insomnia, confusion and behavioural changes progressing to unconsciousness and eventually death.
- Tachycardia and increased cardiac output; however, impending respiratory arrest may be preceded by bradycardia.
- Increased ventilation.
- Cyanosis (see Chapter 5).

Hypercapnia Again the clinical features are non-specific and must be assessed directly by blood gas measurement. However hypercapnia may be suspected clinically by a flapping tremor, vasodilatation manifested by warm peripheries, a bounding pulse, papilloedema, drowsiness, confusion and headache.

> **Practical Point**
>
> Many patients will have received supplementary oxygen, especially en route to hospital, which may obscure signs of previous hypoxaemia (e.g. cyanosis). Patients with chronic obstructive pulmonary disease should not be deprived of supplementary oxygen.

Revision Panel 12.3

Causes of respiratory failure

Gas exchange failure

Hypoxaemia without hypercapnia:

- Airways disease – asthma, emphysema, chronic bronchitis.
- Vascular disease – thromboembolism.
- Disease of lung parenchyma – pneumonia, pulmonary fibrosis, pulmonary oedema, active alveolitis.

Failure of ventilation

Hypercapnia usually with hypoxaemia:

- Chest wall problems – trauma, deformity.
- Central drive problems – self-poisoning, neurological disorders.
- Neuromuscular disease – poliomyelitis.
- Mechanical load abnormalities – severe obstruction.

POISONING

Self-poisoning

This is one of the most common causes of admission to the acute medical wards of hospitals in the Western world. Whilst the pattern of presentation varies widely depending on the type and amount of drug taken, you must always bear in mind the possibility of drug overdose when dealing with an acutely ill patient with disturbed consciousness. The clinical patterns seen in the UK are shown in Revision Panel 12.4.

Other forms of poisoning

Doctors may forget the possibility of poisoning (whether accidental, occupational or malicious) when seeing an acutely ill patient. These highly toxic substances include cyanides, arsenic, thallium, carbon monoxide and pesticides such as paraquat and the organophosphatides. The clinical features of poisoning of all these substances are beyond the scope of this book but consider poisoning in any severely ill patient in whom you cannot establish a diagnosis.

Revision Panel 12.4

Clinical patterns of poisoning in the UK

Type of drug taken	*Groups affected*	*Clinical presentation*
Alcohol	All ages from teenagers upwards.	Ataxia, dysarthria, nystagmus progressing to coma. Problems related to aspiration of vomit.
Non-opioid analgesics	All ages, accidental poisoning in children.	
■ Aspirin	More in older age groups.	Hyperventilation, vasodilatation, sweating, tinnitus, deafness, coma rare.
■ Non-steroidal anti-inflammatory agents	More in older age groups.	Nausea and vomiting, severe toxicity unusual.
■ Paracetamol	All ages.	With as little as 10–15 g there may be severe hepatocellular necrosis.
Opioid analgesics	Drug addicts.	Respiratory depression and coma.
Anti-depressants	Those with chronic depression on therapy.	Hypotension, hyperreflexia, convulsions, dysrhythmias.
Beta-blockers	May be taken accidentally by children.	Variable with different preparations but massive overdosage causes bradycardia and hypotension.
Iron salts	May be taken accidentally by children.	Nausea, vomiting, gut bleeding, coma, hepatocellular necrosis.
Hypnotics and anxiolytics		
■ Barbiturates	Now being prescribed less often and consequently less self-poisoning.	Drowsiness, respiratory depression and coma.
■ Benzodiazepines	All groups.	Drowsiness and ataxia, long-term coma unusual.
Theophylline	All groups but availability tends to be limited to those with access i.e. those on treatment for asthma.	Vomiting, restlessness, agitation, tachycardia, later dysrrhythmias.
Phenothiazines	Particularly psychotic patients on long-term therapy.	Arrhythmias and hypotension, dystonic reactions.

Practical Point

Always consider poisoning in:
Any seriously ill patient in whom you cannot make a diagnosis.
Any acutely ill patient with disturbed consciousness.

The poisoning may be:
Self-induced.
Accidental.
Occupational.
Malicious.

ACUTE AND CRITICAL ILLNESSES WHICH MAY NEED INTENSIVE CARE

As well as being able to recognize features that identify the critically ill patient, you must be aware of those circumstances or conditions in which intensive care advice should be sought (Revision Panel 12.5). This does not necessarily mean that ventilation will be required but highlights extremely dangerous situations.

Revision Panel 12.5

Patients who require intensive care advice.

All with suspected meningococcal septicaemia (Fig. 12.3).

Poisoned patients with altered levels of consciousness and arrhythmias, including tachycardia (> 120/minute).

Patients in status epilepticus.

Victims of near drowning.

Patients with signs of inhalation injury.

Cerebrally agitated patients with brain contusion, undiagnosed hypoxia, or poisoning.

Head injuries with Glasgow coma scale 10 or rapidly falling.

Asthmatic patients not responding to maximum therapy, becoming exhausted, or high/normal carbon dioxide pressure.

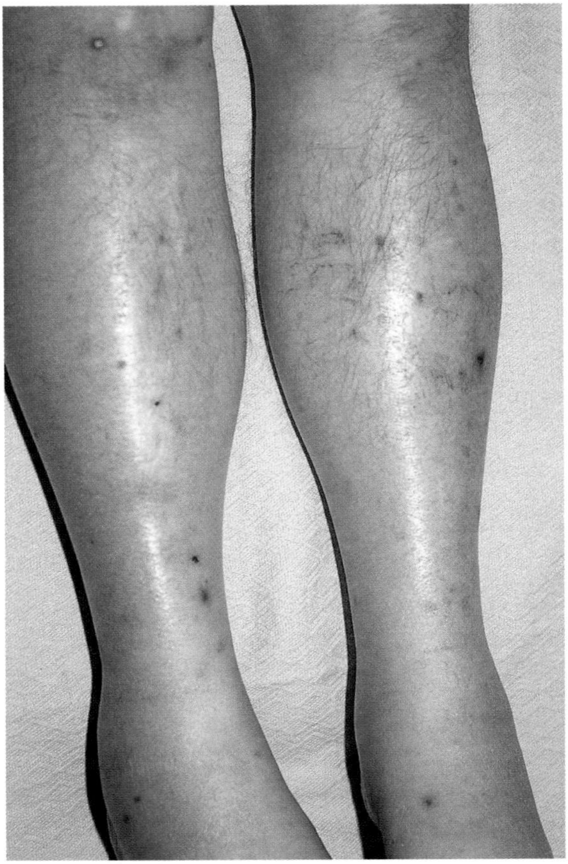

FIG. 12.3 Purpura in meningococcal septicaemia. This was the only pointer to the diagnosis in a patient with a high fever.

The elderly patient who seems muddled

13

SOME GENERAL ADVICE

Keep an open mind. When a 'confused old person' is admitted to hospital, minds snap shut, the main thought often being how to prevent a bed being blocked. Yet life or death may depend on correct appraisal.

When reviewing a patient who appears muddled, the differential diagnosis comes down to:

- Transient confusional state – while this at first sight resembles dementia, it may be reversible.
- Dementia – even when this is established, much can be achieved by defining what can and what cannot be mended.

Confusion or delirium is a non-specific reaction of the brain to a wide variety of noxious stimuli (Fig. 13.1). In old age (as in very young children), confusion may develop at a lower threshold than normal.

You should consider a confused state in the elderly as a common non-specific presentation of almost any physical or mental disorder. Many old people are slower mentally as well as physically and may also be deaf and sometimes dysphasic, leading to the suspicion that they are confused when they are not.

> **Practical Point**
>
> Elderly people easily become confused as the result of illness or drugs.

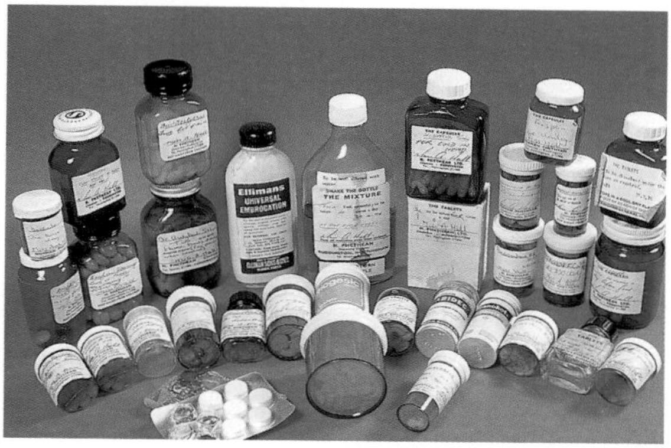

FIG. 13.1 Medicines prescribed or self-administered are among the most common causes of confusional states. This collection of tablets 'accompanied' an elderly woman admitted in a muddled state.

Because most confused old people are *very old*, and because most very old people are *women*, the feminine gender will be used throughout this chapter.

HOW TO BEGIN – SOME DOS AND DON'TS

As people get old they find it harder to assimilate new information or to become accustomed to new faces and surroundings. Take your time. Don't rush through your patient's history or examination. When assessing an old person, ensure that:

- Whenever possible the assessment is conducted in the patient's home or normal setting.
- She is warm, comfortable and appropriately positioned.
- She has clean spectacles and any hearing aid is working.
- She has had the opportunity of emptying her bladder.

See also Revision Panel 13.1.

Revision Panel 13.1

How to ensure your assessment is reliable

DO

Introduce yourself and explain who you are.

Speak clearly, remembering that not all very old people are deaf.

Be prepared to repeat any question that appears not to be fully understood.

Address your patient courteously, using her correct name.

DON'T

Presume to be familiar by addressing her by her first name or by calling her Gran.

Be afraid to establish physical contact by holding her hand.

THE EXAMINATION

Traditionally this comes after the history but with a muddled elderly patient it is useful to do a quick examination first, to get an approximate frame of reference against which to gather the history. In addition, much of the history will be obtained from sources other than the patient.

Start by setting the scene by a few simple opening remarks, enquiring where she is, where she lives and about her family and neighbours? Without having to resort to standard formal questions, you will very quickly be able to establish information about her cognitive state.

Practical Point

Older people expect courtesy and not trendy familiarity.

The aims of your examination are to assess:

- Whether your patient is acutely confused or delirious.
- How good is her comprehension.
- How good is her cognitive function.

Delirium

Delirium is a level of awareness which fluctuates to and fro along a spectrum between, at the two extremes, full alertness and coma. At times clouds seem to float across the patient's thinking and awareness; one minute she is with you, the next she has gone. In the more severe forms there may be illusions, delusions and hallucinations. Acute confusional states are almost always due to specific, commonly physical, derangements, which are often reversible. Assessing delirium may be difficult, especially in mild or subacute forms.

Comprehension

It is essential to assess comprehension. Consider if there is any deafness or dysphasia. Sometimes an elderly patient may have difficulty in understanding a thick local accent or the perhaps limited English of a doctor from overseas.

Cognitive function

Assess cognitive function by a series of focussed and standard questions. These may sound odd to some patients, so dress them up with a few introductory words such as 'I am going to ask you some questions that may sound silly, but I want to check how good your memory is'. A short list of standard questions is given in Revision Panel 13.2. A widely used and simple, but fuller, test is the 'Mini Mental State' questionnaire (Fig. 13.2).

Always pay attention to the way the patient tackles the tasks but don't forget the possible effect of sedating or befuddling drugs. Look for:

(A) *MINI MENTAL STATE*

Patient ....
Examiner ....
Date ....

Maximum Score	Score	
		ORIENTATION
5	( )	What is the (year) (season) (date) (day) (month)?
5	( )	Where are we: (country) (county) (town) (hospital) (ward)?
		REGISTRATION
3	( )	Name 3 objects: 1 second to say each. Then ask the patient all 3 after you have said them. Give 1 point for each correct answer. Then repeat them until he/she learns all 3. Count trials and record. Trials ....
		ATTENTION AND CALCULATION
5	( )	Serial 7s. 1 point for each correct. Stop after 5 answers. Alternatively spell 'world' backwards.
		RECALL
3	( )	Ask for the 3 objects repeated above. Give 1 point for each correct,
		LANGUAGE AND COPYING
9	( )	Name a pencil and watch. (2 points)
	( )	Repeat the following: 'no ifs, ands or buts'. (1 point)
	( )	Follow a 3-stage command: 'Pick up a paper with your right hand, fold it in half and put it on the floor'. (3 points)
	( )	Read and obey the following: 'Close your eyes'. (1 point)
	( )	Write a sentence. (1 point)
	( )	Copy design. (1 point)
30		Total Score
		ASSESS level of consciousness along a continuum

Alert	Drowsy	Stupor	Coma

A score of 20 or less strongly suggests dementia or other significant impairment.

(B) *INSTRUCTIONS FOR ADMINISTRATION OF MINI MENTAL STATE EXAMINATION*

ORIENTATION

(1) Ask for the date. Then ask specifically for parts omitted e.g. 'Can you also tell me what season it is?' One point for each correct answer.
(2) Ask in turn 'Can you tell me the name of this hospital?' (town, county, etc.) One point for each correct answer.

REGISTRATION

Ask the patient if you may test his memory. Then say the names of 3 unrelated objects, clearly and slowly, about one second for each. After you have said all 3, ask him to repeat them. This first repetition determines his score (0–3) but keep saying them until he can repeat all 3, up to 6 trials. If he does not eventually learn all 3, recall cannot be meaningfully tested.

ATTENTION AND CALCULATION

Ask the patient to begin with 100 and count backwards by 7. Stop after 5 subtractions (93, 86, 79, 72, 65). Score the total number of correct answers.

If the patient cannot or will not perform this task, ask him to spell the word 'world' backwards. The score is the number of letters in correct order, e.g. dlrow = 5, dlorw = 3.

RECALL

Ask the patient if he can recall the 3 words you previously asked him to remember. Score 0–3.

LANGUAGE AND COPYING

Naming: Show the patient a wrist watch and ask him what it is. Repeat for pencil. Score 0–2.
Repetition: Ask the patient to repeat the sentence after you. Allow only one trial. Score 0 or 1.
3-Stage commands: Give the patient a piece of plain blank paper and repeat the command. Score 1 point for each part correctly executed.

FIG. 13.2 The Mini Mental State questionnaire. Reproduced, with permission, from Folstein MR *et al. Journal of Psychiatric Research* 1975; **12**: 189–198.

- Very easy distractibility – suspect acute confusional state.
- Apparent concentration but simple mistakes made – suspect dementia.
- Slowed response – suspect depression.

Examine for dyspraxias. Ask the patient to perform simple tasks which you have demonstrated e.g. folding a piece of paper.

In addition to the standard tests for dysphasia and dyspraxia, consider the disorders of body and space image which originate from lesions of the non-dominant parietal lobe such as dressing apraxias, or anosognosia or hemiagnosia.

Clock drawing

A useful test of visuospatial and general cognitive function is the clock test. Draw a large

> **Revision Panel 13.2**
> **Ten simple questions**
>
> Age
> Time (hours)
> Year
> Name of place
> Recognition of two people
> Date of birth
> Date of beginning of World War II
> Monarch
> Counting backwards from 20 to 1
> Five minute recall – 26 Mulberry Close

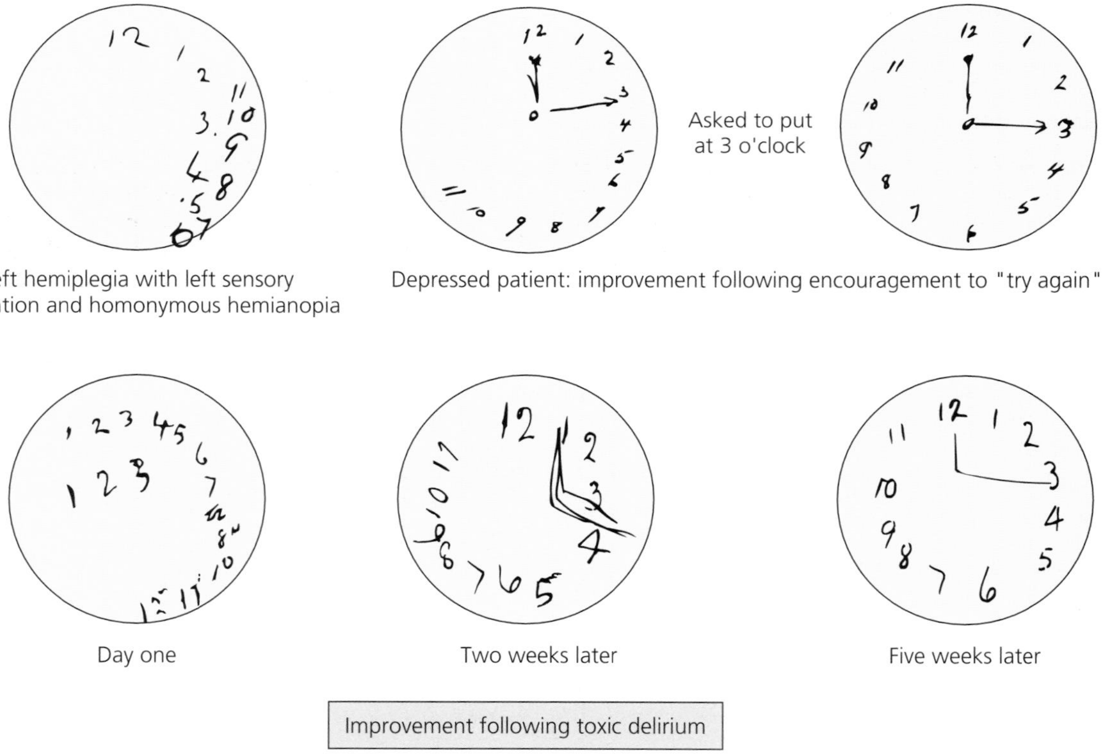

FIG. 13.3 Some examples of clock drawing. The changes following delirium are reproduced, with permission, from Schulman KI *et al. International Journal of Geriatric Psychiatry* 1986; **1**:135–140.

circle on a piece of paper and then ask the patient to put in the face of a clock. You may need to repeat this, as it is a somewhat odd request. This test may detect subtle and specific impairments (e.g. hemi-inattention). Go on to ask the patient to put in the hands at a fixed time e.g. twenty minutes to three. Samples of some of these responses are shown in Fig. 13.3.

Though you are assessing confusion and cognitive impairment do not neglect the other aspects of the Mental State examination such as whether your patient is depressed, elated, anxious, deluded, obsessional or hallucinated, etc.

THE HISTORY

The patient may give a good history but mostly it is the history from other sources which is paramount. When the patient has been brought to hospital make sure that you speak with accompanying people – be they family, neighbours, carers or policemen. Key points, listed as 'Hows' are as follows:

- How long has the patient been like this? – i.e. when was the patient last normal? If the history is short, days or weeks, the patient is unlikely, in the absence of an obvious physical cause, to be suffering from a dementia. You are much more likely to be dealing with an acute confusional state or a depressive 'pseudodementia'.
- How did it begin? – suddenly or gradually? Was the onset related to some relevant event such as illness, injury or fall? Or was it related to a major life event such as bereavement or change of home? These latter events are particularly potent precipitants of depressive states, which in the elderly may present as confusion.
- How often? What were previous circumstances and what was the outcome? What treatment was given?
- How has the illness progressed?
- How has she been treated? What drugs has she been taking? Remember that medicines, prescribed or self-administered, are among the most common causes of confusional states. Particular offenders are the cholinergic drugs and alcohol.
- How bright was she before? Your examination may be complicated by the fact that the patient was not particularly intelligent previously. Past jobs and reports from friends and neighbours may help here.

IN SUMMARY

Not all muddled old people are demented. To give them the benefit of meticulous appraisal is not only their right, but makes work with this growing group of almost all doctors' patients more interesting and more satisfying.

14 Special difficulties with the elderly

Most people aged between 65 and 75 years are generally fit and active. After 75, with increasing age, they commonly have multiple diseases which may present atypically and often lead to progressive disability and dependence. This chapter deals with the over 75-year-olds and, as most of these are women, the female gender is used throughout. (See also Chapter 13.)

Much of the examination technique you have learned applies equally to young and old. Examining a very elderly patient may be more complicated because:

- Each patient may have multiple medical problems (see Revision Panel 14.1).
- Presentation of disease may be 'atypical'.
- Complications following the primary illness are more common.

TAKING THE HISTORY AND DIAGNOSTIC TRAPS

Interview the patient in a well-lit, quiet room, making sure that you are both relaxed and that the patient can clearly see your face. Do listen carefully, as the chance remark often provides you with the initial clue as to what is really going on.

When taking the history from an elderly patient remember that:

- She may be slow to respond. Parkinson's disease, depression, and myxoedema are common so allow plenty of time for answers.
- She may be deaf. Do not confuse this with dementia.
- She may be confused. Try to gain an impression early on if this is so.
- Obtain a 'collateral' history from relatives, carers, friends, neighbours, social workers and the General Practitioner.
- The history from patients and relatives may not be entirely reliable.
- Iatrogenic disease, usually related to medication, is common due to polypharmacy and confusion over dosing and frequency (see Fig. 13.1).
- High-tone deafness is common. Speak clearly and in a low-pitched voice and make sure that any hearing aid is switched on and working (or ask the ward staff if there is a special amplifier available).

First, you should try to get an early impression of whether the patient is confused; a formal test of cognitive function is not necessary at this stage as you may insult someone who is cognitively intact. Look for subtle clues – inconsistencies in dates, what the patient says she can do compared with the amount of help she is having – or less subtle clues such as referring to deceased relatives as if they are still alive. When you have gained the patient's confidence you may introduce questions from the Mini Mental Test (Chapter 13) with the comment 'I am now going to ask questions which may seem very simple to you, but they are an important part of my examining you; I hope you don't mind'.

Good memory for events long past may be misleading – this often forms the basis for the

Revision Panel 14.1

Factors complicating the examination of elderly patient

Multiplicity of disease (co–existing acute and chronic illnesses)

Acute conditions e.g.
- chest infection,
- myocardial infarction,
- pulmonary embolus,
- stroke.

Chronic conditions e.g.
- arthritis,
- previous stroke,
- dementia.

Atypical presentations of acute illness
- falls,
- immobility,
- incontinence,
- confusion,
- acopia* (carers no longer able to cope),
- hypothermia (usually secondary to illness/drugs),
- iatrogenic illness (e.g. drug-induced postural hypotension or confusion).

Increased complication rate
- mild stroke, leading to a fall, fractured femur, bedsores and incontinence is one example.

patient or her relatives claiming that she has a 'wonderful memory'. She may have clear childhood memories but no recollection of what she ate half an hour ago. Long-term memory is often well preserved in early dementia, whereas short-term memory is lost. Specific questions to relatives, carers or friends about the patient's current daily activities, for example, may reveal that she forgets to turn off the gas or burns pots and pans. Such 'collateral' history helps to build a complete picture of the individual in the home environment.

Ensure that points elicited in the history refer to the current illness and not to the past. A confused patient easily muddles things that happened last week with those that happened last year, leading to as much confusion in the doctor as in the patient.

The time course of symptoms is very important. Sudden deterioration in health indicates an acute illness (e.g. myocardial infarction, pulmonary embolus, stroke or infection). Is the presenting symptom (including falls, incontinence, confusion or 'acopia'*) recent or long-standing and gradually getting worse?

A statement that a patient or relative 'is doing OK' may reflect low (or declining) expectations so you will need to ask specific questions about washing, dressing, toileting, shopping and cooking to find out much more about what she is really like. Most elderly people are independent but needing a community care assistant, meals on wheels, district nurse and day centre or day hospital points to varying degrees of dependence. Falls, incontinence and confusion are often regarded as inevitable and hence are not readily mentioned. Ask relatives about them specifically.

Ask about her state a few weeks before. This will help with realistic rehabilitation targets. If she was fully independent then the current illness is the likely cause of her present disability and the latter is therefore potentially remediable.

Multiple diseases lead to multiple medications. More drugs mean more side-effects. About 10–15% of elderly patients admitted to medical wards have iatrogenic illness as either a primary or secondary diagnosis. You may think that your patient is only taking two or three drugs but she may also be taking drugs hoarded from previous illnesses. Ask the relatives to bring all her drugs to the hospital and clarify what she is or is not taking.

Dizziness

Dizzy patients refer to a variety of sensations and it is important not to be misled by your own preconceived ideas. One patient may mean *rotatory* vertigo, the sensation that she or her surroundings are spinning. Other patients may mean something different – 'light-headedness', headache, 'a fuzzy feeling in the head', a vague sense of unsteadiness or 'weakness in the knees'. Ask the patient exactly

---

*Acopia is an ugly piece of shorthand meaning 'inability to cope'.

Revision Panel 14.2

Episodic dizziness – a simple guide (see Chapter 33)

Symptom	*Time course/precipitants*	*Underlying cause*
Vertigo: rotatory.	More than 10 seconds and precipitated by movement or position.	Vestibular.
	Very brief (2 or 3 seconds) precipitated by movement.	Cervical mechanoreceptor dysfunction especially spondylosis.
Vertigo: non-rotatory or dizziness.	Very brief (2 or 3 seconds) precipitated by movement, standing up or turning.	Cervical mechanoreceptor dysfunction. Cerebrovascular disease. Postural hypotension.
Either of above plus loss of consciousness.		Cardiac dysrhythmia. Epilepsy.

what she means by 'dizziness'. Find out what precipitates the attack and how long it lasts. Is it associated with any other symptoms? How long has the problem been going on and what else was happening at the time e.g. other illnesses or trauma to the head? Sorting out dizziness and vertigo can be complicated but a few simple guidelines will define the cause in many cases (see Revision Panel 14.2).

Loss of consciousness and 'blackouts'

If a patient says she has become unconscious she probably has. If, however, she says she did not, this may not be true. About one-third of patients losing consciousness due to carotid sinus hypersensitivity do not remember it – this is called retrograde amnesia. Failure of the patient to confirm loss of consciousness must be further pursued if other evidence suggests that she probably did lose consciousness. An independent witness is vital in this situation (see Revision Panel 14.3).

THE EXAMINATION

As in younger patients a thorough physical examination is essential. Certain features of particular importance are discussed here.

Revision Panel 14.3

Loss of consciousness (syncope) in the elderly

Vasovagal syncope (vasovagal syndome, neurocardiogenic syncope) – fear, pain, prolonged standing, heat, large meals, excess alcohol.

Micturition syncope – elderly men, at night, micturition whilst standing.

Defaecation syncope – elderly women, constipation, local painful conditions of anus.

Cough syncope – chronic obstructive pulmonary disease.

Orthostatic hypotension – see Revision Panel 14.4.

Carotid sinus syndrome.

Epilepsy.

Transient cerebral ischaemic attacks (TIAs).

Subclavian steal syndrome – associated with arm exercise.

Pulmonary embolus.

Myocardial infarction.

Mechanical obstruction to cardiac outflow – aortic stenosis, hypertrophic obstructive cardiomyopathy.

Cardiac dysrhythmias.

Hyperventilation – anxiety states, agitated depression.

The environment

The condition of the patient's dwelling not only indicates her previous abilities but also the effectiveness of the support being given. The state of dress and standard of cleanliness are also useful clues.

Hearing, vision and speech

Problems with any of these can lead to isolation in old age. Varying the volume of speech gives a useful indication of the patient's hearing. Check for earwax. With normal hearing, wax is unlikely to cause much impairment, but may lead to critical further hearing loss in someone who has impaired hearing. If the patient has a hearing aid make sure it is working. Know how to change a battery and what the switch positions mean.

> **Practical Point**
>
> *Hearing aid switch positions*
>
> **O**: Off.
> **M**: Microphone for person-to-person conversation.
> **T**: Inductive loop aerial pick-up used in theatres, cinemas, churches and telephone boxes.
> **M & T**: Microphone and inductive loop together – increases flexibility of use in particular situations.

If vision is poor examine the patient with an ophthalmoscope, a 'pin-hole' and Snellen's chart. The pinhole acts as a perfect lens and corrects refractive errors; improved vision using this technique indicates a need for formal refraction. Dirty spectacles commonly cause poor vision; washing them may improve things considerably!

Speech disorders arising from neurological conditions are dealt with in Chapter 7. Speech may become unclear in an elderly person as a result of ageing processes, dental trouble or ill-fitting dentures. With ageing, speech becomes slower, lower in volume and higher in pitch. Often the voice is querulous though whether due to ageing or to psychological factors is unclear.

Dental caries may be a focus for acute or chronic infection or may lead to ulceration. Poor-fitting dentures may cause ulceration and poor nutrition. The 'portcullis' sign (the upper denture falling on to the lower one when the mouth is opened) may be due to poor fitting, but if developed recently may indicate dehydration or a stroke leading to loss of tone in buccal musculature (Fig. 14.1).

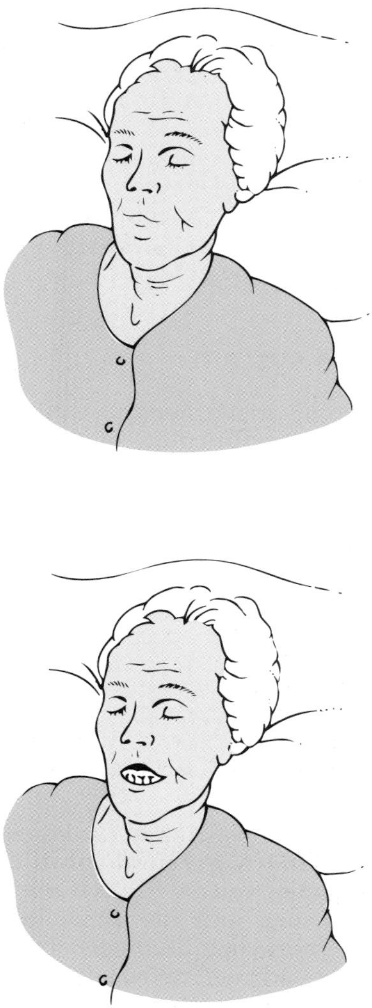

(a)

(b)

FIG. 14.1 The 'portcullis' sign may indicate dehydration or a stroke leading to loss of tone in buccal musculature.

Orofacial dyskinesia (tardive dyskinesia), characterized by chewing movements of lips and jaws, is due to major tranquillizers or occasionally extrapyramidal disorders and may cause dysarthria.

An oral lesion which causes considerable anxiety to both patient and relatives is 'caviar tongue' – clusters of sublingual varicosities; these are not due to serious pathology and reassurance can be given.

Nervous system

Examination of the nervous system may be complicated by difficulties of obtaining a clear history and by the effect of age on normal neurological examination.

A history of sudden change in physical capacity or behaviour may be all that is available. The patient with a stroke may show only minor physical signs – slight facial asymmetry, mild slurring of speech, slight changes of tone. These subtle changes may only be apparent to a doctor or nurse who has known the patient for a long time. Her relatives should be asked 'Has there been any change in speech or walking recently, or does her face look different?'

Small muscle wasting in the hands, without other evidence of neurological disease, is common in the frail elderly. Reflexes generally are diminished and the ankle jerk may be absent in normal individuals. Brisk reflexes commonly indicate underlying neurological disease, as do positive finger and pectoral jerks. The pectoral jerk is elicited by the examiner placing one hand over the lower border of the pectoralis major and tapping the back of the hand with a tendon hammer. A positive jerk is found in young individuals but, with age, it tends to disappear, usually reappearing in the presence of cerebrovascular disease.

The pupils may be small and dilate poorly in a darkened room. Pupillary-dilating drugs can facilitate fundal examination: do remember that there is a small risk of such drugs precipitating glaucoma. Occasionally the pupils may be unequal in size or irregular in shape from scarring due to previous iritis.

Practical Point

Neurological examination in the elderly

Pupils are often small and dilate poorly.

Small muscle wasting in the hands is common in the frail.

Ankle jerks may be absent.

Feet

The feet are important because of:

- Peripheral vascular disease.
- Neuropathy.
- Overgrown toe-nails.

Patients with poor vision, difficulty in bending or clumsy hands may have difficulty in cutting nails, which then cause pain on walking or even immobility. With prolonged neglect, onychogryphosis (overgrown, claw-like nails) may develop, requiring expert chiropody (Fig. 14.2). Footwear influences mobility: ancient, poorly fitting slippers should be replaced by well-fitting shoes. The pattern of wear on the sole of a shoe is useful diagnostically; a patient with foot-drop due to a minor stroke may have increased wear over the outer, anterior aspect of the sole on the affected side.

Gross swelling of the legs may be due to immobility rather than heart failure. The 'armchair legs' syndrome of the elderly (Fig. 14.3) responds better to mobilization than to diuretics.

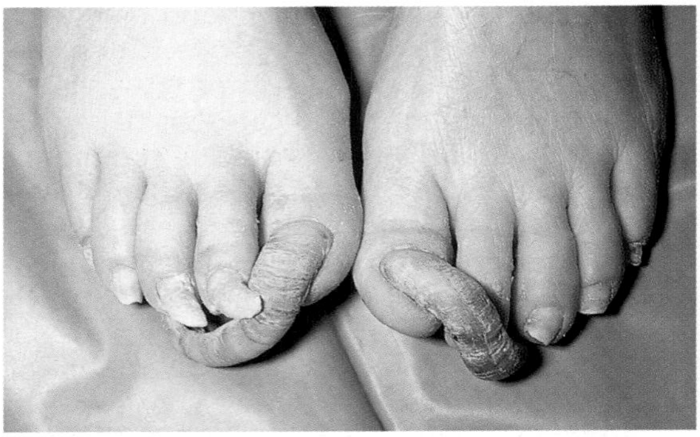

FIG. 14.2 Onychogryphosis requiring expert chiropody.

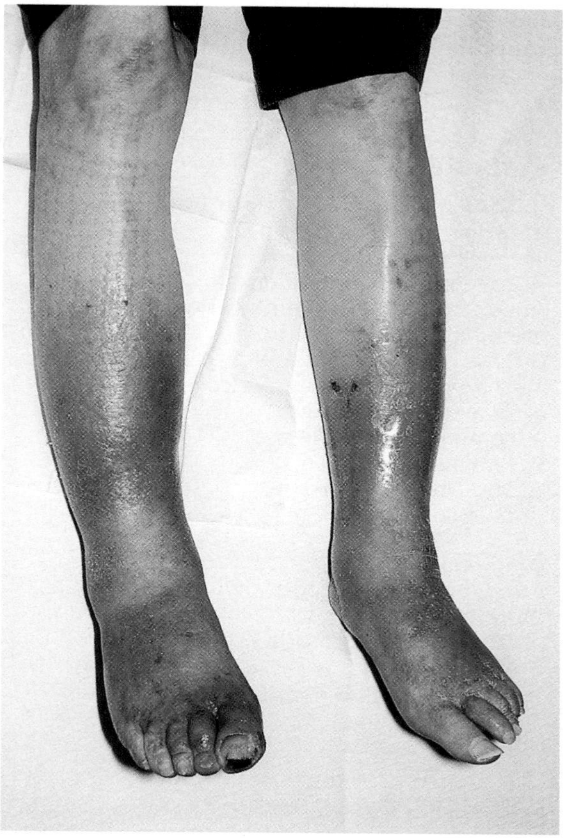

FIG. 14.3 'Armchair legs' syndrome of the elderly. Gross swelling of the legs may be due to immobility rather than heart failure.

Skin

With age the skin becomes thinner and less elastic, the capillaries are more fragile and in malnutrition there is decreased subcutaneous fat and less collagen. Senile purpura and increased skin looseness are the result, the latter making particularly difficult detection of dehydration by assessment of skin turgor over the forearm or anterior abdominal wall. The best area for assessing turgor is the forehead where the skin is closely anchored to underlying fascia (see Revision Panel 11.6).

Particular attention should be given to skin over the 'pressure areas' (bony prominences over which pressure may develop). Reddening of the skin warns of possible undue pressure. If redness is accompanied by surrounding induration there is pressure necrosis of subcutaneous tissue. The 'iceberg' phenomenon may be present – a small superficial area of necrosis, with a much larger underlying area of induration. The latter is easily overlooked but indicates the true extent of necrotic tissue. Nursing staff may be worried that ulceration is extending and view this as a failure of nursing care. What is usually happening is that the ulcer enlarges as an inevitable part of the evolution of the pressure sore, indicating the full extent of necrosis.

A pressure sore is a disaster for the patient; it is a source of sepsis, a metabolic drain and hinders rehabilitation (Fig. 14.4).

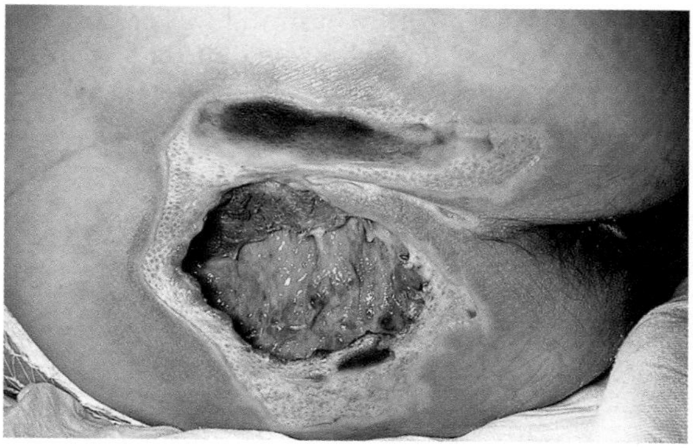

FIG. 14.4 Bedsore.

Temperature

A single temperature reading is of little use unless the patient is hypothermic (aural or rectal temperature below 35°C) or pyrexial (above 37.5°C). Because of the risk of missing a patient with hypothermia the patient's temperature should always be taken with a thermometer with a range extending down to at least 30°C (see Fig. 12.2).

'Normal' temperatures vary widely even in younger individuals; in elderly patients temperatures recorded 6-hourly for 2 or 3 days give the best information. Occasionally elderly patients have systemic infections but normal temperatures. The temperature chart usually shows a rise in base-line temperature.

Blood pressure

There is increasing evidence that treating hypertension in elderly patients helps to prevent cardiac disease and strokes. The acute phase of many illnesses, particularly left ventricular failure and stroke, leads to a sharp rise in blood pressure, which is not an indication for antihypertensive treatment. In acute stroke such treatment may result in reduced cerebral blood flow and a consequent risk of further cerebral thrombosis. In acute stroke antihypertensives should generally be withheld for 2 weeks and then only instituted if hypertension persists.

Of particular importance in the elderly is orthostatic hypotension – a fall in systolic blood pressure of greater than 20 mmHg when the patient rises from lying to standing. There are many causes and the condition may be multifactorial (Revision Panel 14.4). It is useful to take the blood pressure after the patient has been recumbent for 10 minutes and then 30 seconds, 1 minute and 2 minutes after standing. In autonomic failure the pressure at 30 seconds is lowered and remains so at 1 and 2 minutes or may drift even lower due to failure of compensatory peripheral vasoconstriction. If autonomic function is intact the pressure at 30 seconds may be significantly lowered, whereas at 1 and 2 minutes after standing it may be similar to the lying pressure; this may be found with drug-induced hypotension or dehydration and implies that the autonomic system can still compensate. Such a patient may complain of symptoms very soon after standing which settle if the patient holds on to something for about a minute. Characteristic symptoms of orthostatic hypotension are dizziness and faintness on standing; even when these features are absent the patient may exhibit postural unsteadiness and falls. In the early stages of the condition the pressure fall may only be present early in the morning, when circulating blood volume is at its lowest. If the patient has early morning symptoms the blood pressure should be measured when the patient first gets up.

Revision Panel 14.4

Causes of orthostatic hypotension in the elderly

Autonomic dysfunction due to
Age-related changes in physiological mechanisms.
Disease causing change in physiological mechanisms such as:
- diabetic neuropathy,
- cerebrovascular disease,
- Parkinson's disease,
- Shy–Drager syndrome,
- polyneuropathy.

Drug-related
Antihypertensive agents.
Diuretics.
L-Dopa-containing drugs.
Phenothiazines.
Tricyclic antidepressants.
Benzodiazepines.
Nitrates.

Other illnesses
Myocardial infarction.
Pulmonary embolus.
Dehydration and sodium depletion.
Infection.

Incontinence

Any immobile patient unable to ask for help to get to the toilet, due, for example, to dysphasia, fear or dementia, will be incontinent of urine. Two-hourly toileting usually restores continence. Persistent incontinence requires investigation. Common causes of incontinence in the elderly are listed in Revision Panel 14.5.

Bladder size should be assessed. Palpation may suffice, but, in many patients, measurement of the post-micturition volume i.e. after the patient has emptied the bladder, by ultrasonography, either in the X-ray department or with a portable bladder scanner, will be needed to assess impaired bladder emptying.

Revision Panel 14.5
Causes of incontinence in the elderly

Urinary incontinence
Unstable bladder.
Prostatism.
Atrophic vaginitis.
Pelvic floor disease.
Retention with overflow
- faecal impaction,
- drugs,
- prostatism,
- urethral stricture,
- atonic neurogenic bladder.

Acute urinary tract infection – in the presence of one or more of the above factors predisposing a normally continent patient to urinary incontinence.

Acute confusional state.

Psychological factors – e.g. a 'dirty' protest at a social situation that the patient finds unbearable.

Faecal incontinence
Abnormal intestinal activity
- diarrhoea,
- faecal impaction.

Abnormal neurological control
- dementia – unstable rectum, loss of social awareness, neglect of the call to stool with secondary impaction.

Neurological damage to
- spinal cord,
- cauda equina,
- peripheral nerves.

Abnormalities of the pelvic floor
- stretching of the pelvic floor – chronic constipation with straining, longstanding damage from multiple childbirths in women,
- trauma to the anal sphincter.

Psychological factors – e.g. a 'dirty protest'.

The patient may have retention with overflow; this may be due in men to prostatic disease, and in both sexes to faecal impaction. Rectal examination can detect both but if the rectum is empty exclude 'high constipation' by abdominal palpation and X-ray.

Apart from overflow the most common cause of urinary incontinence is the 'unstable bladder', due to loss of higher neurological control in cerebrovascular disease or senile dementia. The incontinence is unpredictable, the patient getting little warning. In multiparous women distinguishing this problem from stress incontinence due to pelvic floor weakness can be difficult, because the unstable bladder often contracts under the stimulus of coughing or standing up ('pseudostress' incontinence). Ask the patient to cough while standing and observe the perineum. In simple stress incontinence only brief leakage occurs while the abdominal pressure (and hence intravesical pressure) exceeds sphincter-closing pressure – the bladder does not contract. In 'pseudostress' incontinence the cough triggers contraction of the unstable bladder resulting in a prolonged urine stream which stops slowly as bladder pressure drops below sphincter pressure.

Faecal incontinence often accompanies the unstable bladder but comes later in the course of the patient's underlying illness. Any patient with faecal incontinence should be examined for faecal impaction and given treatment leading to control of incontinence even in demented patients. Faecal incontinence unassociated with urinary incontinence is usually due to local bowel pathology, most commonly constipation and impaction as well as acute infective diarrhoea, colonic tumours, diverticular disease, inflammatory bowel disease, anal stricture, anal prolapse and malabsorption.

Mobility and gait

Diminished mobility is a major problem for elderly patients. Early gait assessment is invaluable for diagnosis and in defining a baseline to measure progress. Many neurological conditions have characteristic gaits, some of which are described elsewhere. Some changes are very subtle. Slight dragging of a foot may be the only sign of a pyramidal lesion, most commonly a stroke. The dragging may be heard rather than seen – but check that the noise is not due to poorly fitting footwear. An early sign of Parkinson's disease is failure to swing one or both arms when walking.

A useful test of balance is the 'heel–toe' walking test. Get the patient to walk across the room placing the heel of the leading foot in contact with the toes of the trailing foot as if walking a tightrope. The patient should look directly ahead and she must not hang on to any support. In patients who stagger the commonest cause is cerebrovascular disease though other neurological conditions e.g. neuropathies, cerebellar disorders, must be excluded. The patient will stagger to the side with the lesion: for example a patient will stagger towards the side affected by a stroke.

The 'walking-talking' test is useful to determine the likelihood of falling. Get the patient to walk alongside you in an uncluttered area, down an empty corridor. Walk in silence for a few moments to ensure the patient can walk steadily. Then ask the patient a question to which she has to respond. Normally the patient can do so and continue walking. If she has to stop walking while answering she is at significant risk of falling.

In planning rehabilitation the amount of help a patient needs to walk is important: how many helpers are needed, the extent of physical or psychological support they give and what walking aids are required. If the patient cannot walk, can she transfer from bed to chair and back again, and from a wheelchair to the toilet and how much help is required?

Revision Panel 14.6

The Barthel activities of daily living (ADL) index

Activity	*Score*	
Bowels	0	Incontinent or needs enema.
	1	Occasional accident (once a week or less).
	2	Continent.
Bladder	0	Incontinent or catheterized and unable to manage catheter.
	1	Occasional accident (not more than once in 24 hours).
	2	Continent or able to manage catheter unaided.
Grooming	0	Needs help with personal care (face, hair, shaving, teeth).
	1	Independent.
Toilet	0	Dependent.
	1	Needs some help.
	2	Independent (on and off toilet, wiping and dressing).
Feeding	0	Unable.
	1	Needs some help (e.g. cutting up, spreading butter).
	2	Independent.
Transfers	0	Unable – no sitting balance.
	1	Major help (physical from one or two people), can sit.
	2	Minor help (verbal or physical).
	3	Independent.
Mobility	0	Unable.
	1	Wheelchair independent (able to negotiate corners, doors etc.).
	2	Walks with help of one person (verbal or physical).
	3	Independent (with or without walking aid).
Dressing	0	Dependent.
	1	Needs help (can do about half unaided).
	2	Independent (including buttons and zips).
Stairs	0	Unable.
	1	Needs help (verbal, physical or carrying walking aid).
	2	Independent (both up and down).
Bathing	0	Dependent.
	1	Independent (bath and shower unsupervised).

Practical Point

Commonly used aids for the elderly: basic points to note

Walking frames

- For some patients a wheeled frame may be more suitable – less danger of falling backwards – e.g. Parkinson's disease.
- Height of frame – hand grip should come to level of ulnar styloid when patient stands with arms down by sides.

Walking sticks

- Height of stick – handle of stick should come to level of ulnar styloid when patient stands with arms down by sides.
- Tip of the stick should have an unworn rubber ferrule to prevent slipping on the floor.

Wheelchairs

- If the chair has a pneumatic tyres make sure they are fully inflated otherwise it will be difficult to push and the brakes may not work correctly.
- Make sure the brakes are working properly on both sides of the chair. A loss of braking may make the chair unstable and tip over when the patient tries to get out of it.

Activities of daily living

Multidisciplinary assessment of the patient's ability to perform tasks, essential to independent living, aids the planning of rehabilitation and discharge. The Barthel ADL Index is commonly used (Revision Panel 14.6); it measures increasing independence on a scale of 0 to 20. The Index can be used to assess premorbid and current function and to monitor progress during rehabilitation.

Aids and appliances

No examination is complete without assessment of the aids being used: are they the most suitable, safe, and of the correct size? The Practical Point above gives a checklist of common aids.

Revision Panel 14.7

Examination and diagnosis of the elderly

Initial examination of a very elderly person requires great attention to detail and is time-consuming: quite small, simply resolved factors may make the difference in achieving independence.

Even if the patient does not become independent the information collected inevitably plays a vital role in planning on-going care.

Most elderly patients have multiple diseases and problems.

Much of what is important in the care of the elderly centres on solving problems such as falls, immobility, confusion, incontinence, dizziness and the difficulties faced by carers.

Although accurate diagnosis is important, optimizing function, if necessary using aids, appliances and prostheses, is paramount.

15 How to deal with the unconscious patient

Throughout this book, the importance of the history as a major contributor to the final diagnosis has been repeatedly emphasized. When dealing with the unconscious patient, however, the doctor starts at a distinct disadvantage. There is usually no history available from the patient and often little from family and friends. In addition, the relevancy (and reliability) of much of the information which is obtained is difficult to establish. It may be several hours or even days before full and accurate details are known.

In these circumstances, it is essential that the doctor not only remains open-minded about possible diagnoses but also modifies the usual examination routine by:

- Trying to *establish exactly what happened* from a wide range of sources.
- Conducting an *immediate assessment* to rule out life-threatening conditions.
- Conducting a *general examination* looking for specific physical signs.
- Arranging *appropriate investigations* to exclude potential causes for the collapse.
- Proposing a *'working diagnosis'* as the most likely explanation for the collapse.
- *Monitoring* regularly to assess for any change in the patient's status.
- Devising a suitable *management plan* specific to the patient's needs. These seven points will be discussed in detail below.

ESTABLISH EXACTLY WHAT HAPPENED

It is crucial to get as much information as quickly as possible. Much depends on an accurate account of the sequence and timing of events leading up to the collapse and the previous medical history must not be ignored. All possible sources of information must be contacted – friends, relatives and neighbours are obvious examples, but members of the emergency services may also make an important contribution, providing details of the scene of the collapse and any developments while en route to hospital.

Some simple ground rules should be applied (see Revision Panel 15.1).

> Revision Panel 15.1
>
> **Establishing exactly what happened: some ground rules**
>
> *DO*
>
> Ask others to ferret out as much as they can of the circumstances of the episode.
>
> Ask about any recent illnesses.
>
> Enquire about previous complaints and episodes of collapse, however brief.
>
> Look for clues such as hospital out-patient cards or Medi-Alert bracelets or cards.
>
> Keep any tablets or empty bottles that may have been near the patient.
>
> Seek out ambulance crew or police for information they may have.
>
> Contact the patient's family doctor to discuss past history and any recent visits.
>
> *DON'T*
>
> Let witnesses, friends or relatives leave until you have interrogated them fully.
>
> Forget to record their observations.

Revision Panel 15.2
Immediate assessment

Always

Assess A-B-C of airway, breathing and circulation.

Check blood pressure, pulse and respiration.

Make sure gag reflex present.

Commence resuscitation if necessary.

Look for trauma, especially to the head.

Assess depth of unconsciousness.

Check temperature rectally.

Take 5 ml venous blood for a rapid glucose check.

INITIAL IMMEDIATE ASSESSMENT

Always carry out an immediate assessment (see Revision Panel 15.2) as soon as you see the patient. It need only take a few seconds but it will establish the need for prompt life-saving action. Take blood samples at the first opportunity, as later circulatory collapse makes blood taking more difficult. A blood glucose greater than 3 mmol/litre rules out hypoglycaemia; lower than this, give glucagon.

GENERAL EXAMINATION (Fig. 15.1)

You may already have made some useful observations during your initial assessment but now accuracy rather than speed must take over. There are many causes of unconsciousness, but there are a few common ones you should suspect first – drug overdose (whether intentional or not), hypoglycaemia, respiratory failure with carbon dioxide (CO_2) retention, stroke and epilepsy.

General observations

Always check body temperature using a rectal thermometer, or an aural version if one is available. Remember that *hypothermia* is not restricted to winter months in the UK but may be a sign of systemic disease such as hypothyroidism. *Hyperthermia* is a frequent sign of fever but elderly patients may have overwhelming infection without a rise in temperature.

Check the skin for evidence of:

- Cyanosis associated with poor cardiac output or respiratory disease.
- Markers of liver disease such as spider naevi, portal hypertension and jaundice.
- Pigmentation of hypoadrenalism.
- Striae of Cushing's disease.
- Rashes suggestive of septicaemia.
- Cherry-red colour of carbon monoxide poisoning.
- Blisters on the legs induced by barbiturate poisoning (rare today).
- Coarse and dry skin of untreated hypothyroidism.
- Injection sites on abdomen and legs suggestive of insulin treatment in diabetes and forearm 'needle tracks' as evidence of intravenous drug abuse.
- Bee and wasp stings (hard to see) causing profound hypotension and collapse.

Respiration is often depressed in the unconscious. Distinctive respiratory patterns may be seen in systemic disease localized to the brain stem:

- In Cheyne–Strokes respiration, breathing starts quietly, increases gradually, reaches a peak and then stops abruptly for a few seconds before the cycle starts again. This may be the result of dysfunction within the cerebrum or the brainstem, CO_2 retention from chronic lung disease, coma due to a metabolic disorder such as diabetes mellitus or left ventricular failure.
- Deep, sighing hyperventilation may occur in diabetic ketoacidosis and in uraemia where it is acidosis-driven (Kussmaul respiration) or in neurological disease affecting the pons.
- Shallow, inconsistent breathing indicates disease affecting the respiratory centre in the brainstem and is pre-terminal.

While watching the pattern of breathing, the distinctive 'pear drops' smell of ketones may become apparent. The ability to smell ketones is genetically acquired and you either can or you can't! Also obvious may be the characteristic smell of alcohol and the sweet breath of liver failure.

Cardiovascular status

Blood pressure, heart rate and rhythm and jugular venous pressure should be checked. Coronary disease and cerebrovascular disease are closely associated, so if there is a sternal scar, consider a stroke resulting from an embolus from atrial or ventricular thrombus in those with coronary disease, or resulting from over- or under-anticoagulation after valve replacement.

Neurological status

Neurological examination is part of the routine medical examination. Brain dysfunction is a frequent cause of collapse and unconsciousness, so there is no room for short cuts. Neurological examination must be complete and thorough.

Starting at the head, check for trauma and check the ears and nose for signs of bleeding.

A stiff neck indicates meningeal irritation from meningitis or subarachnoid haemorrhage.

Careful examination of pupil size and reaction to light is important (Fig. 15.2).

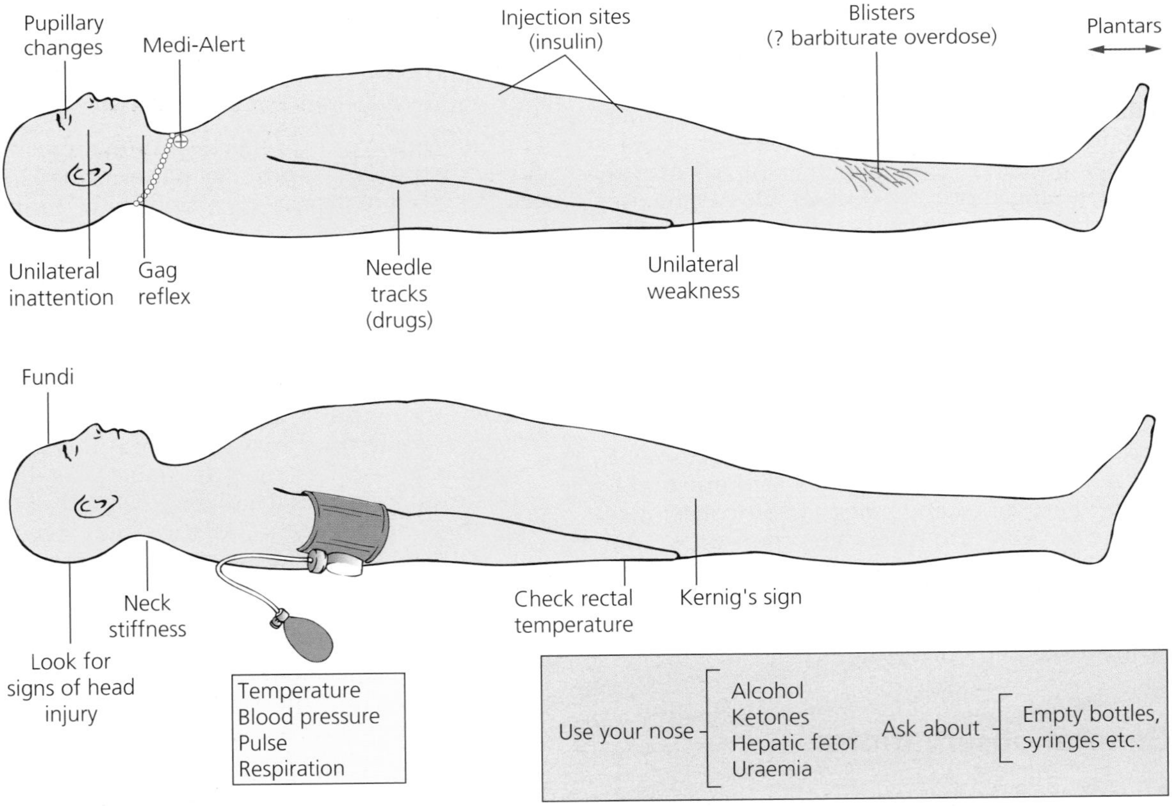

FIG. 15.1 Diagram of what to look for in the unconscious patient.

- A single pupil which does not respond to light is a neurosurgical emergency. The brain is under increased pressure and the brainstem and cerebellum forced ('coned') through the foramen magnum, stretching the IIIrd cranial nerve (hence the dilated pupil).
- Both pupils appearing as 'pinpoints' may indicate haemorrhage into the pons or overdose with opiates such as heroin.
- Both pupils mildly dilated but unresponsive to light means damage to the midbrain so that the pupillary light reflex is interrupted.
- A single constricted pupil with eyelid drooping ('ptosis') is Horner's syndrome which follows disruption of the sympathetic nerve supply to the eye.
- Fixed dilated pupils are seen in deeply unconscious patients in barbiturate overdose and in hypothermia. They are also one of the signs of brain death.

Practical Point

A warning

Get expert help at once if you suspect 'coning'.

Eye movements should be checked carefully:

- Slow and roving eyes are seen in light coma.
- Sustained ('conjugate') gaze to one side is obvious when damage is confined to a single hemisphere. The eyes look towards the damaged hemisphere (and so towards the normal limbs) in lesions affecting the supranuclear pathways and away from the affected hemisphere (and so towards the paralysed side) in lesions of the pons.
- Doll's head reflex is a normal response. When the head is turned passively to one side, both eyes turn in the opposite direction. This reflex is lost in deep coma and brainstem lesions. It is also absent in brain death.
- Caloric vestibular-ocular reflex is also a normal response. When ice-cold water is poured into the external auditory meatus, both eyes turn towards the side being irri-

Practical Point

A warning

Never give drugs which may affect pupil reflexes in patients with any impairment of consciousness until you have sought expert advice.

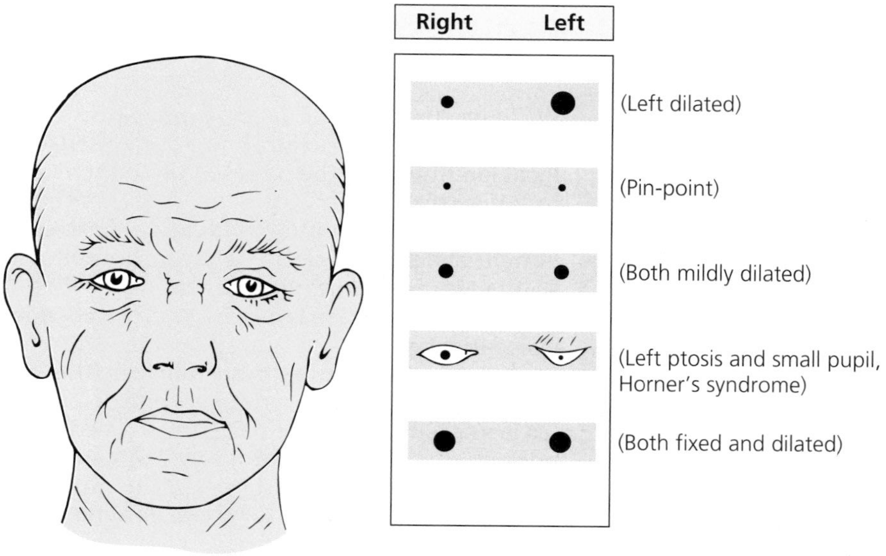

FIG. 15.2 Pupillary changes in the unconscious patient.

gated. In brainstem disease, the reflex is lost. It is also absent in brain death.

- Sudden downward bobbing eye movements are seen in bleeding into the pons or cerebellum.

Motor responses are difficult to assess in the unconscious patient but there are several simple tests which are useful:

- Facial droop implies a hemiplegia.
- Muscle tone may be increased or decreased on one side suggesting damage to one hemisphere.
- Response to painful stimuli may be greater on one side than the other.
- Visual threat by rapidly moving the hand towards one side of the face as if to strike it usually invokes a blink response. If this is lost, the patient has at least visual attention on one side and so has a hemianopia.
- Tendon reflexes may be absent on one side indicating a hemiplegia.
- Plantar reflex is often extensor in coma.
- Abnormal postures may be adopted in response to painful stimuli. A patient who extends both arms and both legs in response to pain is more deeply unconscious than a patient who responds by flexing all the limbs.

'Surgical' causes of collapse should also be considered. Always check the abdomen for tenderness and bowel sounds – perforated ulcer, pancreatitis and ruptured abdominal aneurysm may present with collapse.

APPROPRIATE INVESTIGATIONS

The purpose of investigations is to establish a cause for the collapse. Knowledge of the most common causes makes ordering of tests easier than speculative and wasteful investigation. The following is a brief list only:

- Full blood count – a raised white count may indicate infection.
- Urea, sodium, potassium, calcium and liver function.
- Drug screen – paracetamol and salicylates, and an extra 20 ml for more tests if needed.
- Cortisol and thyroid function.
- Blood cultures.
- Lumbar puncture – only if meningitis or encephalitis is suspected and brain scan has excluded an intracranial mass. This avoids precipitating lethal coning.
- CT (computed tomography) or MRI (magnetic resonance imaging) brain scan may be necessary. A patient on a ventilator can still undergo a brain scan.

Monitoring progress

It is important to have a means of determining whether the patient is improving or deteriorating. Repeating all the above tests every hour or so would be too time-consuming so the Glasgow coma scale, shown in Revision Panel 15.3, has been devised and has been widely adopted. By checking specific responses to command or to painful stimuli, it is easy to document the patient's clinical state and to recognize any change, whether for better or worse. Painful stimuli include extreme pressure on the sternum or nail beds and pressure over the supraorbital ridges.

Recording is straightforward and provides an instant visual presentation of the patient's recent and current status. A patient may be admitted deeply unconscious with an initial coma score of 3, but over the next few hours, the patient's condition may improve, reflected in an increasing coma score.

MANAGEMENT PLAN

Whether the patient is best managed on a medical or neurosurgical ward depends on local facilities and the needs of the patient, but in all cases, careful nursing and continual monitoring are essential to identify changes in patient status, especially deterioration of consciousness level and vital functions.

Particularly important are care of the skin, eyes and mouth. Fluid replacement can be assessed by estimating insensible loss (this can be in excess of 2 litres a day) and urine output (catheterization will be necessary). Feeding is not usually necessary for a few days.

If a cause is identified, appropriate treatment can be commenced but for some patients, little is required other than nursing care.

Revision Panel 15.3
The Glasgow coma scale

ASSESSMENT	*SCORE*
Eye movements (E)	
Spontaneous	4
In response to speech	3
In response to pain	2
None	1
Motor response (M)	
Obeys command	6
Localizes	5
Withdraws	4
Abnormal flexion	3
Extensor response	2
None	1
Verbal response (R)	
Orientated	5
Confused	4
Conversation	3
Inappropriate words	2
Incomprehensible sounds	1
None	

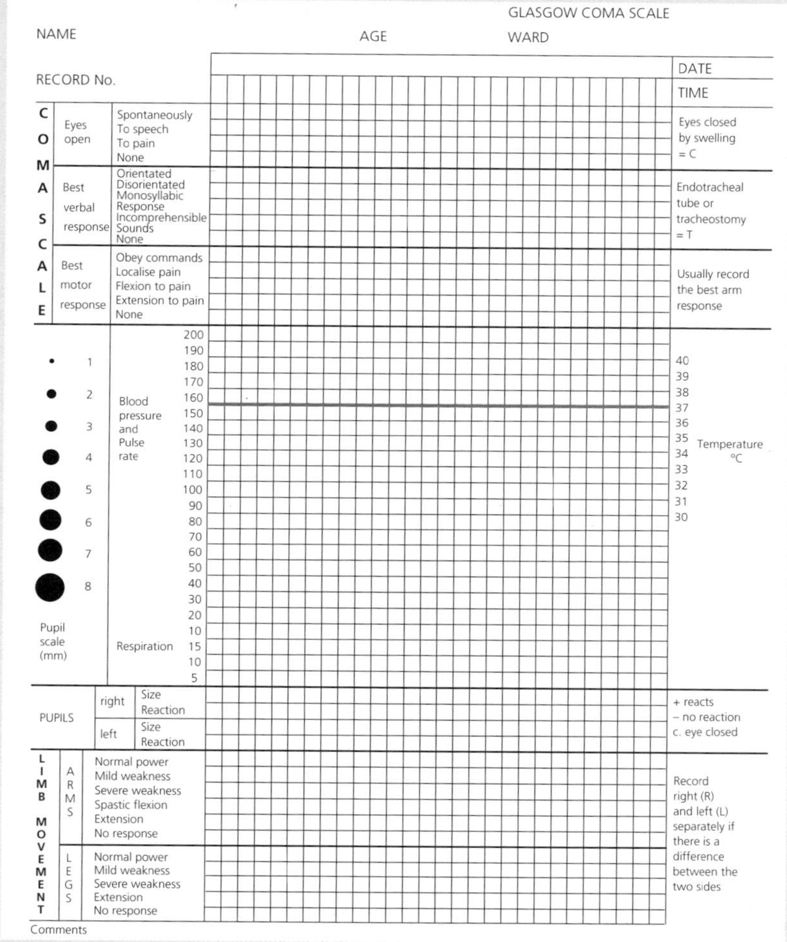

GLASGOW COMA SCALE
NAME
AGE
WARD
RECORD No.
DATE
TIME
COMA SCALE
Eyes open
Spontaneously
To speech
To pain
None
Eyes closed by swelling = C
Best verbal response
Orientated
Disorientated
Monosyllabic Response
Incomprehensible Sounds
None
Endotracheal tube or tracheostomy = T
Best motor response
Obey commands
Localise pain
Flexion to pain
Extension to pain
None
Usually record the best arm response
1 2 3 4 5 6 7 8
Pupil scale (mm)
Blood pressure and Pulse rate
200 190 180 170 160 150 140 130 120 110 100 90 80 70 60 50 40 30 20 10
Respiration
15 10 5
40 39 38 37 36 35 34 33 32 31 30
Temperature °C
PUPILS
right
left
Size
Reaction
+ reacts
– no reaction
c. eye closed
LIMB MOVEMENT
ARMS
Normal power
Mild weakness
Severe weakness
Spastic flexion
Extension
No response
LEGS
Normal power
Mild weakness
Severe weakness
Extension
No response
Record right (R) and left (L) separately if there is a difference between the two sides
Comments

Major causes of unconsciousness

- With drug overdose and poisoning, 20% of patients are unconscious on arrival at hospital. Most take any drugs lying around, washed down with alcohol. Aspirin, paracetamol, hypnotics and antidepressants are widely available.
- Hypo- and hyperglycaemia and metabolic acidosis.
- Major organ failure (liver, kidney and respiratory failure with CO_2 retention).
- Meningoencephalitis, trauma, abscess, haematoma, hypoxic, ischaemic and hypertensive cortical and midbrain injury and subarachnoid haemorrhage.
- Demyelination, neoplasm and haemorrhage affecting the brainstem.
- Disturbances of calcium, sodium and potassium.
- Pituitary, adrenal and thyroid disease.
- Hypothermia.

BRAIN DEATH

Brainstem functions are essential to support life. At some point, doctors may decide to determine whether the brainstem is functioning and can maintain life. Patients who remain unconscious and unresponsive and who are being ventilated may be thought to have sustained 'irreversible loss of the capacity for consciousness combined with the irreversible loss of the capacity to breathe'.

Irreversible brain damage may leave a patient 'brain dead' but with a beating heart capable of maintaining the circulation.

Certain preconditions must be met before any tests for brain death can be considered:

- The cause of coma must be known and be irreversible.
- Hypothermia and metabolic and pharmacological (including muscle relaxants and alcohol) causes of coma must be excluded.

Two tests are conducted 24 hours apart by senior doctors (those who have been registered for five years or more). One doctor must be independent of the team looking after the patient.

To make a diagnosis of brain death, the doctor will check the following:

- Absence of response to pain both peripherally and centrally.
- Pupils will be fixed in response to a bright light.
- Eye movements are absent both on turning the head (see the doll's head manoeuvre) and when the ears are irrigated with cold water.
- Corneal reflex is absent.
- On stimulating the pharynx with a suction tube, the gag reflex is absent.
- On stimulating the larynx with a spatula, there is no cough reflex.
- There are no respiratory efforts.

Artificial ventilation is switched off and the partial pressure of CO_2 allowed to rise to provide a stimulus to the brainstem, but note that:

- Before the test, ventilation for 5 minutes with 5% CO_2 and 95% O_2 is given to ensure adequate stimulation to the respiratory centre while avoiding hypoxia;
- Oxygen must be given during testing via a tracheal cannula at 6 litres per minute.

Once brain death has been confirmed, the ventilator may be switched off. Your responsibility is now to support the family as much as you can and allow them to sit at the bedside as long as they wish.

Revision Panel 15.4

Summary: Assessing the unconscious patient

Try to establish history using information from all available sources.

Make a quick initial assessment to see if cardiopulmonary resuscitation is needed.

Carry out a more detailed general examination looking for specific causes.

Investigate for most frequent causes of unconsciousness first.

Assess and record degree of unconsciousness on Glasgow coma scale.

Propose a 'working diagnosis' based on the most likely cause of collapse.

Monitor changes in conscious level on the Glasgow Coma Scale.

Devise a suitable management plan.

Eye problems for the non-specialist

16

The eye may be the site for early signs of disease elsewhere in the body. This is because you can examine directly nerve tissue and blood vessels in and around the eye. However, before making a diagnosis of systemic disease from eye signs it is often important to exclude disease limited to the eye itself. For example, before embarking on invasive investigations of an unusual defect in the visual field, you must exclude the possibility of a retinal detachment.

Many sophisticated and ingenious instruments are now part of the ophthalmologist's armamentarium, but it is still possible for you to make useful observations without any instruments apart from the ophthalmoscope. In this chapter the types of systemic disease that manifest themselves in the eye are considered, but you need to remember that many eye signs may be due to disease of the eye itself, such as cataract, glaucoma and macular degeneration. These three conditions are very common in elderly patients and their recognition can lead to cure of blindness or preservation of vision.

Practical Point

Cataract, glaucoma and macular degeneration are common in the elderly and their correct evaluation can lead to preservation of vision.

EYE SIGNS WITHOUT INSTRUMENTS

Changes in the eyelids

Swelling of the eyelids may be:

- The result of oedema occurring overnight in a middle-aged person without obvious systemic upset.
- Due to either hypo- or hyperthyroidism (see Fig. 10.6).
- A feature of renal disease, heart failure or superior vena caval obstruction.
- The result of an acute systemic hypersensitivity reaction, for example after an injection of penicillin.
- A rare complication of sarcoidosis or lymphoma (where the swelling is firm).
- Atopic eczema and psoriasis where they are usually part of a more obvious generalized skin disease.
- Occasionally erysipelas, a rare but potentially serious cause of bilateral lid swelling with inflammation.

Xanthelasma (see Fig. 4.4) is a common yellowish deposit seen in the elderly usually affecting the skin of the eyelids and may be associated with hypercholesterolaemia.

Staphylococcal infection of the lash follicles and accessory glands of the lid margins can commonly cause lid swelling and redness. A 'stye' is an infection of the lash follicle and a 'chalazion' is a small cyst in the eyelid resulting from infection of a meibomian gland.

Herpes zoster should always be kept in mind especially if there is associated headache, but the development of a rash usually accompanies or precedes the swelling (see Fig. 7.10).

A capillary haemangioma of the eyelids and side of the face known as the 'port wine stain' may be part of the Sturge–Weber syndrome. Such individuals suffer glaucoma in association with meningeal haemangiomata and need specialist investigation (Fig. 16.1).

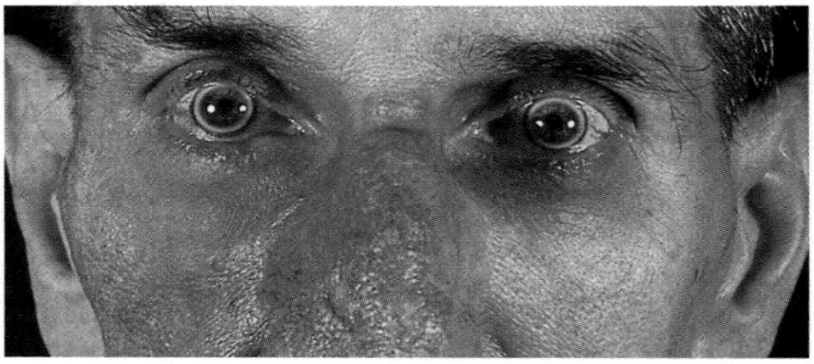

FIG. 16.1 Sturge–Weber syndrome. When the 'port wine stain' covers the upper part of the face the eyes should be examined for glaucoma. Note also the arcus senilis.

Proptosis and exophthalmosis

Forward protrusion of the globe is called proptosis. There are many causes of proptosis, hyperthyroidism being common, but symptomless unilateral proptosis should alert you to the possibility of an orbital neoplasm (Fig. 16.2). Sometimes one eye is larger than the other giving the false impression of proptosis. The larger eye is myopic and thus the diagnosis of an abnormally large eye can be made by refraction (measurement for spectacles).

Exophthalmos also means forward protrusion of the eyes but the term is usually restricted to the appearance seen in ophthalmic Graves' disease.

You should assess proptosis by standing behind the seated patient and looking down and comparing the position of the globes from above. This simple method avoids mistaking widening of the eyelids on one side from true proptosis. Remember that the palpebral aperture becomes narrower with age and the position of the lids becomes lower in relation to the globe (see Revision Panel 16.1).

Practical Point

Symptomless unilateral proptosis may be due to a retro-orbital tumour.

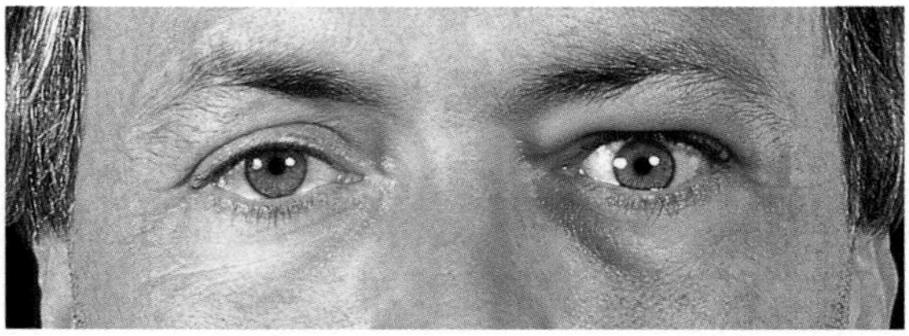

FIG. 16.2 Unilateral proptosis due to a retro-orbital tumour.

Revision Panel 16.1
Causes of proptosis

Basic disorder	*Features*
Muscle palsy	About 1–2 mm of proptosis accompanies palsies of the extraocular muscles.
Infection	Orbital cellulitis is usually secondary to adjacent sinusitis. Needs urgent investigation.
Thyrotoxicosis	Commonest cause of unilateral or bilateral proptosis; look for other eye signs.
Trauma	Retro-orbital haemorrhage.
Tumour	Haemangioma commonest but other tumours such as meningiomas may occur.
Pseudotumour	A localized, chronic, inflammatory swelling of unknown cause.
Mucocele of sinuses	
Lymphomatous tumours	

Swellings of the lachrymal glands and sac

Unilateral swelling of a lachrymal gland may be caused by neoplasms, for example carcinoma or lymphoma. Bilateral swelling is not uncommon as with Sjogren's syndrome (dry eyes and rheumatoid arthritis) or sarcoidosis. Dacryocystitis or inflammation of the lachrymal sac causes a red tender swelling below the inner canthus (Fig. 16.3).

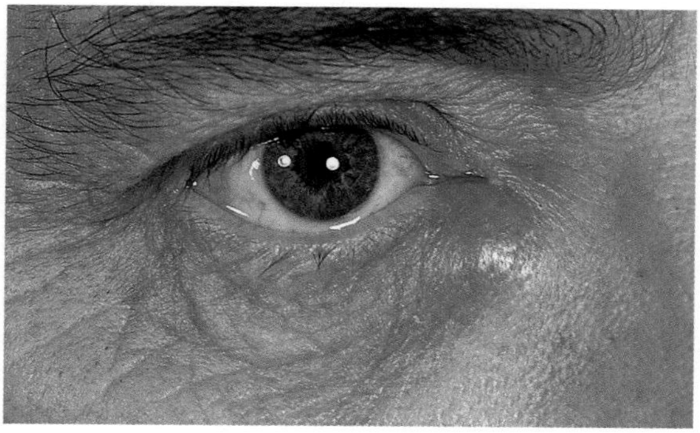

FIG. 16.3 Acute dacryocystitis. Note the redness and swelling at the inner corner of the eye.

Changes of the conjunctiva and sclera

Remember that the appearance of the 'white' of the eye is not only dependent on the colour of the sclera but also on changes in the overlying bulbar conjunctiva. The bulbar conjunctiva covers the globe of the eye and is continuous with the palpebral conjunctiva which lines the inside of the eyelids.

The palpebral conjunctiva of the lower eyelid can give some indication of anaemia. Jaundice even when slight may be evident as yellowing of the bulbar conjunctiva and of the sclera. When the conjunctiva is oedematous, the thickened, glistening membrane can bulge slightly at the lid margin giving the impression that the eyes are brimming with tears (chemosis). This 'tear that never drops' is seen in thyrotoxicosis and in other oedematous states such as heart failure.

The red eye in systemic disease

Subconjunctival haemorrhage Spontaneous leakage of blood subconjunctivally is a common cause of a sudden red eye; usually the individual is otherwise healthy. Recurrent subconjunctival haemorrhages should make you suspect diabetes mellitus or blood dyscrasias. Vomiting, strangulation or extreme respiratory effort may cause subconjunctival haemorrhages (Fig. 16.4).

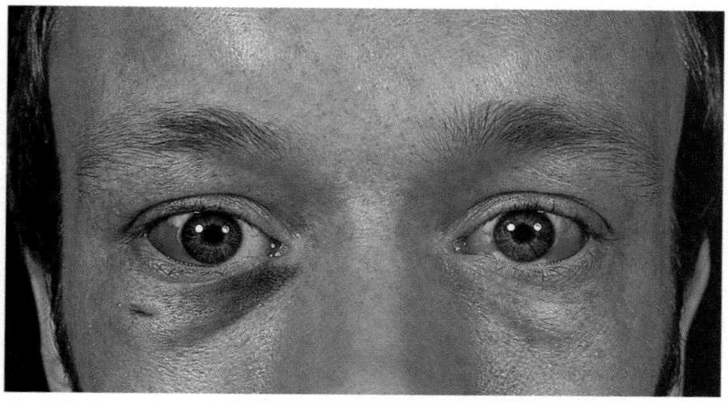

FIG. 16.4 Subconjunctival haemorrhages after an episode of cardiorespiratory arrest.

Episcleritis This terms refers to an inflammation of the connective tissue underlying the conjunctiva. It tends to be more painful than conjunctivitis and there is no purulent discharge. Episcleritis may be an important sign of rheumatoid arthritis. It is seen in certain other diseases of joints and connective tissue, in particular Reiter's syndrome. Less commonly the sclera may be involved in a similar inflammatory process known as scleritis. This tends to be very painful and in severe cases may lead to necrosis of the sclera. After healing, the thin areas of sclera appear bluish black.

Associated with skin diseases, red eye may occur with:

- Atopic eczema which may be associated with disease of the skin of the eyelids and occasional involvement of the eye itself.
- Allergic conjunctivitis. The eyelids thicken and the lashes disappear after years of recurrent irritation and scaling of the skin.
- Acne rosacea.

Keratoconjunctivitis This is inflammation of the cornea and conjunctiva, which may be due to inadequate tear secretion or failure to close the eyes properly when blinking or during sleep. This can happen in thyrotoxic eye disease or with a VIIth cranial nerve palsy.

Other miscellaneous causes of red eye include

- Polycythaemia.
- Chronic alcoholism (due to dilatation of the conjunctival vessels).
- Renal failure.
- Attacks of migraine (on the affected side during attacks of headache) (see Fig. 26.2).
- Permanent telangiectasia of the conjunctiva as in ataxia telangiectasia and the Osler–Weber–Rendu syndrome (see Fig. 6.4).

> **Practical Point**
>
> Never forget the possibility of intraocular causes, for example glaucoma and iridocyclitis, causing red eye. These may lead to blindness unless treated promptly.

Blue sclera

The normal white of the eye takes on a bluish hue if the sclera is thin allowing the underlying dark pigment to show through. Patients with severe rheumatoid arthritis and previous scleritis can be seen to have bluish slightly raised areas on the sclera. This is usually seen by raising the upper eyelid. A general bluish appearance is sometimes seen in the Ehlers–Danlos syndrome, a generalized inherited disorder of connective tissue, causing hyperelasticity of the skin and hypermobility of the joints. Blueness of the sclera is also a feature of fragilitas ossium or brittle bone disease.

Brown sclera and conjunctiva

Diffuse flat, brown pigmentation may be due to precancerous melanosis of the conjunctiva. In fact this type of pigmentation may be observed for many years without evidence of malignancy. Ochronosis is an exceptionally rare disorder of the metabolism of homogentisic acid. A brown black pigment derived from homogentisic acid is deposited in the tissues including the cornea and sclera.

Extraocular muscle weakness

Test eye movements by asking your patient to follow a light or the tip of a pencil into the cardinal positions of gaze. One eye may appear to be off-line and the eyes may fail to move together i.e. a squint becomes obvious but this does not necessarily indicate any muscle weakness. In fact most cases of childhood squint show a full range of eye movements and are due to a failure of coordination between convergence and accommodation.

When a patient presents with a squint due to eye muscle weakness then a more serious underlying cause must be suspected.

> **Practical Point**
>
> An acute squint developing in adult life is likely to be due to serious underlying disease.

Squint occurring suddenly in adult life may occasionally be due to the breakdown of a longstanding muscle balance problem but it is more likely to be due to a cranial nerve palsy and demands urgent investigation. Such squints of sudden onset are accompanied by diplopia. If the diplopia becomes worse during the day or when tired then myasthenia gravis may be the underlying cause especially if accompanied by ptosis. Systemic causes of acquired weakness of eye muscles are shown in the Revision Panel 16.2.

Revision Panel 16.2

Systemic causes of acquired weakness of eye muscle

Muscle disease
Thyrotoxic eye disease.
Myasthenia gravis.

Nerve lesions
Vascular, hypertension, diabetes.
Intracranial space-occupying lesion.
Non-localizing effect of raised intracranial pressure.
Trauma.
Multiple sclerosis.

Nystagmus (see also Chapters 7 and 17)

Simple testing of eye movements will reveal the presence of nystagmus if this was not evident on first seeing the patient. In general terms:

- Nystagmus of an irregular type, rotary or horizontal, present in all positions of gaze, without the subjective sensation of movement is congenital in type. Further ophthalmological examination is needed because there are often other abnormalities in the eyes.
- Nystagmus on lateral gaze may indicate muscle weakness but unsustained nystagmus in extremes of gaze may be seen in otherwise normal individuals.
- Persistent nystagmus on lateral or vertical gaze is always a suspicious sign of more generalized neurological disease.

Ptosis

Drooping of one or both eyelids (ptosis) is commonly congenital but acquired ptosis is often an important sign of systemic disease (see Fig. 16.5). The main causes are summarized in Revision Panel 16.3. The ptosis associated with sympathetic nerve damage is very slight (as in Horner's syndrome) and may be missed unless you look carefully.

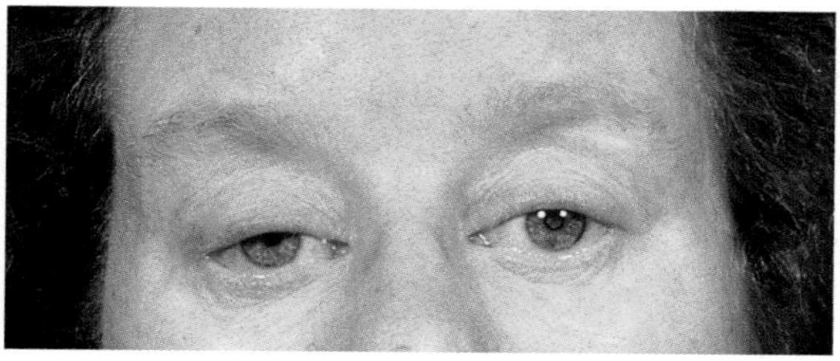

FIG. 16.5 Ptosis in a patient with myotonic dystrophy.

Pupillary changes

An abnormal pupil reaction is perhaps the most important of all systemic signs in the eye (Fig. 16.6). The normal pupil reaction is present at birth but the small pupils in early infancy make testing difficult. Older children have larger pupils and the size then diminishes slowly into old age. The pupils dilate with excitement and constrict during sleep or general anaesthesia. Morphine addicts have small pupils.

When testing the pupils look for:

- Initial size and any irregularity.
- Reaction to direct light and consensual stimulation.
- The reaction to accommodation.

Revision Panel 16.3

Causes of ptosis

Congenital	
Myogenic	Myasthenia gravis (and other myopathies).
Neurogenic	Sympathetic (Horner's). IIIrd nerve palsy. Any lesion in the pathway of these nerves.
Mechanical	Inflammation, redundant skin.
Pseudoptosis	Small eye, atrophic eye, lid retraction on other side.

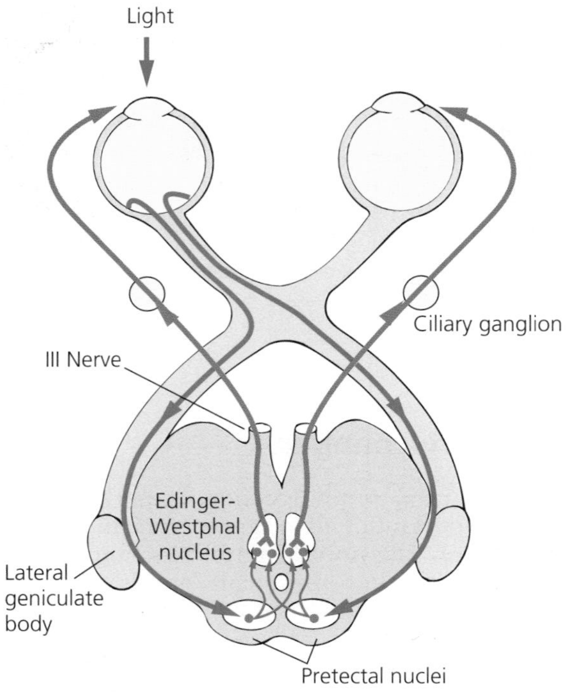

FIG. 16.6 The pupillary pathway. The afferent fibres for the pupillary light reflexes (dark red/brown) run in the optic nerves and the optic tracts. They synapse in the pretectal nucleus where the second neuronal fibres arise. These then link with the ipsilateral and contralateral Edinger–Westphal nuclei. The pupilloconstrictor fibres (green) then pass in the IIIrd nerve to the ciliary ganglion.

The pupil reaction can be an important measure of conduction in the optic nerve. A unilateral afferent defect is best detected by swinging the light from normal to affected eye. The pupils will dilate as the light is moved across. This is sometimes called the 'swinging flashlight test'. Since the direct pupil reaction is a response to light rather than one to formed images, it is unimpaired by opaque media in the eye. Localized retinal damage may not impair the pupil reaction unless it is localized to the macular region. Optic nerve damage on the other hand may cause an afferent pupillary defect out of proportion to the loss of vision. It is an important sign in the diagnosis of optic neuritis.

The non-reactive pupil

When a pupil fails to react, test it in a dark room. It is worth remembering that:

- The small pupils of an elderly patient may appear to be non-reactive to the naked eye when tested in daylight.
- The pupils of diabetic patients may be small and show little reaction owing to autonomic degeneration.
- Patients who have suffered chronic iridocyclitis may have adhesions between iris and lens, which prevent the normal movement of the iris.

The abnormally dilated pupil

Unilateral mydriasis may be due to:

- Locally administered eye drops – the commonest cause.
- Holmes–Adie syndrome. This condition is most common in young women. The affected pupil is usually dilated and contracts very slowly in response to direct and indirect stimulation. In bright light the pupil may be constricted on the affected side and take up to half an hour to dilate in the dark. This tonic pupil reaction may be combined with absent tendon jerks in the limbs. After a delay of months or years the other eye may become affected. The overall disability is minimal.
- Acute narrow-angle glaucoma which can occasionally present as a dilated pupil without very much pain in the eye.
- IIIrd nerve palsy. Since the nerve fibres, which cause constriction of the pupil, are conveyed in the oculomotor nerve, oculomotor palsy if complete is associated with mydriasis. For this reason dilatation of the pupil may be a sign of raised intracranial pressure after head injury.
- One pupil being larger than the other as a congenital anomaly. Both usually react normally under these circumstances.

The abnormally constricted pupil

Possible causes are:

- Use of miotic drops for glaucoma. These are still used occasionally for the treatment of glaucoma though most current treatments do not constrict the pupil.
- Horner's syndrome. The total syndrome comprises miosis, narrowing of the palpebral fissure owing to paralysis of the muscle in the eyelids, loss of sweating on the affected side of the forehead and a slight reduction of the intraocular pressure. When a constricted pupil on one side is seen always check carefully the position of the eyelids. Horner's syndrome may be caused by a wide diversity of lesions anywhere along the sympathetic pathway but quite often it is seen without any detectable underlying cause.
- The Argyll–Robertson pupil – a rare but well known example of the small pupil which responds to accommodation but not to direct light. This type of pupil reaction was originally described as being due to neurosyphilis but now is much more frequently seen in diabetics.

Iris colour

The normal iris may vary in colour from blue or green to brown and the exact pattern of pigmentation is a subtle facial characteristic. At birth the iris has a slate grey colour achieving its adult colour after about 6 months. Heavily pigmented irises are brown and minimally pigmented ones are blue.

Changes in colour of the iris are usually significant. The blue iris may turn brown after treatment for glaucoma with latanoprost eye drops and the brown iris may turn blue/grey after chronic iridocyclitis. Certain other disease states can alter the iris colour. Intraocular haemorrhage can give the iris a green tinge and siderosis from a retained intraocular foreign body may turn the iris brown. A severely ischaemic eye as seen occasionally in diabetes or following a retinal vein occlusion may show a pinkish coloured iris due to the spread of fine new vessels across its anterior surface (rubeosis iridis). Albino subjects have blue eyes but the irides can be shown to transilluminate by shining a torch along the line of view through the pupil. In Down's syndrome a series of white nodules are usually seen arranged around the iris. They are known as Brushfield's spots and are occasionally seen in normal subjects. Patients with Von Recklinghausen's disease (neurofibromatosis) show a number of brown, neurofibromatous nodules on the iris known as Lisch nodules.

EYE SIGNS WITH BASIC INSTRUMENTS

Visual acuity measurement

The non-specialist sometimes overlooks this basic and important test of vision and yet the patient's own report of visual status may sometimes be proved to be erroneous once the visual acuity has been measured. A series of different sized letters are presented on a chart at 6 metres. A normal-sighted person at 60 metres should see the largest letter at the top. If a patient can only see the top letter, the vision is denoted as '6/60'. A normal-sighted person would be expected to see the smaller letters at 6 metres, the visual acuity being given as 6/6 or even better at 6/5 or 6/4. It is obviously important to quantify a patient's visual symptoms in this way, but quite often the eyesight is threatened by loss of the peripheral field of vision. When this happens the visual acuity may remain normal even with gross constriction of the field. This is because the central five degrees of the field is specialized to detect fine detail.

Visual field testing

The simplest way to test the field is by confrontation. Tell your patient to cover one eye with a hand and then cover your own eye with your hand so that the patient's field can be compared with your own. Ask the patient to say 'yes' if he can see fine movements of your fingers. The test can be made more accurate by using a pin with a red head on it as a target.

However, none of the confrontation techniques can match the accuracy of formal perimetry. The Humphrey perimeter is the most widely used and versatile instrument in hospital practice. The pattern of a visual field defect gives useful localizing information for lesions in the visual pathway and retina (see Fig. 7.5).

- Lesions in the optic nerve anterior to the chiasma cause unilateral defects because the right half of each retina is linked by nerves to the right half of the occipital cortex and because fibres from the nasal half of each retina cross at the optic chiasma.
- Lesions posterior to the chiasma produce hemianopic or quadrantic defects.
- Lesions of the occipital cortex tend to be more congruous i.e. similar on each side. Cortical lesions also show better preservation of central vision (macular sparing).
- With expanding pituitary tumours, the resulting pressure on the centre of the chiasma produces a bitemporal defect.

Localized defects in the retina produce equivalent localized defects in the visual field. Defects due to retinal disease are relatively common, for example due to glaucoma in the elderly. It is surprising how patients may fail to notice quite extensive loss of the peripheral field. Hemianopic patients may continue to drive in spite of the risks to life and limb because they are unaware of the extent of their problem.

Ophthalmoscopy

The study of eye disease was revolutionized by the invention of the ophthalmoscope in 1850 by Herman Von Helmholtz. The problem may seem simple enough to us today; it is that of trying to look into a dark cupboard through the keyhole. As soon as one's eye is placed in front of the keyhole no light enters the cupboard. The secret is to look along a beam of light. This can be achieved by looking through a hole in a tilted mirror. The modern instrument (Fig. 16.7) incorporates a battery, preferably rechargeable, a bulb preferably halogen, a small mirror and a set of minute lenses which can be interposed to allow for the spectacle correction of patient and observer. Rotating the knurled rim of a disc in which the lenses are fitted does this.

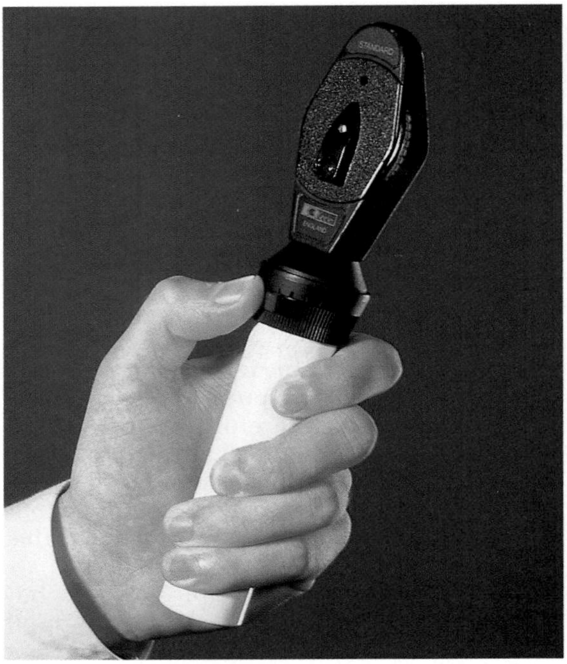

FIG. 16.7 The ophthalmoscope.

You must learn how to use the ophthalmoscope efficiently and effectively:

- Ask your patient to sit in a chair and to look straight forward.
- Hold the instrument vertically and at first view the eye from a distance of about 2 feet.
- Then go close in (Fig. 16.8).
- Hold the instrument in your right hand and using your right eye view the patient's right eye.
- Conversely, use your left hand and left eye to view the patient's left eye.

Learn to do it this way; otherwise noses come into contact in an embarrassing way. You need to start the examination at a distance to view the optical media against the red reflex. This is

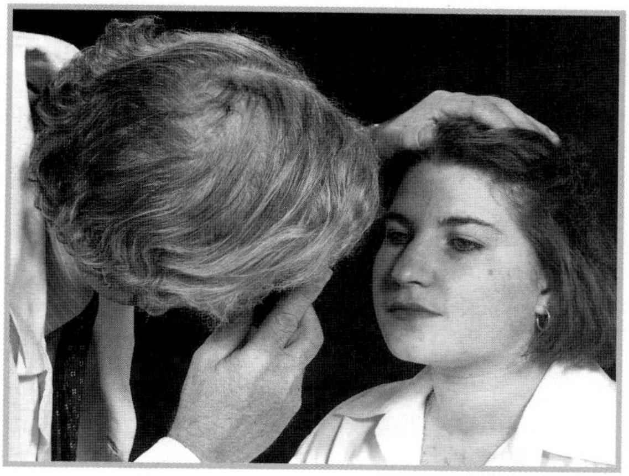

FIG. 16.8 Ophthalmoscopy. Note, right eye to patient's right eye; left eye to patient's left eye.

the best way of detecting opacities in the cornea, lens or vitreous and especially cataract.

It is useful to have a routine method of examination:

Look for the optic disc This is situated slightly medial (nasal) to the posterior pole of the eye and slightly above the horizontal meridian.

Follow the vessels Upper and lower branches of the central retinal vessels divide into nasal and temporal so that each of the four branches should be followed out to the periphery in turn.

Look at the fovea Simply ask the patient to look at the light. The fovea can only be properly seen with the pupil dilated. It appears as a minute dot with yellowish surrounding pigment.

Look at the background Scan the optic fundus between the vessels noting any abnormalities such as haemorrhages, exudates or abnormal pigmentation. The choroidal vasculature outside and beyond the retinal vessels can be seen in many normal fundi.

Look at the periphery Ask the patient to look to the extremes of gaze and dial a 'plus lens' on the ophthalmoscope. The examination of the peripheral fundus is critical in routine ophthalmoscopy but demands more time and skill than examination of the posterior pole.

When learning ophthalmoscopy there are two main problems. First, the field of view is quite small and serial pictures of the fundus must be put together in one's mind. Second, reflections of light from the cornea can seem a nuisance and at first interfere with the view. Practice and proper coordination of hand and eye gradually eliminate these difficulties.

The laser-scanning ophthalmoscope is now available. This instrument gives a television picture of the fundus of the eye which can be stored on disc and studied on a visual display unit (VDU); the student of the future may not even need to learn ophthalmoscopy once such instruments become readily available.

OPHTHALMOSCOPIC APPEARANCES OF SYSTEMIC DISEASE

Cardiovascular system

Changes in the retinal vessels reflect the rate of progression and severity of systemic hypertension. Irregularity of arteriolar calibre and tortuosity of the perimacular arterioles is an early sign. The light reflex from the walls of the arterioles is heightened giving the description of 'silver wiring'. Nipping of the veins at the point of crossover of an arteriole is also an important early sign. In patients with accelerated hypertension the retinal arterioles become more markedly narrowed and irregular, and hard exudates may appear radiating from the macular to give the appearance of a macular star. Soft exudates (cotton wool spots) indicate the presence of infarcts in the nerve fibre layer. Papilloedema is present in severe cases (see Fig. 2.14).

Central retinal artery occlusion (Fig. 16.9) presents as sudden loss of vision in one eye and the retina looks pale and oedematous with grossly narrowed arterioles. The macular region may stand out as a normal red colour

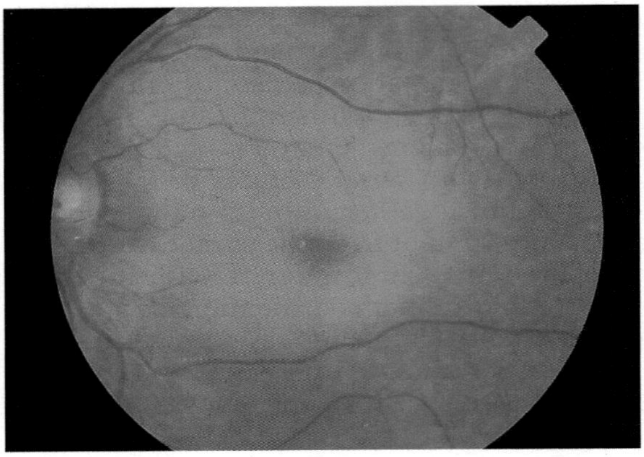

FIG. 16.9 Central retinal artery occlusion. Note the grey area of oedema around the normal red colour of the fovea.

against the surrounding oedematous retina. The condition may be secondary to vascular disease and hypertension or may be due to emboli from the heart or internal carotid arteries.

Central retinal vein occlusion (Fig. 16.10) presents as blurred vision rather than loss of vision and the most striking feature in the fundus is the multiplicity of haemorrhages with engorgement of the veins. The condition may be associated with hypertension or hyperviscosity of the blood; however, in many instances the underlying cause cannot be demonstrated. There is an association

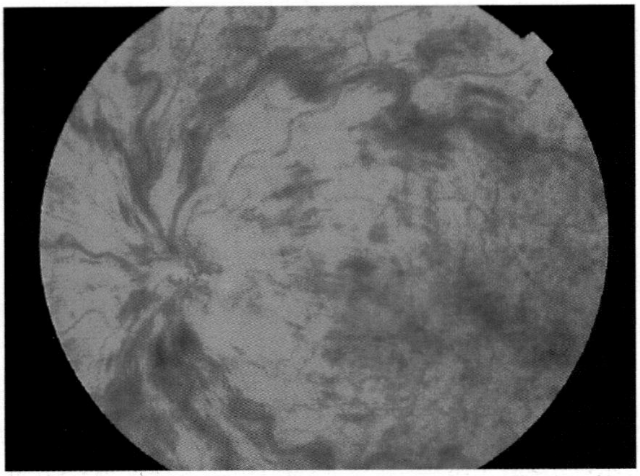

FIG. 16.10 Central retinal vein occlusion.

between central retinal vein occlusion and primary open-angle glaucoma.

Cranial or temporal arteritis (see also Chapter 26) is a cause of sudden loss of vision in the elderly; the second eye may subsequently be involved causing complete blindness. This not uncommon disease of the elderly usually presents with severe headache and tenderness over the extracranial arteries. The latter become inflamed, tender and often occluded and pulseless. The visual loss is due to arterial insufficiency and inspection of the fundi may reveal papilloedema and marked narrowing of the arterioles. The picture of central retinal artery occlusion is also sometimes seen.

Inflammatory changes in the retina and retinal vessels are seen in a wide variety of systemic diseases. They may take the form of venous engorgement and sheathing with leakage of blood into the vitreous or arterial narrowing with consequent retinal ischaemia. **Systemic lupus erythematosus** may produce multiple cotton wool spots in the fundi and **Behçet's syndrome** similarly may be associated with retinal ischaemia although here the presence of recurrent hypopyon (pus in the anterior chamber) may obscure the fundus. The presence of cotton wool spots in a young person should raise the suspicion of self-injection of drugs and human immunodeficiency virus (HIV) infection. Severe and often poorly controlled diabetics may show cotton wool spots. The characteristic features of diabetic retinopathy are also described elsewhere (see Figs 10.1, 10.2).

Diabetes

This is still the most common cause of blindness in young people in this country; particularly vulnerable are insulin-dependent patients who have previously had indifferent control of their diabetes. The onset of **proliferative retinopathy** (new vessel formation and leaking of blood into the retina and vitreous) can occur rapidly over 2 or 3 months. These patients require urgent laser treatment and sometimes vitreous surgery (Fig. 16.11a).

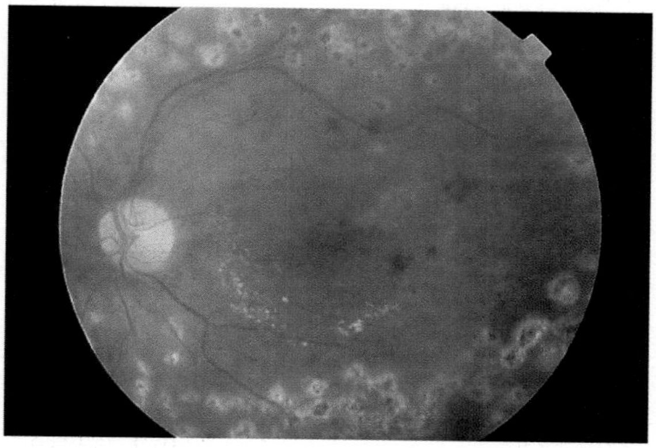

FIG. 16.11a Proliferative diabetic retinopathy. This fundus has been treated with laser and the laser marks are seen as pigmented areas. Only some residual evidence of the active disease remains as new vessels on the optic disc.

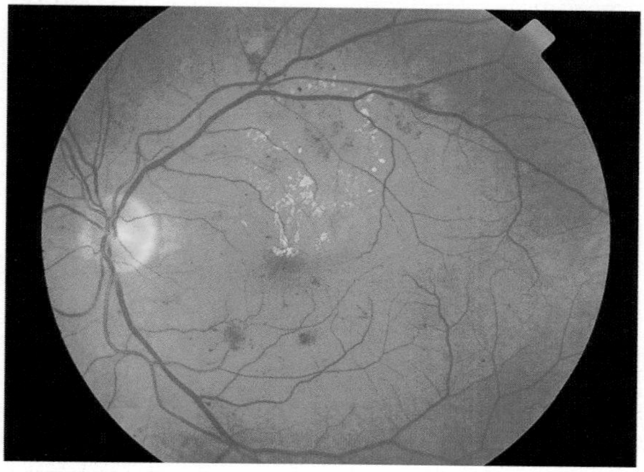

FIG. 16.11b Diabetic retinopathy. The typical changes of background are easily seen – retinopathy, hard exudates and haemorrhages.

Patients who have had diabetes for many years very often show **background retinopathy** (microaneurysms and hard exudates) which in turn can involve the macular region and consequent loss of reading vision (Fig. 16.11b). Venous engorgement and soft exudates herald the onset of severe proliferative retinopathy. The prognosis for background retinopathy is much better as long as the macula is not involved.

Respiratory system

In severe cases of respiratory insufficiency papilloedema may be present due to **hypercapnia** and consequent increased cerebral and retinal blood flow (see Fig. 5.20). The retinal veins may be engorged and central cyanosis may be evident on ophthalmoscopic examination. Specific chest diseases, which produce ophthalmoscopic signs are **tuberculosis** and **sarcoidosis**. Miliary tuberculosis can sometimes be diagnosed by discovering the miliary tubercles in the choroid. They are seen typically in the severely ill patient as discrete, slightly raised, whitish-yellow lesions at the posterior pole which fade and become pigmented. Sarcoidosis may present as acute iridocyclitis or as lachrymal insufficiency causing a dry eye. The fundoscopic changes include periphlebitis. The retinal vessels become sheathed and careful examination may reveal small white patches in the internal limiting membrane of the retina known as candle wax patches.

Haemopoietic system

Severe anaemia from whatever cause may be associated with scattered haemorrhages, some of which have a white centre. Soft exudates may also be present. These changes are most marked in pernicious anaemia and the acute leukaemias. Retinal haemorrhages may be seen in **thrombocytopenia** of any cause.

In sickle cell disease eye changes are due to vascular occlusion rather than anaemia. These are seen most often in sickle cell haemoglobin C disease (SC) but also in homozygous sickle cell disease (SS) and in sickle cell thalassaemia. Vascular occlusions are seen in the peripheral retina with unusual looking haemorrhages and subsequent tendency to peripheral neovascularization.

Central nervous system

Papilloedema is an important ophthalmoscopic sign in central nervous system disease which has already been discussed in Chapter 7.

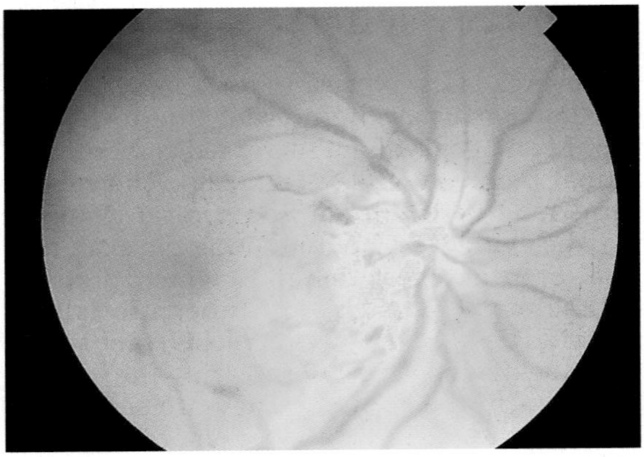

FIG. 16.12 Papilloedema.

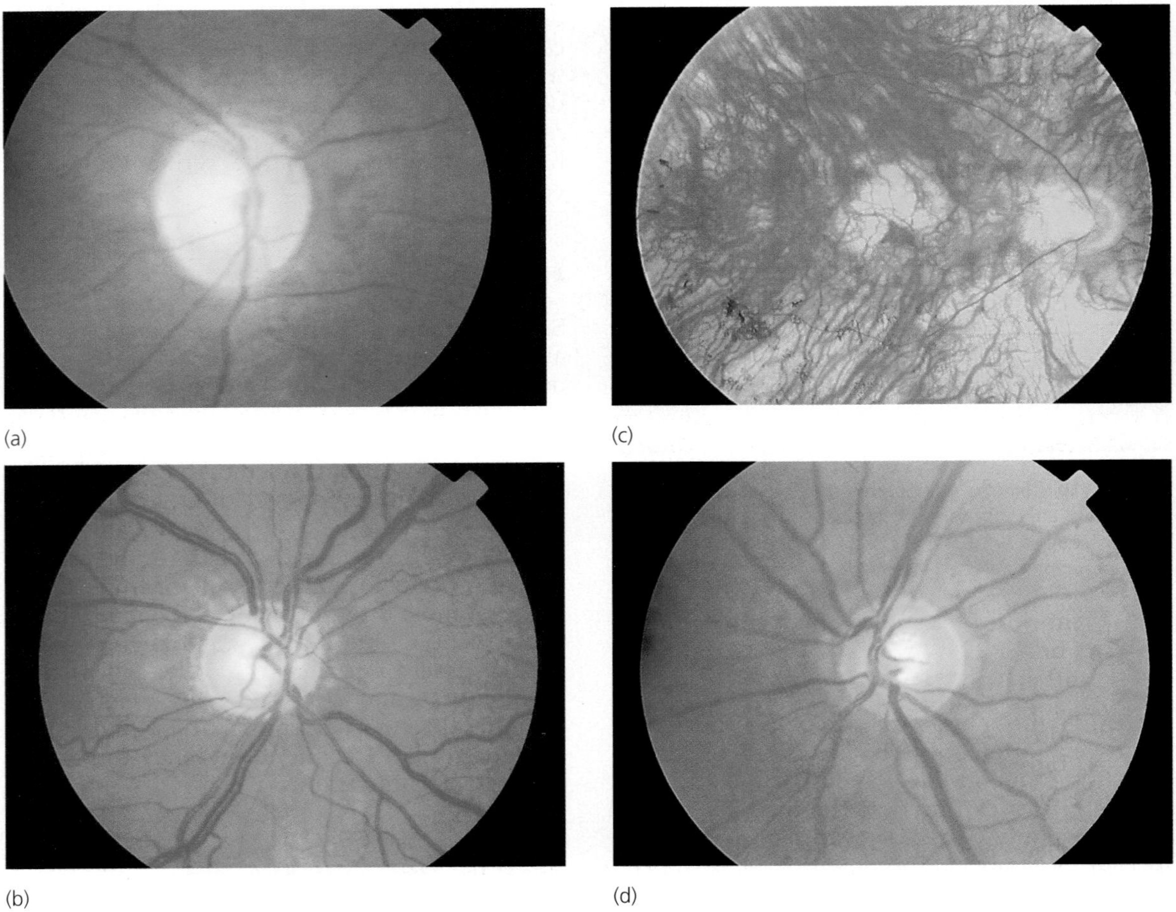

FIG. 16.13 Examples of optic atrophy. (a) Optic atrophy after vascular occlusion. (b, d) Left and right eyes of a patient with glaucoma more advanced on one side. (c) Optic atrophy in retinitis pigmentosa.

Revision Panel 16.4
Causes of papilloedema

Raised intracranial pressure.
Severe accelerated hypertension.
Central retinal vein thrombosis.
Cranial arteritis.
Hypercapnoea.

Be careful to distinguish true swelling of the optic disc (Fig. 16.12) from apparent swelling as is sometimes seen in hypermetropic (long-sighted) eyes.

The main causes of papilloedema are listed in Revision Panel 16.4.

Optic atrophy When nerve fibres in the optic nerve become atrophic, the optic disc becomes abnormally pale.

The following may be associated with optic atrophy.

- Previous obstruction of the central retinal artery or vein (Fig. 16.13a).
- Compression of the optic nerve by an aneurysm or tumour.
- Retrobulbar neuritis: rapid loss of central vision in one eye of a young person with pain on eye movement is characteristic. The fundus at this stage is usually normal but optic atrophy may begin to appear after 2 or 3 weeks. An afferent pupillary defect is present. About half of the patients with retrobulbar neuritis subsequently develop demyelinating disease in other parts of the body after a delay of some years.
- Resolution of papilloedema.
- Inherited retinal degenerations such as retinitis pigmentosa (Fig. 16.13c).
- Toxins: a number of poisons can specifically damage the optic nerve. Methanol and also quinine are classic examples.
- Trauma.
- Glaucoma (see Figs 16.13b, d).

DRUGS AFFECTING THE EYESIGHT

Many drugs can cause transient blurring of the vision and this effect may be more evident in patients approaching the age when reading glasses are needed (about 45 years). Any drug which has a potential for dilating the pupil has a theoretical risk of causing narrow-angle glaucoma in a susceptible subject. Narrow-angle glaucoma occurs in middle-aged, long-sighted individuals. If a patient is already known to have glaucoma and is undergoing treatment, there is little cause for concern. Chloroquine is a drug which can cause blindness if the recommended maximum dose is exceeded but small doses appear to be perfectly safe even when administered over several years. Amiodarone can sometimes cause blurring of vision because it is deposited in the cornea. The effect is reversible. Steroids when administered in drop form or by mouth can cause glaucoma and they can also increase the rate of formation of cataracts.

17 The absolute minimum on ear, nose and throat

Diseases of the ears, nose and throat (ENT) comprise more than 10% of all general practice consultations so an understanding of their symptoms and an ability to carry out a basic ENT examination is necessary for all doctors. For the non-specialist a suitable auriscope will allow examination of the ears, the throat and the anterior part of the nasal cavity.

As with all medical practice clinical evaluation starts with a well-taken history. Quality of voice, its timbre and degree of nasality and any hearing disability will quickly become apparent.

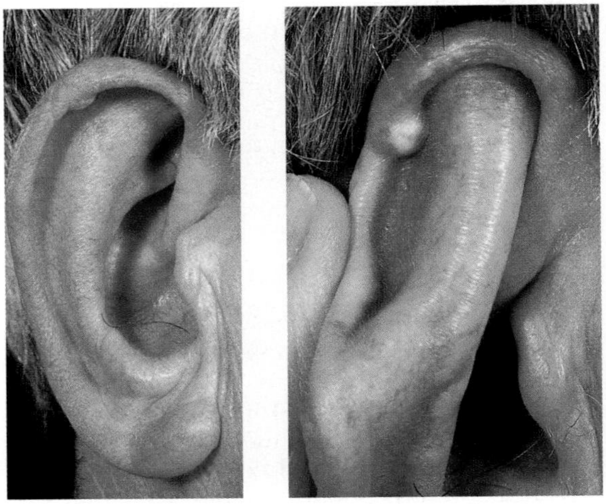

FIG. 17.1 A gouty tophus. Note that such a lesion may be missed unless the ear is examined carefully.

THE EAR

Symptoms commonly include:

- Deafness.
- Discharge.
- Pain.
- Tinnitus.
- Fullness in the ear.
- Dizziness.

Examining the ear

Formal examination of the ear (Revision Panel 17.1) starts with an inspection of the outer ear; gross abnormality and absence or malposition of the pinna will be readily noted as seen either as an isolated lesion or as part of a syndrome such as Treacher–Collins.

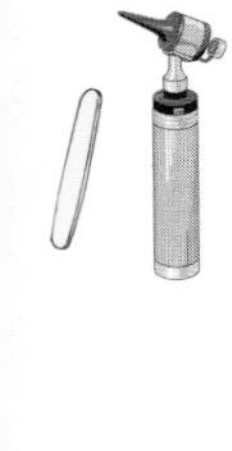

Practical Point

The only instruments required for the non-specialist are a simple tongue depressor and a suitable auriscope (Fig. 17.3).

Note the presence of pre-auricular tags and pits or sinuses and other abnormalities such as gouty tophi or other lesions on the pinna itself (Fig. 17.1). Swelling and tenderness occur with cellulitis, chondritis or perichondritis of the pinna. Ear lobe clefts are associated with coronary artery disease (Fig. 17.2). Deflect the pinna forwards and examine for scars, postaural swellings such as sebaceous cysts and possible carcinomas. Examine for preauricular and postauricular lymph nodes.

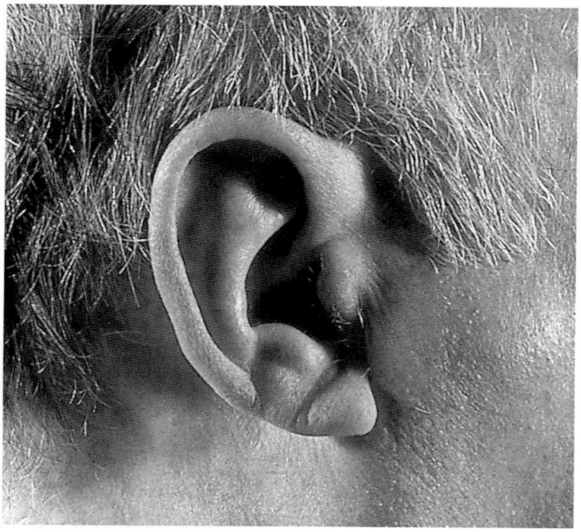

FIG. 17.2 A deep earlobe cleft. These lesions, though occasionally congenital, are associated with coronary artery disease.

Having checked the outer ear, inspect the opening of the external auditory meatus, looking particularly for signs of discharge and note its nature. Next, use the auriscope with an appropriate size speculum to examine the deep ear canal and the tympanic membrane. Correct technique will enable an optimum view of these structures while minimizing discomfort. For the *left* ear, hold the instrument in the *left* hand; rest the ulnar side of your hand on the patient's cheek and straighten the ear canal by pulling gently on the pinna with the right hand (Fig. 17.3).

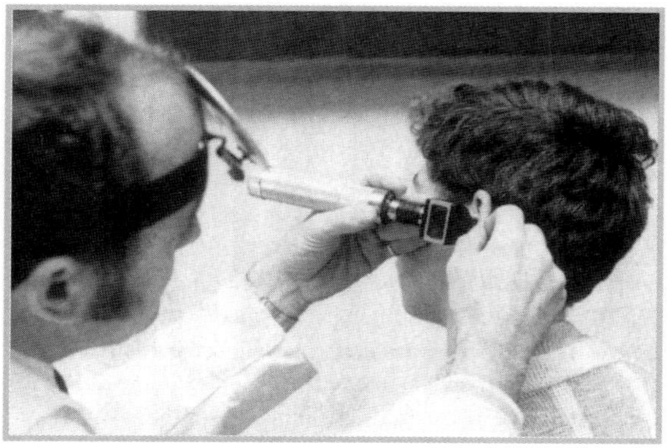

FIG. 17.3 The correct use of the auriscope.

Revision Panel 17.1
Examination of the ear

Assess hearing during history taking.

Note the presence and position of the pinnae.

Examine the postaural region.

Before introducing a speculum into the ear canal examine its opening.

Use the appropriate size speculum and introduce it gently.

Examine the deep ear canal and the tympanic membrane.

Carry out tuning fork tests and more formal tests of hearing including spoken voice testing.

While introducing the speculum, note any abnormalities of the canal such as otitis externa, a furuncle and exostoses. If present, wax may need to be removed by gently syringing. If otitis externa or a furuncle is present, be very gentle as the ear canal may be extremely tender.

The normal eardrum presents as a shallow cone with an anteroinferior reflection from the examining light, the cone of light. The handle of the malleus is seen projecting down towards the umbo and the incus-stapes assembly may just be seen through the semi-translucent normal membrane (Fig. 17.4).

Previous inflammatory disease of the ear may cause a thickened appearance. If there is an effusion in the middle ear then the drum

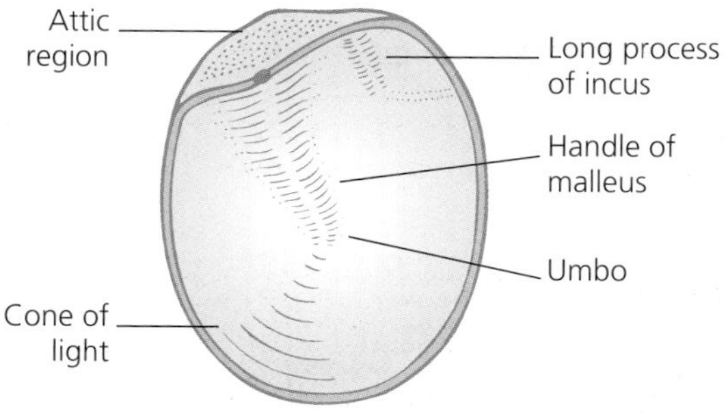

FIG. 17.4 The appearance of the normal left eardrum.

POINTS

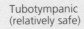

Attico antral (unsafe)	Tubotympanic (relatively safe)
Scanty offensive discharge	Discharge profuse and mucopurulent, rarely offensive
Cholesteatoma	Mucosal disease
Perforation/defect in attic region may be hidden by overlying crust.	Perforation in membrana tensa
Membrana tensa may be normal.	Attic normal

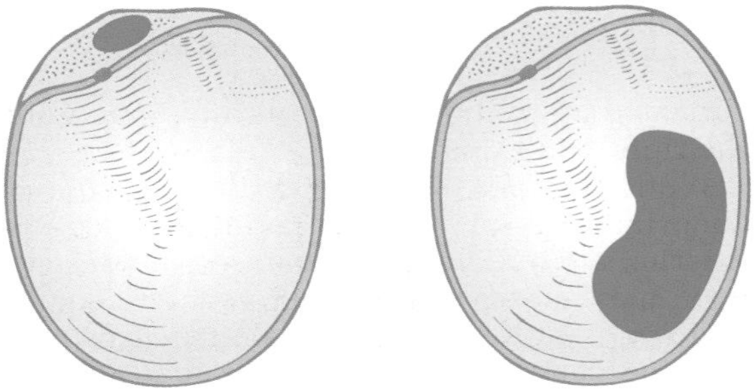

FIG. 17.5 Points about perforation of the eardrum.

may have a yellowish appearance. A perforation of the pars tensa or central part may be identified. Perforations of the attic may be much more difficult to see and may be hidden by a small overlying crust. Features of perforations are shown in Fig. 17.5.

Hearing may be tested by simple voice tests but the Rinne and Weber tests of air and bone conduction require a 512 Hz tuning fork (Fig. 17.6).

Rinne test

Air conduction is tested by presenting the fork approximately 2.5 cm from the ear with the tines parallel to the ear canal (Fig. 17.6a); bone conduction is assessed by pressing the fork firmly against the mastoid process (Fig. 17.6b). Ask the patient in which position the tuning fork is louder.

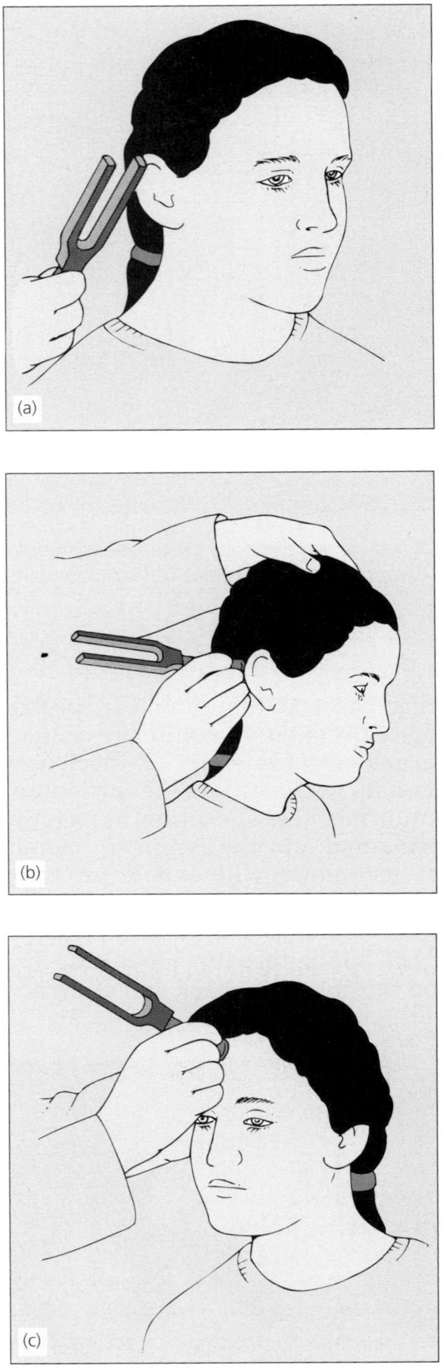

FIG. 17.6 (a), (b) The Rinne test. (c) The Weber test. It is essential to support the head with the examiner's hand to obtain firm bony pressure when carrying out bone conduction tests.

Revision Panel 17.2

Interpreting Rinne and Weber tuning fork tests

Rinne	*Weber*	*Meaning*
R + ve L + ve	Central	Normal, mild, moderate or severe bilateral sensori-neural loss.
R + ve L − ve	To left	Left conductive or mixed loss.
R − ve L − ve	Central	Bilateral mixed or conductive loss.
R + ve L − ve	To right	Left severe or profound sensori-neural loss.

R: right; L: left

Weber test

Press the fork firmly on the patient's skull in the midline and ask whether the patient can hear the tuning fork and if so whether it seems louder on one side or lateralizes (Fig. 17.6c).

Absolute bone conduction may be assessed by comparing the patient's bone conduction with that of the examiner. The significance of the results is summarized in Revision Panel 17.2.

THE NOSE

Symptoms

Symptoms of nasal and sinus disease include:

- Blockage.
- Discharge.
- Postnasal drip or catarrh.
- Bleeding.
- Headache.
- Cheek swelling.

Examining the nose

Note first of all whether the patient is mouth breathing or even gasping for breath. Check for dry lips, indicating nasal obstruction. The first clue suggestive of a cleft palate may be a hyper-nasal-sounding voice (Revision Panel 17.3).

Next examine the external nose for gross abnormalities of size, shape and position, features such as rhinophyma, and the nature of any nasal discharge.

You can get a reasonable view of the anterior part of the nasal cavity by lifting the tip of the nose and using a good torch; for a more detailed view use either a Thudichum speculum or a large aural speculum on an auriscope. Points to note on anterior rhinoscopy include the position of the septum and the nature of the nasal mucosa (usually pink in health). The inferior and middle turbinates are easily seen, the former often mistaken for a nasal polyp. Little's area, the most common bleeding site, lies on the anterior part of the septum.

Revision Panel 17.3

Examination of the nose

During the history assess for any hyponasality or hypernasality.

Check for visible nasal discharge.

Examine the external nose noting any lateral deviation.

Carry out intranasal examination with a good light and an appropriate speculum.

Note the position of the septum and the nature of the nasal mucosa.

Important signs are:

Cheek swelling (Fig. 17.7).

Unilateral bloodstained discharge.

Unilateral nasal polyp.

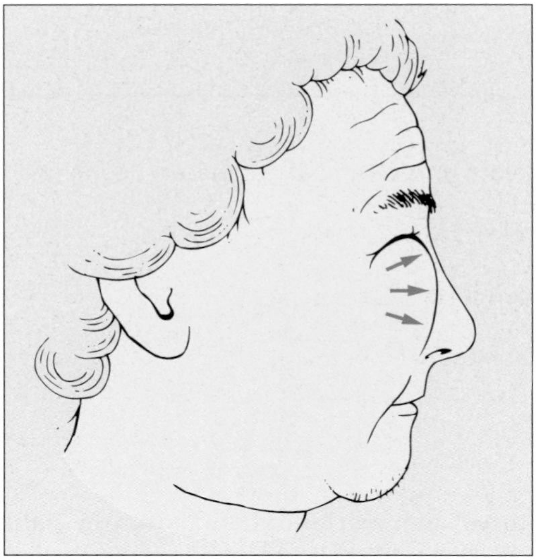

FIG. 17.7 Cheek swelling is a possible sign of sinus cancer.

Examination of the oropharynx may yield clues about nasal disease, for example the presence of mucopurulent postnasal discharge, perhaps with a secondary pharyngitis.

Check the nasal airway by placing a metal tongue depressor under the nostrils and noting the degree of misting on expiration through the nose.

Finally palpate the nose for any structural abnormalities and tenderness over the maxillary and frontal sinus areas, noting particularly any cheek swelling, a sign of possible carcinoma of the maxilla.

> **Practical Point**
>
> Cheek swelling is rarely due to infection, and is a sign of possible carcinoma of the maxilla.

PHARYNGEAL AND LARYNGEAL DISEASE

Symptoms

Symptoms of laryngeal and pharyngeal disease include:

- Hoarseness.
- Sore throat.
- Dysphagia.
- Lump in the throat.
- Neck swelling.
- Noisy breathing due to stertor or stridor.

Examining the mouth

Every doctor should be able to examine the mouth, pharynx and neck but laryngeal examination usually requires special facilities and training. Even so, you can get some idea about laryngeal disease from a good history and by listening to the voice (Revision Panel 17.4). A weak breathy voice may indicate a recurrent laryngeal nerve palsy, especially if there is a bovine cough.

Note any signs of other central nervous system disease such as palatal or tongue paralysis, or stigmata of systemic disease such as myxoedema. Any patient with a hoarse voice for more than three weeks should be referred for a formal laryngoscopy by an otolaryngologist.

> Revision Panel 17.4
>
> **Examination of mouth, pharynx and larynx**
>
> Note voice quality during history.
>
> If the voice sounds hoarse, check for a bovine cough and observe the vocal cords for paralysis.
>
> Check for stridor or stertor.
>
> Examine the mouth and pharynx with a good light, with any dentures removed.
>
> Examine the tonsillar region, fauces, palate and posterior pharyngeal wall.
>
> Asymmetry or irregularity of the tonsils suggests carcinoma.

Noisy breathing may be due to stertor, an inspiratory sound arising from disease in the pharynx causing airway obstruction, or stridor, a crowing sound due to airway obstruction in the larynx, trachea or main bronchi. Stridor may be inspiratory in laryngeal obstruction or biphasic if the lesion is in the lower trachea or main bronchi.

Practical Point

Any patient with a hoarse voice for more than three weeks should be referred for a formal laryngoscopy by an otolaryngologist.

Remember finally to examine the mouth with dentures (if worn) removed; these may obscure carcinoma in the back or floor of the mouth.

Examining the pharynx

You will need a good light and a tongue depressor. The fauces should be inspected followed by the tonsils if present. Enlarged tonsils are not necessarily a sign of disease. Tonsillar crypts filled with debris constitute a *tonsillolith*. Gross tonsillar swelling with a white membrane often indicates glandular fever (Fig. 17.8). Be alert to any tonsillar asymmetry or irregularity as evidence of a possible neoplasm. Check the palate for possible paralysis and also for evidence of a repaired cleft. Examine the posterior wall of the oropharynx, noting the presence of any inflamed lymph follicles.

Examining the neck

No examination of the upper respiratory and alimentary tracts and ears, nose and throat is complete without formal examination of the neck (Revision Panel 17.5).

Ensure the patient sits upright, stripped to the waist (a woman being allowed to retain her brassiere) with the neck very slightly flexed and in a good light. Palpate gently in turn the

Practical Point

Do not forget the possibility of acute leukaemia in a patient with a foul ulcerated throat and bleeding infected gums.

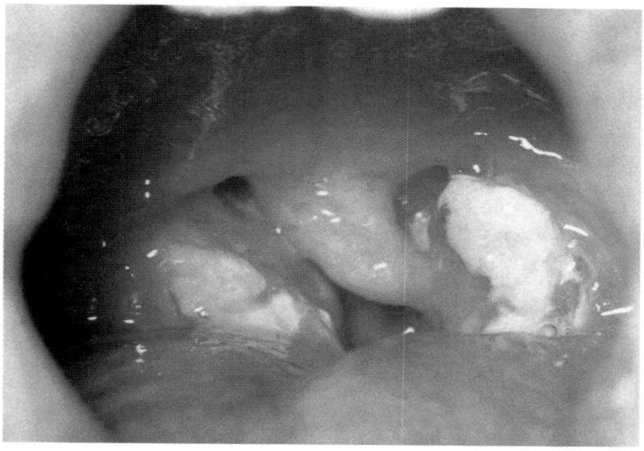

FIG. 17.8 The throat in glandular fever. A nasty sore throat, with a white membrane over the enlarged tonsils should alert you to this diagnosis.

submental, submandibular region and then posteriorly to the angle of the mandible; follow down the jugular chain to the clavicles and then laterally into the posterior triangle. The anterior triangle may then be thoroughly examined, taking care to examine in the midline down to the suprasternal notch and then finally the suboccipital region. In some instances as with a thyroid swelling or possible carotid body tumour, auscultation may be required.

If the submandibular or parotid salivary glands are swollen, then intraoral and bimanual examination is indicated, looking especially for any abnormality of, or discharge from, the opening of Wharton's duct or Stensen's duct. Then palpate for any possible stone in the duct itself.

Revision Panel 17.5

Examination of the neck

Sit the patient upright with the neck slightly flexed and the upper body appropriately unclothed.

Be methodical and gentle.

Do not forget to examine midline structures.

If salivary glands are swollen examine the intraoral opening of the salivary ducts and carry out a bimanual palpation.

Auscultate thyroid swellings and possible carotid body tumours.

18 Illness contracted abroad

With increasing international travel and wider access to exotic locations, there is an increasing requirement for doctors to be aware of illnesses that may be contracted abroad. Travellers may have a serious, rapidly progressive illness rarely seen in the UK, requiring specific diagnostic tests and treatment, or which may prove a danger to health care workers or other staff.

The most frequently encountered clinical problem will be an acute illness in a returned traveller, but you may come across some patients, usually immigrants, refugees or long-term travellers, who have acquired a chronic illness in another country as a result of longer term exposure to the causative agents. Always enquire about travel whenever a clinical history is being taken.

ILLNESS IN THE RETURNED TRAVELLER

Your first priority is to identify the seriously ill patient for whom emergency treatment is required. Remember that the returned traveller may present with a severe illness that could have been acquired at home, such as:

- Meningococcal septicaemia.
- Bacterial meningitis.
- Toxic shock syndrome.
- Staphylococcal septicaemia.

Illnesses that could have been acquired abroad include:

- Malaria.
- Rickettsial disease.
- Viral haemorrhagic fever.

In considering illnesses acquired abroad, the usual list of possible causes should be supplemented by causes rarely or never seen in the UK but relatively common in tourist destinations. More than half the illnesses seen in returned travellers will have been acquired locally at home.

Your history should include very specific documentation of the places visited and the duration of stay. You must also establish the date of onset of symptoms as this helps with the differential diagnosis. For example, an incubation period of 4 days excludes malaria, but an incubation period of 2 weeks excludes dengue (Revision Panel 18.1).

It is important to determine what vaccinations were taken prior to travel, whether prophylaxis was used for diarrhoea or malaria and whether antibiotics or other medications were consumed in the course of the illness (Revision Panel 18.2).

You should also enquire about exposure to animals, ticks, mosquitoes, or sandflies and about illness in other members of the party. The patient is likely to remember exposure to uncooked foods, especially seafoods, and whether there were opportunities for exposure to blood-borne viruses (Revision Panel 18.3).

Practical Point

In every history, always ask
'Have you travelled away from home?'
Also ask of immigrants
'Have you been home?'

Revision Panel 18.1

Usual (approximate) incubation periods of imported infections[a]

Less than 10 days	*Intermediate (up to 21 days)*	*Greater than 21 days*
Dengue	Malaria	Malaria
Yellow fever	Viral haemorrhagic fever	Hepatitis A,B,E
Tick typhus	Scrub typhus	Rabies
Plague	African trypanosomiasis	Visceral leishmaniasis
Paratyphoid fevers	Typhoid	Amoebic liver abscess
Sandfly fever	Brucellosis	Filariasis
Legionnaire's disease	Q fever	Tuberculosis
	Relapsing fever	Q fever
	Hepatitis A	Acute schistosomiasis

[a]Modified from Yung AP, Ruff TA. Travel Medicine 2. Upon return. *Med J Aust* 1994; **160**, 206–212.

The efficacy of vaccination does vary a lot:

- Vaccines for yellow fever, rabies, tetanus and hepatitis A and B are quite effective.
- Vaccines for typhoid and cholera have incomplete efficacy.
- Immunization against diphtheria may not provide life-long immunity.

Revision Panel 18.2

Key points in assessing illness in the returned traveller

Always ask about places, contact, illnesses.
Was prophylaxis taken as prescribed?
Any possibility of malaria?
Is isolation required?
Any skin lesions?

Pay special attention to animal bites (and need for post-exposure rabies vaccination), significant contact with fresh water in regions endemic for schistosomiasis, risk of sexually transmitted diseases and history of previous illnesses.

In an ill patient with a history of travel, two important questions need to be answered immediately:

- Could this be malaria?
- Is isolation necessary?

Could this be malaria?

Fever and rigors are classical symptoms of malaria but episodic fevers are neither necessary nor sufficient to make the diagnosis. Whereas a history of fever is to be expected, the patient may be afebrile at presentation and atypical symptoms can occur. It is worth remembering that malaria can be a great mimic. Fever in any patient returning from an endemic area should be considered to be due to malaria until proved otherwise. A blood smear should be taken and examined the same day (Fig. 18.1).

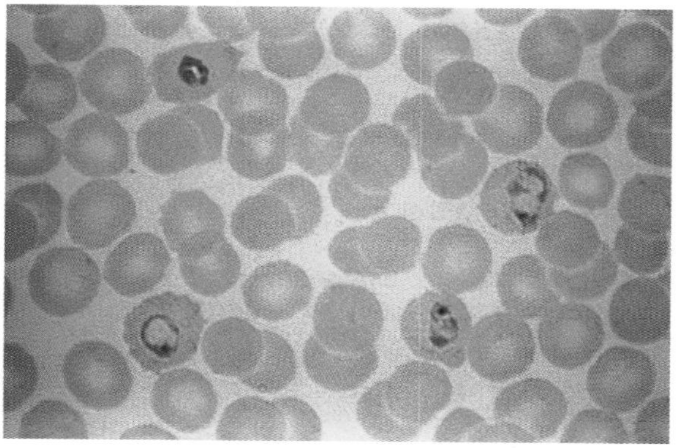

FIG. 18.1 A blood film showing *Plasmodium vivax* malaria.

Practical Point

Fever in a returned traveller:

The diagnosis is malaria until disproved.
A blood smear should be taken and examined the same day.

It is also important to remember that no prophylaxis is completely effective and that 'atypical' symptoms are common in malaria, easily leading to misdiagnosis. Former residents of endemic regions may not be aware that immunity wanes rapidly, so they may be at risk when returning to their country of origin for a holiday.

Is isolation required?

Isolation or other special nursing precautions may be required while excluding diagnoses of potentially transmittable diseases such as viral haemorrhagic fever, cholera, typhoid or tuberculosis.

You should have a low threshold for admitting for a period of observation and for requesting specialist advice for a patient with rigors, severe myalgia, impaired conscious state or unexplained rash.

Fever, sore throat, rash or haemorrhage in a traveller returning from an area with an outbreak of viral haemorrhagic fever (most commonly Central or West Africa) also warrant isolation and urgent consultation with an infectious disease specialist.

Revision Panel 18.3
Special points from the history

- Specific details of places visited, duration of stay and date of return.
- Specific date of onset of symptoms to calculate incubation period.
- Details of illnesses while abroad and relationship to presenting symptoms.
- Prophylaxis used (drugs, vaccines, bednets).
- Exposure to animals, insects, uncooked food.
- Illnesses in fellow travellers.
- Consider malaria.

Headache and mild alteration of conscious state may occur with many acute infections but in a returned traveller should increase the suspicion of malaria or typhoid.

Neurological disturbance may be a feature of Legionnaire's diseases, Lyme disease, brucellosis or leptospirosis and a rapidly progressive deterioration should suggest meningitis, especially meningococcal.

SPECIAL POINTS ON EXAMINATION

After general examination for shock or dehydration, pay special attention to the following points:

Neurological status

Could this be cerebral malaria or meningoencephalitis? Confusion may be a feature of typhoid fever, malaria or legionnaire's disease.

Mouth

If the tonsils are affected, consider diphtheria.

Eyes

Check for evidence of jaundice or conjunctival injection suggestive of leptospirosis. In acute viral hepatitis, fever has usually settled by the time jaundice is apparent. Jaundice in the presence of ongoing fever makes viral hepatitis an unlikely diagnosis; ascending cholangitis or leptospirosis may need to be considered.

Skin

Rash or petechiae may be seen only with meticulous examination in a good light, with special attention to lower limbs and buttocks. Remove all clothing to examine for the eschar of tick bite (Fig. 18.2). The rash of meningococcal septicaemia may be maculopapular or

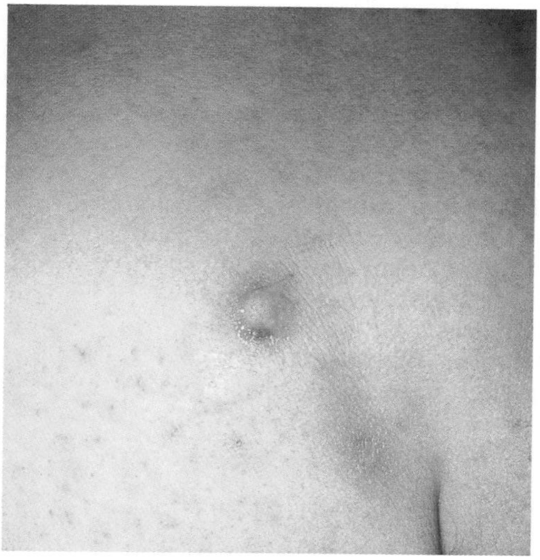

FIG. 18.2 The eschar on the lower back in a patient with scrub typhus.

petechial (see Fig. 12.3). The rash of dengue may resemble sunburn or photosensitivity to tetracyclines before petechiae are noted.

Chest

Do not rely on auscultatory signs as these may be virtually absent in the early phases of atypical pneumonia, including legionella.

Generalized lymphadenopathy

This may be present in acute viral illness (including Epstein–Barr virus (EBV) or human immunodeficiency virus (HIV) seroconversion) and regional lymphadenopathy may follow bites or accompany tuberculosis.

Abdomen

Mild-to-moderate hepatomegaly is present in hepatitis but may occur with malaria, amoebic liver abscess or brucellosis. Liver tenderness without jaundice is typical of a liver abscess. Splenomegaly may occur in malaria, typhoid fever, brucellosis, leptospirosis or acute viral illness.

COMMON CLINICAL PRESENTATIONS IN RETURNED TRAVELLERS

Diarrhoea and abdominal pain

Diarrhoea is the most common presenting illness, with high attack rates occurring in travellers from developing countries. The common causes of acute diarrhoea include *Escherichia coli*, *Campylobacter*, *Shigella* and *Salmonella* species but a small proportion result from *Entamoeba histolytica* that is diagnosed by examination of a fresh faecal specimen.

Most episodes are mild and self-limiting but fever, and abdominal pain, associated pus or blood in the stools occurs in a proportion of episodes. Severe diarrhoea with dehydration could point to a diagnosis of cholera. Pain in the right upper quadrant associated with fever is consistent with amoebic abscess (even in the absence of diarrhoea).

The most common cause of persistent diarrhoea and intermittent cramping abdominal pain (usually without blood in stool) is *Giardia lamblia*. Some patients with travellers' diarrhoea progress to chronic symptoms that require more intensive investigations. Travel-associated diarrhoea may be the first presentation of irritable bowel syndrome.

It should be noted that constipation, not diarrhoea, is a common feature of patients presenting with enteric fever (typhoid fever caused by *Salmonella typhi*) and that appendicitis could mimic some of the presentations described.

Fever

Malaria, dengue, hepatitis A and enteric fever are common causes of fever in returned travellers. Malaria should be preventable but no prophylaxis is 100% guaranteed; relapsing malaria may occur months or years after exposure. Hepatitis A and enteric fever should be prevented by vaccination. Other causes of fever are shown in Revision Panel 18.4.

Manifestations of malaria can affect every system leading to potentially fatal mistakes. Rigors are common, but there are no diagnostic features about the fever (it may be continuous or absent on presentation) and misleading symptoms such as cough are quite common. Convulsions or coma may be the first presenting symptoms of cerebral malaria.

Revision Panel 18.4

Causes of fever in the returned traveller

The big two
Malaria.
Typhoid and paratyphoid fever.

Treatable causes
Bacterial sepsis (including streptococcus, staphylococcus and meningococcus).
Infectious diarrhoea (including *Campylobacter* and *Shigella* spp.).
Amoebic liver abscess.
Typhus, other rickettsia.
Legionnaire's disease.
Q fever.
Brucellosis.
Psittacosis.
Leptospirosis.

Viral infections
Dengue.
Influenza.
Hepatitis A.
Acute HIV infection.
Viral haemorrhagic fevers.
Other viral infections (including Epstein–Barr virus and cytomegalovirus).

Rare but treatable causes
Melioidosis.
Schistosomiasis.
Leishmaniasis.
Trypanosomiasis.
Plague.
Trichinosis.
Relapsing fever.
Fascioliasis.

Drug fever

Jaundice may be attributed to hepatitis; anorexia and vomiting may be diagnosed as gastrointestinal disturbance or infectious diarrhoea; cough may lead to a diagnosis of bronchitis, and dark urine (haemolysis or haemoconcentration in response to dehydration) may be interpreted as pyelonephritis. On consideration of the diagnosis, a blood slide should be taken and examined at once. In a patient suspected of having cerebral malaria, treatment may be necessary prior to confirmation of diagnosis if delays are anticipated. Repeated specimens may be necessary to confirm the diagnosis.

Respiratory symptoms

Anecdotally, acute respiratory infection is a common occurrence following long haul flights and the possibility of pulmonary embolus should not be forgotten. Legionnaire's disease should be included amongst possible causes of pneumonia.

Rash

This is the leading symptom in some conditions (bites, larva migrans, scabies, fungal infection), but more common as an accompaniment of systemic illnesses such as dengue fever, other viral illnesses or rickettsial infections. In a returning traveller with fever and rash, possible incubation period and other features may help differentiate dengue, other arboviral infection, acute HIV, EBV or rickettsial infection from important cosmopolitan causes such as meningococcaemia, toxic shock syndrome or rubella.

Jaundice

Unvaccinated individuals are susceptible to hepatitis A and risk factors for hepatitis B, C

Practical Point

In diagnostic dilemmas in returned travellers, careful retracing of the history is the most important step in follow-up.

and E should be sought. Jaundice may occur with malaria or leptospirosis.

ASSESSMENT OF IMMIGRANTS OR LONG-TERM TRAVELLERS

These patients may present for 'a check-up' or in a migrant screening programme with illnesses that are prevalent in the country of their former residence. Cultural differences and language barriers may contribute to difficulties in assessment and more than one interview may be essential. Co-morbidity with hepatitis B or C, chronic helminth infection or malaria (in those with some immunity) is common and may be asymptomatic.

Chronic productive cough, with or without haemoptysis, is the usual presentation of acute symptomatic tuberculosis. Symptoms of extrapulmonary tuberculosis may relate to lymphadenopathy or disease of bone. More common than these presentations are abnormalities detected in chest X-ray or 'sterile pyuria'. The possibility of HIV infection should be considered in any patient presenting with tuberculosis.

Presentation with chronic ill health or weight loss should stimulate enquiry and examination for manifestations of:

- Chronic liver disease (hepatitis B, C).
- Tuberculosis.
- HIV infection.
- Schistosomiasis (splenomegaly).
- Kalar-azar (splenomegaly and anaemia).
- Intestinal helminth infection.

Chronic inflammatory bowel disease may first present following an episode of traveller's diarrhoea.

Any skin rash should bring to mind the diagnosis of leprosy and the need for careful neurological examination for reduced sensation to light touch.

Certain abnormal laboratory tests should provoke specific follow up. A history of skin lesions (*Strongyloides*, larva migrans) or contact with fresh water (schistosomiasis) may give clues to the cause of eosinophilia.

Revision Panel 18.5
Summary

Ask all patients about recent travel.

The travel history may be irrelevant to the presenting illness.

No prophylaxis (drug or vaccine) is completely protective.

In a returned traveller, suspect malaria as the cause of any fever until proved otherwise. Check a blood smear the same day.

Malaria may present with atypical symptoms.

Consider the need for isolation pending diagnosis.

Careful history taking and knowledge of incubation periods are essential in establishing differential diagnosis.

19 Renal and genitourinary medicine

Renal medicine and genitourinary medicine have been grouped together in this chapter. Although patients with these diseases are looked after by different sets of specialists in hospital there is considerable overlap in the presentation of symptoms, particularly in relation to the lower urinary tract.

THE KIDNEYS AND BLADDER

Symptoms

There are four main groups of symptoms which may draw attention to disease of the kidneys and bladder:

- Pain.
- Problems with micturition.
- The effects of renal failure.
- Oedema.

Pain

Gross structural disease of the kidney causes pain. This is usually felt in the renal angle which is the region of the loin between the twelfth rib above and the edge of erector spinalis muscle medially (Fig. 19.1). With extensive disease or massive renal swellings the pain may be felt anteriorly. *Ureteric colic* is the term used to describe the passage of stones, debris or blood clot down the ureter. This is usually an excruciatingly severe pain of colicky nature starting in the renal angle and radiating round into the groin and into the penis and scrotum in the male (Fig. 19.2) and the labia in the female. It is a true colic, waxing and waning, but often of such intensity as to cause the patient to roll around in his bed or in the floor in agony. Don't use the term renal colic for this pain; it arises from the contractions of the smooth muscle in the ureter and is therefore correctly termed ureteric colic.

During an attack of renal colic there is often an intense desire to pass urine, even though the bladder is near empty. This symptom is termed *strangury*.

Problems with micturition

These symptoms commonly draw attention to disease of the renal tract. Make sure that you know what your patient actually means before you record in the notes what you think is happening! A few everyday terms may help – but tailor your questioning to your patient's social class. It is easy to offend.

Strictly speaking *dysuria* means difficulty with micturition but in everyday medical usage it is used to describe pain, stinging or scalding on micturition.

Polyuria means the passage of large volumes of urine during the day and at night. This is to be distinguished from *frequency*, which is what it says – the frequent passage of small amounts of urine as occurs in a urinary tract

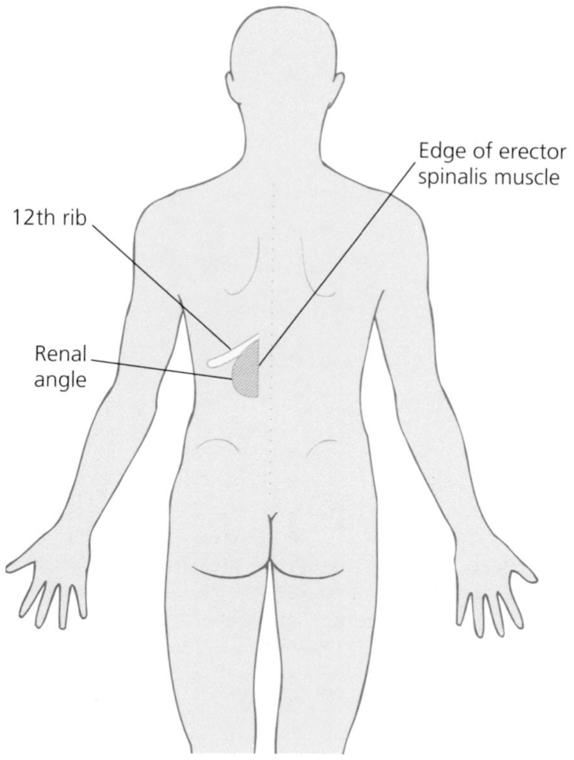

FIG. 19.1 The renal angle.

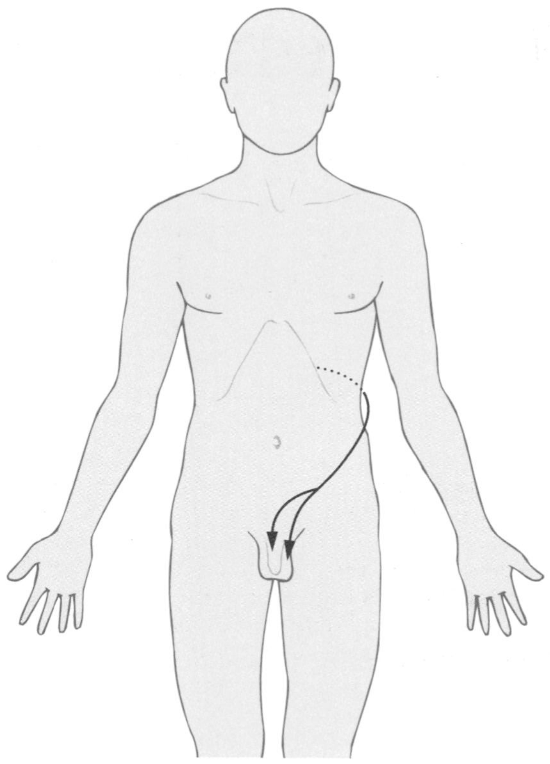

FIG. 19.2 The radiation of ureteric colic in the male.

infection. *Oliguria* is the passage of small volumes of urine in 24 hours; it is usually defined as the passage of less than 400 ml per 24 hours. When no urine is passed the patient is described as being *anuric*. It is essential to distinguish anuria from retention of urine, which is the inability to empty the bladder. *Nocturia* simply means passing urine during the night; this of course inevitably occurs when there is polyuria.

Incontinence is a symptom, which requires careful interrogation. The causes of intermittent incontinence are multiple and include dementia, frailty, cerebrovascular disease, multiple sclerosis, paraplegia and prolapse. Many of these diseases are dealt with elsewhere. Constant dribbling in the female means that there must be a fistula present, usually between bladder and vagina.

Urgency describes the sudden need to micturate often with little or no warning. If the bladder is not emptied quickly urine is voided without control. This relatively common symptom occurs with prostatic hypertrophy and multiple sclerosis.

Some causes of these urinary symptoms are shown in Revision Panel 19.1.

Effects of renal failure

Uraemia is the term used to describe the clinical syndrome of severe loss of renal function. Symptoms appear when the glomerular filtration rate falls below 20–25% of normal. The

Revision Panel 19.1

Renal symptoms and common causes

Frequency
Urinary tract infection.
Irritable bladder.
Small capacity bladder.
Bladder outlet obstruction i.e. prostatism.
Polyuria.
Diabetes mellitus.
Diabetes insipidis.
High fluid intake.
Diuretic therapy.
Chronic renal failure.
Dysuria.
Urethritis.
Prostatitis.

Oliguria/anuria
Dehydration.
Shock.
Acute renal failure.
Bilateral ureteric obstruction.

Haematuria
From kidney: trauma, tumour, tuberculosis, polycystic kidneys, stones, renal infarction, nephritis, pyelonephritis.
From ureter: stones, neoplasms.
From bladder: stones, trauma, acute infections, chronic infections (e.g. bilharzia in tropics), tumours.
From prostate: benign and malignant disease.

Incontinence
Constant dribbling: fistula present, usually vesicovaginal.
Intermittent: dementia and many other neurological disorders, prolapse and perineal weakness.

symptoms are often ill-defined but include tiredness, malaise, anorexia and vomiting. Other patients may be breathless on exertion, have paroxysmal nocturnal dyspnoea and leg oedema. With longstanding renal failure, but not necessarily severely impaired renal function, metabolic bone disease may supervene, giving rise to generalized aches and pains. With end-stage renal failure there is drowsiness and confusion progressing to coma

Oedema

In some patients the appearance of generalized oedema is the first manifestation of a renal problem. Massive leakage of protein into the urine leads to hypoproteinaemia and transudation of fluid into the tissues. This disorder which is termed the nephrotic syndrome may be due to a wide spectrum of renal and systemic disease and renal damage (See Revision Panel 19.2).

In practice the syndrome is defined by the loss of more than 3.5 g protein in 24 hours compared with the normal of less than 250 mg/24 hours.

Revision Panel 19.2

Causes of the nephrotic syndrome

Primary renal disease (glomerulonephritis)

Secondary to systemic disease
Systemic lupus erythamatosis.
Amyloidosis.
Diabetes.
Infections (e.g. malaria, streptococcal).
Myelomatosis.

Drugs
Gold.
Penicillamine.
Captropril.

SIGNS OF RENAL DISEASE

General features

In chronic renal failure the signs are largely non-specific. However, with advancing disease with progression into coma there may be:

- Loss of weight and dehydration.
- Uraemic fetor (a fishy smell in the breath).
- Muscle twitching.
- Rapid acidotic respiration (Kussmaul's breathing).
- Pericardial friction.

- Uraemic frost (now a rare physical sign consisting of a white powdery deposit around the lips and mouth only seen when the blood urea is extremely high).

In association with these signs, and often complicating them, there may be the features of the underlying disease such as diabetes or myelomatosis.

The kidneys

The kidneys are not normally palpable though in a slim person the lower pole of the right kidney may be felt on deep inspiration.

For examination of the left kidney the left hand is placed in the left loin and the right hand palpates anteriorly in an attempt to catch the kidney between the two hands. The right kidney is palpated in a similar way with the left hand in the right loin (Figs 19.3a, b). Percussion over an enlarged left kidney is resonant because the kidney carries the resonant splenic flexure of the colon forwards as it enlarges. This differentiates it from an enlarged spleen which is anterior to the colon.

Bilateral renal swellings (Fig. 19.4) are usually due to polycystic disease but may be due to bilateral hydronephroses when both ureters are obstructed as in retroperitoneal fibrosis secondary to pelvic tumours.

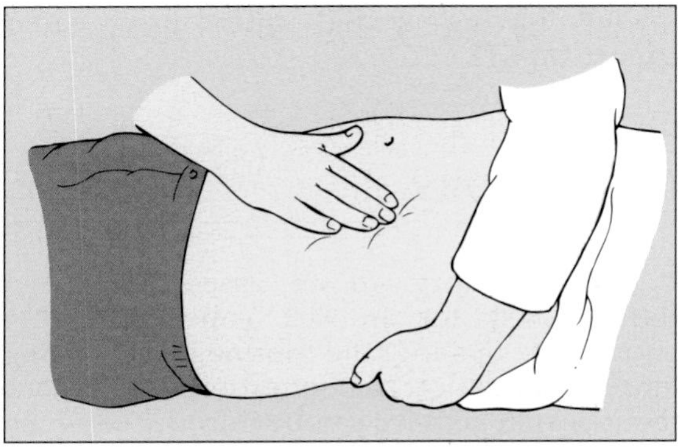

(a)

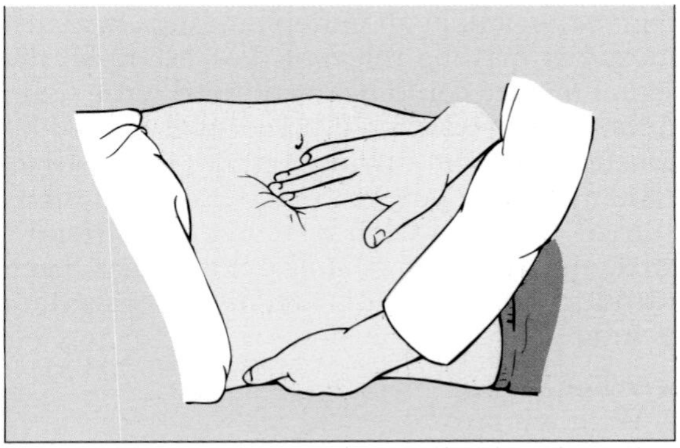

(b)

FIG. 19.3 Palpation of (a) the left and (b) the right kidneys.

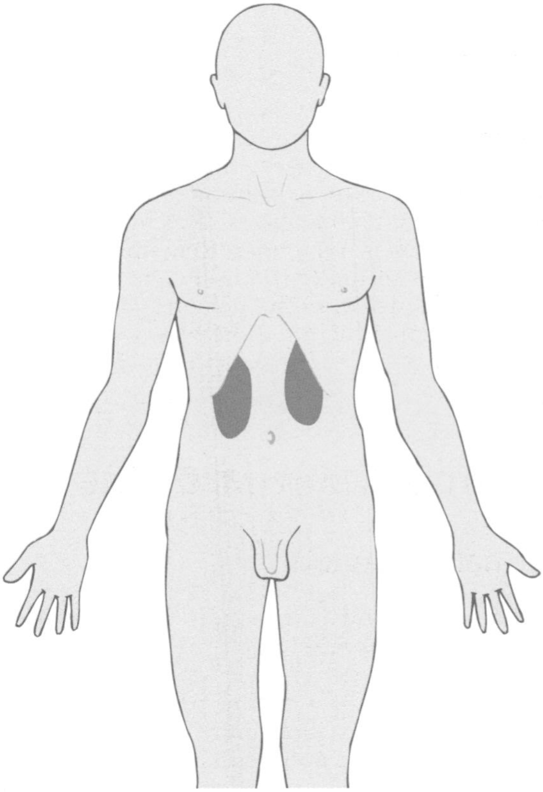

Renal swellings

Palpable from the loin bimanually
Usually resonant to percussion
Move downwards on inspiration

FIG. 19.4 Features of renal swellings. (See also Revision Panel 19.3.)

Revision Panel 19.3
Renal swellings

Unilateral	*Bilateral*
Hydronephrosis.	Polycystic disease.
Pyonephrosis.	Hydronephroses.
Cyst.	
Abscess.	
Tumour.	

The bladder

Acute retention of urine produces an exquisitely painful and tender bladder: pressure on this increases the overwhelming desire to micturate. In contrast chronic retention of urine is characterized by a floppy leaky bladder which is not tender. Remember that in the male it is virtually impossible to assess the size of the prostate in the presence of an overfilled bladder. In women the bladder must be distinguished from the gravid uterus and an ovarian cyst.

GENITOURINARY MEDICINE

Sexual behaviour

Sexual behaviour can significantly impact physical and psychological health and is a factor to consider when assessing every patient. A young woman presenting with acute lower abdominal pain and tenderness may have acute appendicitis requiring surgical intervention; alternatively, she may have acute pelvic inflammation, caused by the spread of a sexually transmitted infection (STI) from the uterine cervix and treated with antimicrobials. The risk of an STI in such a patient can be assessed during the initial history and examination; investigations for infection must be taken if appropriate. Persistent urological or gynaecological complaints, depression and other symptoms may represent covert presentations of sexual difficulties.

What is genitourinary medicine?

Genitourinary medicine focuses on the detection and management of STI, but includes the management of other diseases of the genital tract, notably skin conditions. Sexually transmitted infections:

- Are common, particularly in young adults around 15–25 years old.
- Are often asymptomatic.
- May give rise to symptoms and signs outside the genital tract.

Many sexual relationships are transient; each new partnership affords opportunity for STI acquisition. Doctors need to be aware that anyone having sexual intercourse could acquire an STI.

THE HISTORY

A sexual history allows assessment of a patient's risk for an STI. You can readily incorporate this into the routine history using simple 'matter of fact' questions. Questions about sexual activity can be introduced when you have established a rapport with a patient.

An explanatory comment is usually helpful to give the patient an understanding why such questions may be relevant. For example, the sexual history could be introduced with: 'pain in the lower abdomen is sometimes caused by infection passed during sexual intercourse. Can I ask when you last made love/had intercourse?' or 'Can I ask if you have a boyfriend?' Once the topic of sexual activity has been introduced, areas of detail to ascertain include:

- When?
- With whom?
- Where?
- Contraception?
- Type of intercourse?
- Other partners?

Revision Panel 19.4

Important questions to ask once you have established a rapport

When?
When did you last have sexual intercourse?

With whom?
Was this with a regular partner ? If so, how long have you been making love together?

Was this a casual partner? Do you still have contact with them?

Was the partner male or female?

Where?
Does the partner live locally?
Elsewhere in the UK or abroad?

Contraception?
Did you use any contraception? A condom?

Type of intercourse?
Orogenital or anogenital contact?

Other partners?
When did you have intercourse with someone else?

Appropriate questions that you should ask are shown in Revision Panel 19.4

For patients who are married or in long-standing relationships, asking about other partners is a sensitive issue. An introductory comment can be helpful: 'Please don't feel offended by my next question, which we ask everyone. Have you had intercourse with anyone else recently?'

Some general advice

Even though sex is generally viewed as a private matter, a sexual history is as much a part of the assessment of the possible impact of behavioural factors on health as are questions about alcohol consumption and smoking. In most general medical conditions, there are often no pertinent factors in the sexual history and history taking can quickly move on to another area. When you take a sexual history, you are not prying into a patient's private life but seeking to elicit information relevant to the successful clinical management of your patient.

The main challenges in taking a sexual history are:

- Winning the patient's confidence prior to tackling sexual issues.
- Ensuring confidentiality.
- Careful use of language.

Patients will understandably be reluctant to talk about their sex lives if you display a judgmental attitude or show embarrassment talking about sexual matters yourself. The confidential nature of the doctor–patient relationship must be honoured; in fact, it will probably help if you mention this.

A patient will often feel embarrassed about or ashamed to disclose impotence, an extramarital affair or casual unprotected intercourse. Avoid recording every detail in the case notes – only key factors that are relevant to immediate clinical management.

Practical Point

You do not need to record every detail in the case notes – only key factors that are relevant to immediate clinical management.

Sensitivity is vital when asking personal questions, especially in situations where the consultation might be overheard or a relative is present. It is better to defer taking a sexual history until privacy is assured. The use of vernacular or medical terms to describe genital anatomy and sex needs to be tailored to the individual patient. If a patient uses vague terms when discussing sexual matters you should gently seek clarification of what they mean.

Symptoms

Infection is a major cause of genitourinary symptoms, with a significant proportion attributable to STI, particularly in young adults. Most patients will need tests to establish or exclude infection, as guided by the sexual history, symptoms and signs. The common syndromes in genitourinary medicine and common STIs are listed in Revision Panel 19.5.

Revision Panel 19.5

Common syndromes and sexually transmitted infections

Syndromes

Urethral discharge (Fig. 19.5) with or without dysuria (men).

Vaginal discharge with or without vulval irritation.

Genital ulceration with or without lymphadenopathy.

Pelvic or lower abdominal pain (women).

Epididymal or testicular pain and swelling.

HIV infection and AIDS.

Genital warts.

Infections

Gonorrhoea.

Chlamydial infection.

Urethritis – non-gonococcal.

Trichomoniasis.

Herpes simplex infection (Fig. 19.6).

Genital wart virus infection.

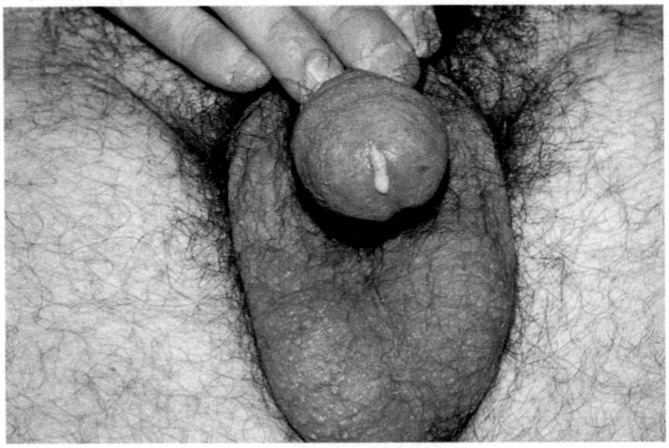

FIG. 19.5 Urethral discharge (gonorrhoea).

Revision Panel 19.6

Risk factors for sexually transmitted infection

Age 15–24.

Previous history of STI.

Single, separated or divorced.

New sexual partner in past three months.

Two or more sexual partners in past year.

Women seeking termination of pregnancy.

Not always using a condom during intercourse.

More than half of all individuals with an STI are free of symptoms. One factor fuelling the continuing spread of STI is the false belief that feeling fine equates with being free of infection. The sexual history is important for identifying individuals at particular risk of STIs and offering advice on sexual health and screening for infection. Major risk factors are listed in Revision Panel 19.6.

THE EXAMINATION

Patients are often anxious and embarrassed at the prospect of their 'private parts' being examined, so tell the patient precisely what you are going to do. Co-operation and the patient's confidence are pre-requisites for an adequate examination. Some patients prefer to the examined by a doctor of their own gender. You should always respect the patient's preference.

Good practice dictates that the presence of a chaperone should always be offered and a male doctor should not proceed with genital examination of a women without a chaperone. Whilst particular emphasis is paid to the genital region when symptoms are confined to this area, a general examination may be relevant, paying particular attention to the skin, mucous membranes of the mouth and eyes, joints and lymph nodes.

The patient should be asked to undress to allow exposure of the genital area. Respect for a patient's dignity dictates privacy whilst undressing or redressing. Do not leave a patient undressed or exposed unnecessarily. Supply a suitable gown or other cover whilst waiting examination.

Practical Point

Pre-requisites for an adequate examination

Gloves.

Chaperone.

Good light.

Suitable chair or couch.

Privacy while undressing.

An adequate gown.

Speculum for female examination.

Proctoscope.

Sample containers and swabs.

Proceed with examination only when the patient is ready. Ensure that you have an adequate source of light to allow inspection of the skin for warts, rashes and lice.

Male genital examination

You should examine carefully:

- Inguinal lymph glands.
- The scrotum and its contents.
- The penis, including the subpreputial area.
- Urethral meatus for discharge by milking the urethra distally from the perineum.
- The perianal area when indicated by the history, followed by proctoscopy.

Female genital examination

Women are usually examined in the lithotomy position. Examine carefully:

- The pubic and perigenital areas as for men.
- The labia majora.
- The labia minora.
- The vaginal introitus.
- The vagina.
- The cervix using a speculum. Always forewarn the patient of your intentions.
- Assessment of uterus and adnexae is made by bimanual palpation.
- The perianal area when indicated by the history, followed by proctoscopy.

Infection cannot be excluded or reliably diagnosed by visual appearances; samples from the appropriate anatomical sites must be taken for microbiological testing.

NOTES ON COMMON CLINICAL SYNDROMES

Urethral discharge and dysuria in men

Discharge from the urethral meatus is often associated with pain on micturition. These symptoms usually occur following intercourse with a new partner and result from inflammation of urethral mucosa. The cardinal sign of urethritis is urethral discharge and the diagnosis is confirmed by either the 'two glass test' (see Practical Point) or simple

Practical Point

The two glass urine test

Ask the man to:

- Start urinating into one clean specimen glass.
- Stop after passing a small quantity.
- Continue urinating into a second glass.

In urethral infection, the first glass will usually have threads in the urine or a haze due to pus cells, which does not clear on adding acid. The second glass will be clear.

Threads may be extracted and examined by microscope to determine whether they contain mucus, sperm, or pus cells.

microscopy of a sample of discharge. Polymorphonuclear leucocytes are usually evident and intracellular diplococci are observed in cases of gonorrhoea. The major infections associated with urethritis in young men are gonorrhoea (Fig. 19.5) and chlamydial infection.

Urethral discharge and dysuria in women

Dysuria in women is usually a symptom of:

- Inflammation of the urethral and bladder mucosa (cystitis).
- Inflammation of the vulva around the urethral meatus.

Urethral gonorrhoea or chlamydial infection in women rarely cause urinary symptoms.

Vaginal discharge

An increased or altered discharge from the vagina is a common presenting symptom in primary care. It is often equated with vaginal infection but may be physiological. The symptom may have relevance to other clinical presentations, including abdominal pain due to pelvic infection and chlamydial conjunctivitis, an eye infection usually caused in the UK by autoinoculation from infected genital secretions. Many episodes of vaginal infection are not caused by sexually acquired infection but it is important to explore risk factors for STIs in women presenting with this symptom. The common causes of vaginal discharge are listed in Revision Panel 19.7.

A women's description of her discharge and the examination findings may suggest the diagnosis, but you should always screen for and exclude STIs, particularly when risk factors are present (see Revision Panel 19.7).

Bacterial vaginosis is characterized by a homogeneous grey/white, malodorous discharge with a raised pH level. It results from a change in the microbial flora in the vagina, with the usually predominant lactobacilli replaced by groups of other bacteria, notably Gram-negative bacilli and anaerobes. Symptoms of vulval itching and signs of inflammation are absent.

Candidosis is inflammation of the vulva and vagina caused by yeasts of the *Candida* species. Common symptoms are vulval irritation and soreness, a thick white odourless discharge and discomfort on intercourse. The diagnosis is established by the demonstration of yeasts and exclusion of other infection.

Trichomoniasis is caused by infection with the flagellated protozoan *Trichomonas vaginalis*. This infection is sexually transmitted and is frequently associated with other STIs. The inflammatory response to the protozoan is variable. Some women experience profuse watery discharge and intense vulval irritation whilst others are asymptomatic.

Endocervicitis characteristically causes a yellow, non-odorous discharge without symptoms of vulval irritation or soreness. A mucopurulent discharge from the cervix may be observed on speculum examination and the cervix may appear hyperaemic and bleed easily to the touch. You should check for infection in women with cervicitis – although chlamydial infection and gonorrhoea are of major concern, these infections are frequently asymptomatic and do not necessarily cause an apparent cervicitis.

Revision Panel 19.7
Common causes of vaginal discharge

Candidosis.

Bacterial vaginosis (anaerobic or *Gardnerella* vaginosis).

Endocervicitis (including chlamydial and gonococcal infection).

Physiological.

Trichomoniasis.

Foreign body, e.g. retained tampon.

Genital skin rashes

These are common and often not related to intercourse or infection. Even so, the presence

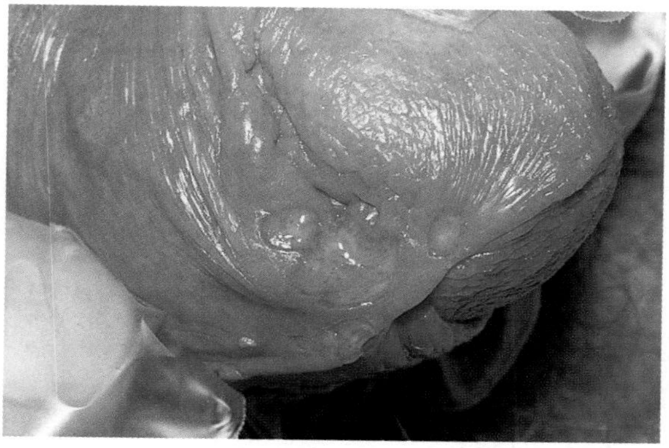

FIG. 19.6 Genital herpes.

of a 'spot on my willie' or a 'sore down below' often triggers a conviction that 'venereal disease' is present. Two conditions will be briefly considered: genital ulceration and genital warts.

Genital ulceration is often caused by sexually acquired infection. Although ulceration can be anywhere on the genital skin or mucosa, it usually occurs on those areas subjected to most friction and trauma during intercourse, namely, the coronal sulcus, fraenum, prepuce and glans in men and the inner labia and fourchette in women. The most common cause of genital ulceration in the UK is infection with herpes simplex virus (Fig. 19.6); other causes are listed in Revision Panel 19.8.

A first episode usually proceeds through the following sequence of symptoms and signs:

- Localized irritation with redness of the skin.
- A cluster of small blisters.
- Tender, shallow, 'punched-out' ulcers.
- Crusting and healing.
- Tender inguinal lymphadenopathy.
- Constitutional symptoms of malaise and fever.

The interval between contracting genital herpes and the development of an episode of ulceration is widely variable, ranging from 24 hours to years. Many patients experience recurrent episodes which are of shorter duration, less painful and have fewer sores than the initial attack.

Syphilis has become an uncommon infection in the UK. The initial genital ulcer of syphilis, or chancre, tends to be non-tender, rounded, has a well-defined margin and a thickened, rubbery base covered with slough though the appearances can vary widely. Inguinal lymph nodes are often moderately enlarged, non-tender and rubbery in texture.

Revision Panel 19.8
Other causes of genital ulcers

Multiple painful genital ulcers (uncommon in UK)
Chancroid: *Haemophilus ducreyi* infection usually seen in tropical countries.
Behçet's syndrome: a chronic, relapsing, multisystem, inflammatory condition of unknown cause.
Drug reactions.
Stevens–Johnson syndrome.

Solitary genital ulcers
Infectious syphilis.
Trauma.
Carcinoma.
Tropical genital infection.

Genital warts are caused by infection with human papilloma virus (HPV). They are transmitted by genital skin–skin contact and are increasing in prevalence. Individuals with subclinical infection substantially outnumber those with visible warts. Those who do develop warts often become aware of non-irritating white lumps or spots in the genital area.

Warts exhibit a range of clinical appearances and are usually multiple. The most familiar form is the condyloma accuminatum, a skin-coloured, pedunculated or sessile papillomatous growth that usually has frond-like surface projections giving a rough appearance. These may enlarge to develop a cauliflower-like appearance. Infection of the vagina and uterine cervix is common, although most cervical infections are inconspicuous and detected on cytology. Genital HPV infection may cause intraepithelial neoplasia.

Perianal warts (Fig. 19.7) are common in gay men but may be seen in both sexes as a result of auto-innoculation from the genital area.

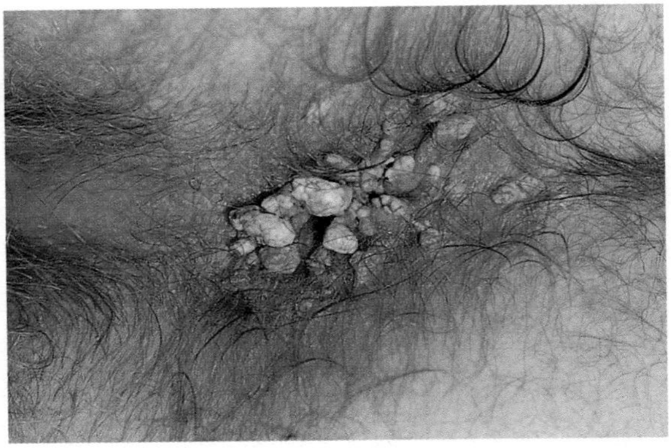

FIG. 19.7 Perianal warts. These are not necessarily indicative of receptive anal intercourse.

Genital infections frequently occur concurrently. It is important to screen for treatable bacterial infection in all patients presenting with an STI, even though the cause of their symptoms may be self-evident. For example, a patient presenting with genital warts should be screened for gonorrhoea and chlamydial infection, and vaginal infection if female.

Another integral element in managing patients with STIs is the management of sexual partners. This is self-evident to prevent:

- Re-infection in an ongoing relationship.
- Morbidity in the partner.
- Further transmission of infection within the community.

A summary of the key steps in managing patients in genitourinary medicine is listed in Revision Panel 19.9.

Revision Panel 19.9

Key steps in managing a patient with sexually acquired infection

Clarify the symptoms.
Take a sexual history.
Establish the diagnosis by examination and investigation.
Treat the patient: appropriate therapy and explanation of their infection.
Manage sexual partner or partners.
Educate about future sexual health.

EXAMPLES

Case 1

Single 19-year-old male student

History

Reports leaking from end of penis for four days and burning on passing urine. No past genital tract symptoms or episodes of infection. No constitutional symptoms. Not taking any medication; no recent antimicrobials.

Sexual history

Intercourse with new girlfriend on four occasions in past three weeks: no condom used. Relationship with previous girlfriend ended three months ago. They regularly had intercourse during their six-month relationship and condoms were always used.

Signs

Mucopurulent discharge from urethral meatus.

Tests

Microscopy of smear of urethral discharge.

Culture of urethral discharge for gonococcus.

Antigen test on discharge/first urine for chlamydial infection.

Diagnosis

Chlamydial urethritis.

Partner management

Advise to refer girlfriend for tests and treatment.

Case 2

Single 19-year-old female student

History

Reports dysuria, frequency and passing small quantities of urine for 24 hours.

Sleep disturbed by need to pass urine.

No past symptoms or episodes of genital infection.

No constitutional symptoms. Oral contraception.

Sexual history

Stable sexual relationship for past 18 months; her only sexual partner.

Signs

Nil.

Tests

Observation of urine: may show haze caused by numerous leucocytes.

Labstix testing for blood, protein, sugar.

Urine culture of mid-stream specimen.

Diagnosis

Acute urinary tract infection (usually enteric bacteria).

Partner management

No action needed.

Comment

Screening for STI might be offered, but no strong indication on clinical and sexual history.

Case 3

Female 32-year-old retail manager

History

Has experienced vulval irritation and soreness together with a heavier vaginal discharge for three weeks. She has had similar symptoms in the past and these resolved with over-the-counter medication for thrush. On this occasion the symptoms had only partially improved with self-medication. She is otherwise well and is not taking any medication

Sexual history

Divorced. Occasional intercourse with male colleague from work during past three months.

Condoms used sometimes.

Casual sexual encounter five months ago whilst on holiday in Spain.

Signs

Nil.

Tests

Tests from vagina for *Candida*, trichomoniasis and bacterial vaginosis. Genital tract tests for chlamydial and gonococcal infection.

Diagnosis

Candidal vaginitis and chlamydial cervical infection.

Partner management

Advise to refer recent partner for tests and treatment.

Comment

History is consistent with candidal infection, but sexual history makes screening for STIs imperative.

20 Musculoskeletal system

INTRODUCTION

The musculoskeletal system concerns muscles, joints and bones – tissues that are linked with support, locomotion and protection. These three tissues are often inextricably linked in the symptoms that they cause, of which pain is the most common.

Symptoms

Pain

Painful joints inflict much misery. On the whole intermittent pain in joints, related to movement, is likely to be mechanical whereas constant aching pain is usually associated with inflammation. Nevertheless there is considerable overlap. Joint pain is often felt over a wide area sometimes well away from the joint involved (Fig. 20.1).

Back pain due to trauma and degenerative disorders is an extremely common symptom in the population being always aggravated by movement and often worsened by periods of enforced immobility. Acquired disease of the skeleton due to osteoporosis and malignant disease is unremitting, being worsened by weight bearing and relieved by rest.

Stiffness

This may have several causes. There may be a bony limitation of movement due to fusion of joint surfaces or calcification of ligaments. Alternatively, associated secondary spasm of muscles due to pain may be responsible or there may be a primary neurological disorder such as Parkinson's disease. Inflammation of the joints such as rheumatoid arthritis is characterized by early morning stiffness which eases with activity.

Swelling

Inflamed joints become swollen as a result of accumulation of synovial fluid within the

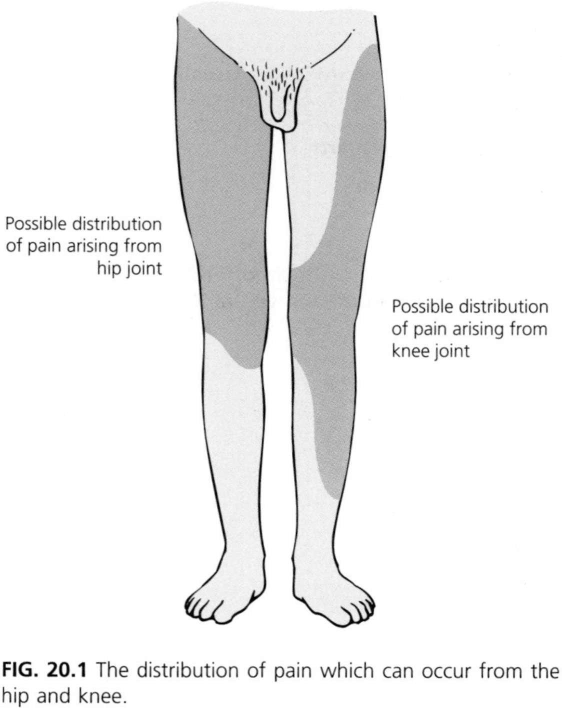

FIG. 20.1 The distribution of pain which can occur from the hip and knee.

joints or swelling of periarticular tissues or a combination of both.

Instability

This is of particular importance with the weight bearing joints. For example a severe tear of a collateral ligament of the knee or depression of a tibial condyle may allow it to angulate sideways.

Locking

There may be a sudden block to movement as with a loose body in the joint.

Signs

> **Practical Point**
>
> *When examining joints:*
>
> Look.
> Feel.
> Move.
> Assess function.

Look

The whole limb must be exposed and compared with the other. Look for:

- Bony deformity.
- Muscle wasting.
- Swelling – is this just due to synovial fluid?
- Scars.
- Other joints that may be involved.

Feel

Watch the patient's face whilst you are palpating, starting where you expect the least tenderness.

Move

Each joint must be put through its full range of movements. The best way to do this is to demonstrate the movements and then to ask the patient to do so (active movement). If your patient cannot do this, take over and put the joint through its full range of movements yourself (passive movement).

Measure movement in degrees using a goniometer and utilizing the *neutral zero* method. In this the anatomical position is zero and flexion is measured from that point (Fig. 20.2).

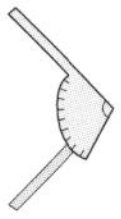

> **Practical Point**
>
> Wherever possible use a goniometer to record joint movement.

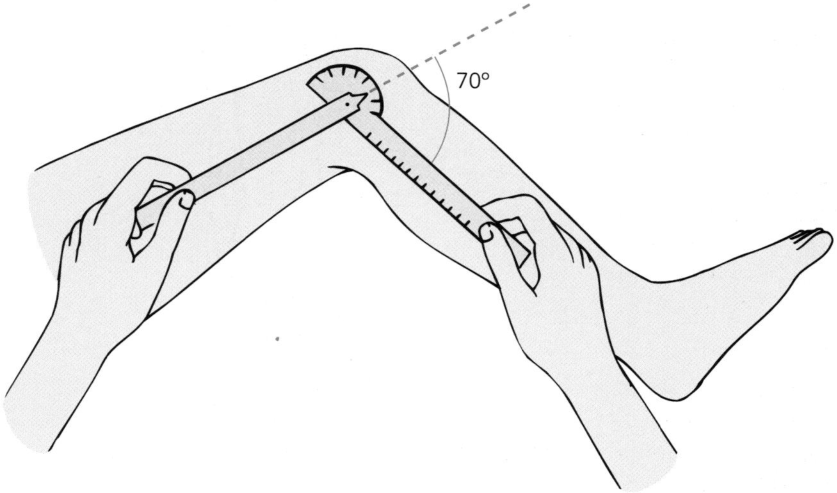

FIG. 20.2 The use of the goniometer to measure joint movement.

Function

For your patient this is the most important factor. The footballer needs his legs for running and kicking; the ballerina needs hers for precise movements and balance. Each patient will present a particular problem and you must use your initiative in testing the functions at fault.

CHANGES DUE TO AGEING

As with the other systems you must be aware of the changes that occur with advancing age. These are illustrated in Fig. 20.3 and are:

- Shortening of the trunk – mainly due to senile osteoporosis and degeneration of the intervertebral discs.
- Increasing kyphosis.
- Limited extension at the hips.
- Flexion at the knees.
- Diminished range of movement of the peripheral joints.

INDIVIDUAL JOINTS

Three important peripheral joints have been selected to demonstrate the basics of examination technique.

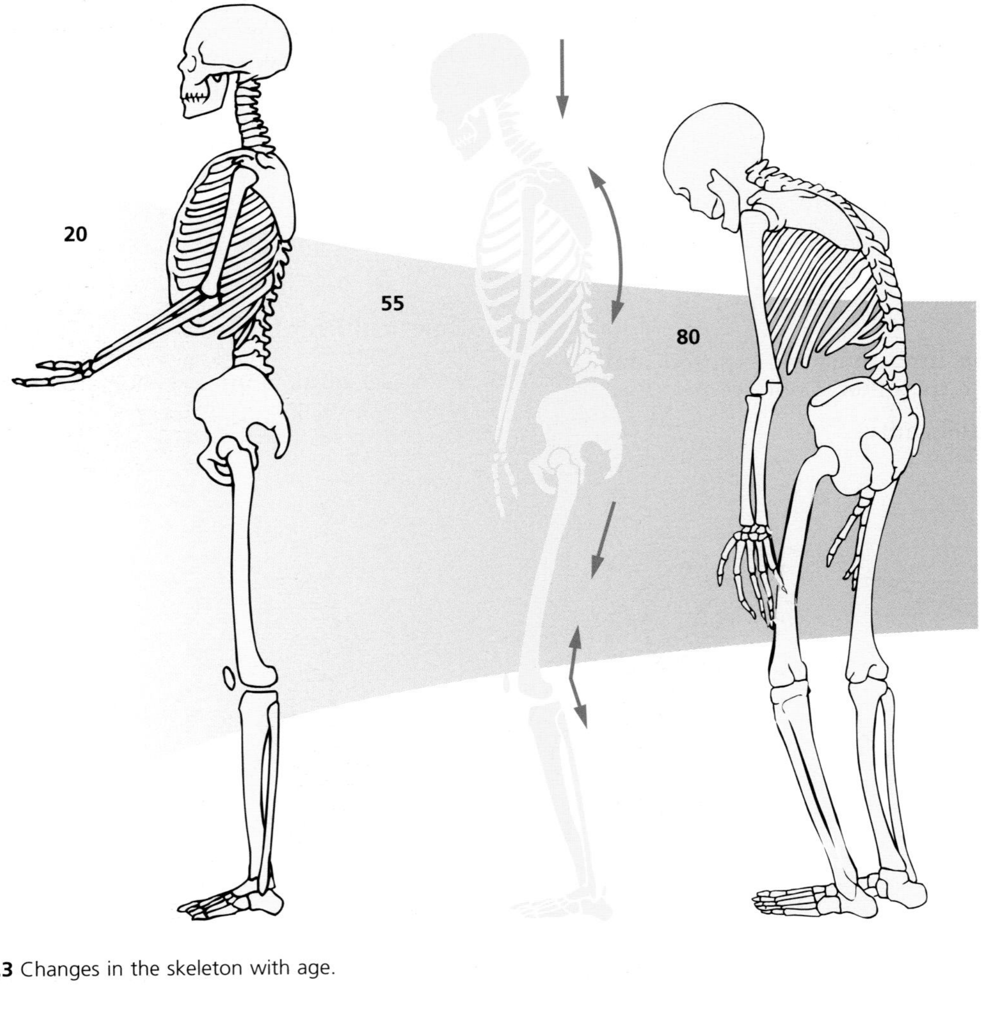

FIG. 20.3 Changes in the skeleton with age.

The shoulder

The shoulder has a very wide range of movement in all directions, which is permitted by a shallow ball and socket joint held in place by a musculocutaneous cuff called the rotator cuff. As well as movement at the gleno-humeral joint further movement is allowed by rotation of the scapula across the thorax. Look particularly for wasting of the deltoid. Test movements (see Fig. 20.4) by asking your patient to:

- 'Lift your arms up like this' whilst you demonstrate full active abduction.
- Hold them up for 10 seconds or so.
- Then allow them down slowly.

Then ask your patient to:

- 'Put your hands behind your head' to test external rotation.
- 'Put your hands behind your waist' to test internal rotation.

Finally test flexion and extension and assess the scapulothoracic component of shoulder movement by repeating abduction with the angle of the scapula fixed.

Frozen shoulder

Frozen shoulder is a very common, but self-limiting, condition occurring from early middle age onwards in which the shoulder stiffens as a result of poorly understood changes in the soft tissues. It is extremely painful, especially at night, and is characterized on examination by very limited movements in all directions. Similar stiffening occurs after immobility due to hemiplegia.

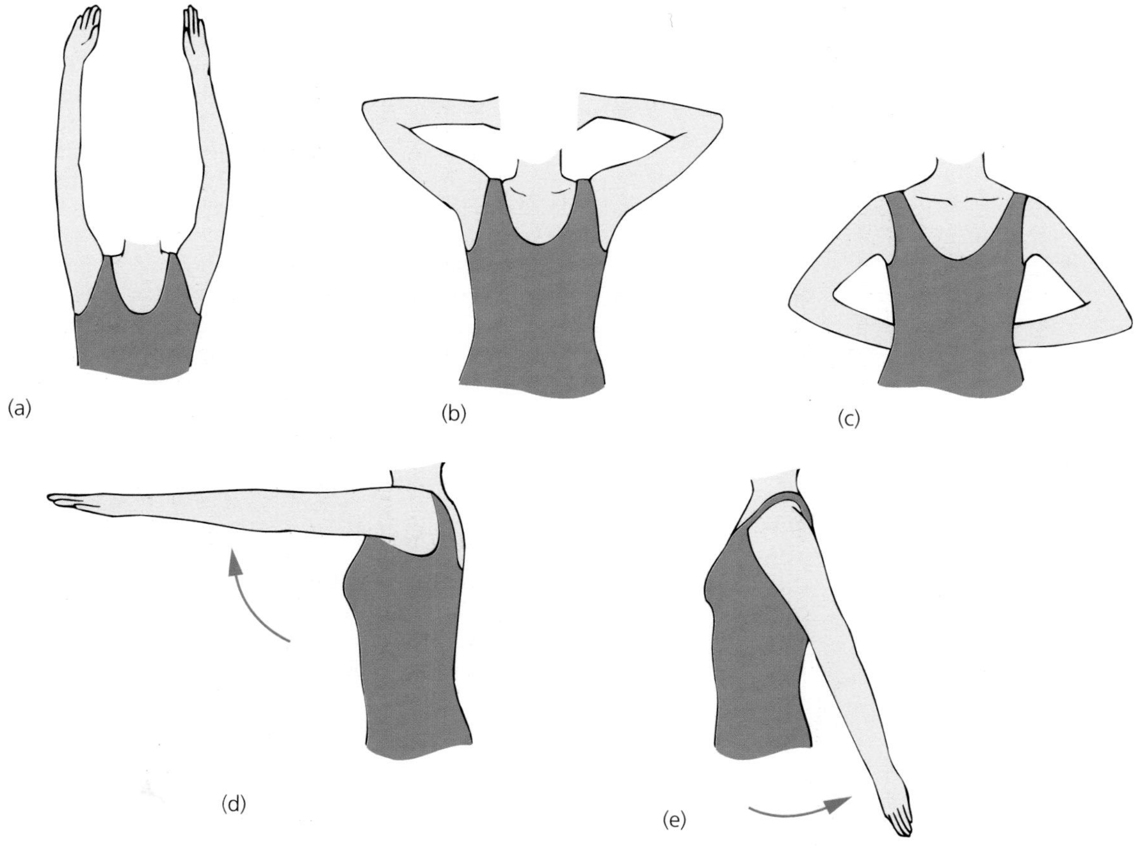

FIG. 20.4 Testing movements of the shoulder. (a) Abduction. (b) External rotation. (c) Internal rotation. (d) Flexion. (e) Extension.

Practical Point

The painful shoulder syndromes are worse at night and prevent sleep.

A rotator cuff or painful arc syndrome

This causes pain on shoulder elevation when the components of the cuff, the tendons of the subscapularis, the supra- and infraspinatus, rub on the under surface of the acromium. Pain is absent initially but develops during further abduction to disappear in the final part of the movement (Fig. 20.5)

The hip

The hip is a ball and socket joint allowing movement in all directions. The joint is deeper than the shoulder, which makes it more stable, but at the same time limits the range of movements. Pain in the hip, usually from osteoarthritis, is felt in the groin or buttock and is worse with movement and weight bearing. The pain from a diseased hip may be referred to the knee and vice versa (see Fig. 20.1). This may give rise to confusion and you must always examine the two joints to define the precise source of the pain.

A limp may be the result of:

- Pain in the hip. The patient quickly moves his weight off the bad leg onto the other.
- A short leg.
- Inefficient abduction of the leg.
- Other mechanical problems in hip, knee, ankle or spine including stiffness, instability or weakness.

The movements you need to test are shown in Fig. 20.6. It is difficult to use a goniometer for this joint so estimates of the range of movement are acceptable. Check the following:

- Extension. It is possible for a patient to lose 30° of extension but still be able to put the thigh flat on the bed or couch. This is because the spine is being extended. To eliminate this put one hand behind the spine and flex the patient's opposite hip with the other hand. This will flatten out the lumbar spine and reveal the true loss of extension (Fig. 20.6a).
- Flexion.
- Abduction (Fig. 20.6b).
- Adduction (Fig. 20.6c). You will have to flex the hip slightly to do this.
- External rotation (Fig. 20.6d).
- Internal rotation (Fig. 20.6e).

Internal and external rotation are assessed with the patient prone.

Osteoarthritis

Osteoarthritis is the commonest cause of pain in the hip in older people. It is associated with limited movements of which the earliest loss is that of internal rotation.

The knee

This is a complex joint in which injuries are common. Much can be learned from inspecting the joint. Look for:

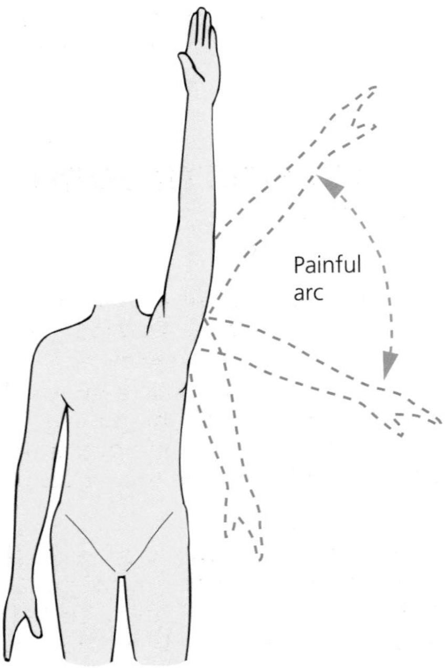

FIG. 20.5 The painful arc syndrome. Note that the pain is usually worse on the downswing.

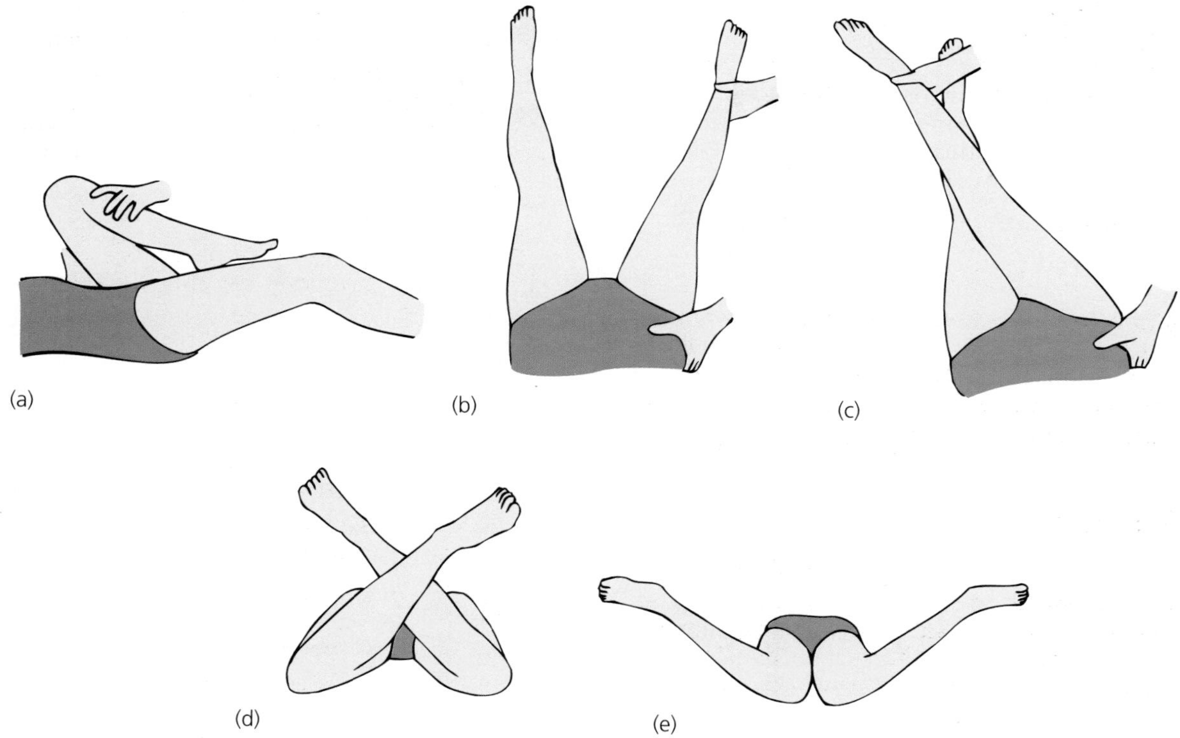

FIG. 20.6 Testing movements of the hip. (a) Note that concealed fixed flexion of the patient's right hip is shown up by placing one hand in the small of the patient's back; (b) abduction, (c) adduction, (d) external rotation, (e) internal rotation.

- Wasting of the quadriceps: measure the circumference of each thigh 10–15 cm above the upper border of the patella.
- Synovial fluid. Does it follow the contours of the synovial cavity which extends 5 cm above the upper border of the patella?
- Sideways angulation. Knock-knee or bow leg? (See Fig. 2.16.)
- Swelling in the popliteal fossa. This is easily missed unless you turn your patient over. A swelling there may be a simple cyst, Baker's cyst or aneurysm.

Measuring flexion and extension is easy. Record using the gonimeter. If the collateral ligaments are torn but the cruciates remain intact, there is no sideways laxity so it is necessary to flex the knee to 20 degrees when testing for lateral stability.

THE DIAGNOSIS OF JOINT PROBLEMS

Joint problems may arise as part of a primary arthritic problem or as a secondary feature of some other disease. This means that when we are examining an abnormal joint we have to take into account a wide range of differential diagnoses. Several factors are of importance in deciding this and you need to take into account:

- Speed of onset.
- The specific joint involved e.g. the first metatarso–phalangeal joint in gout.
- Whether other joints are affected e.g. a polyarthropathy as in rheumatoid arthritis.
- The pattern of joint involvement e.g. symmetrical small joint arthropathy in rheumatoid arthritis.

- Whether a systemic disease is present e.g. sarcoidosis or psoriasis.

It is not the purpose of this book to deal with joint diseases in detail but Revision Panel 20.1 gives some idea of the wide range of diseases that are involved.

Practical Point

Acute septic arthritis demands urgent treatment.

Revision Panel 20.1
Diseases involved in joint problems

Cause	*Age group*	*Joints involved*	*Features*
Infection.[a]	All ages (infection may be superimposed on a pre-existing diseased joint problem such as in rheumatoid arthritis).	Any joint.	Partly dependent on infecting organism (see Chapter 31).
Non-infective inflammatory conditions.			
Rheumatoid arthritis (Fig. 20.7a, b).	Young, middle-aged (females more than males).	Mainly small joints of hands and feet. More proximal joints affected later.	Common. Multisystem disease. Chronic or relapsing. Symmetrical small joint arthropathy.
Psoriatic arthropathy (Fig. 20.8).	All ages.	Mainly hands and feet.	Similar to rheumatoid arthritis but different joints in hand involved.
Ankylosing spondylitis.	Young, middle-aged (males more than females).	Sacroiliac joints. Spine and hips.	Chronic backache with progressive stiffness. Systemic associations such as upper lobe fibrosis and aortic incompetence. HLA B27 positive.
Reactive arthropathy i.e. Reiter's syndrome	Young males.	Mainly joints 'below the belt'.	Usually self-limiting. Associated with urethritis and iritis.
Gout (Fig. 20.9).	Middle and old age	Usually affects first metatarsophalangeal joint initially.	Uric acid arthropathy. Acute very painful attacks progressing to chronic disease.
Osteoarthritis	Increasing with age.	Weight bearing joints: hips, knees and spine.	Common. Wear and tear arthropathy.
Connective tissue disorders, systemic lupus erythematosus, dematomyositis, systemic sclerosis (scleroderma), polyarteritis.	Variable age at onset. All female preponderance except polyarteritis.	Variable joints affected.	Pattern of illness dominated usually by basic disease.

[a]See Practical Point.

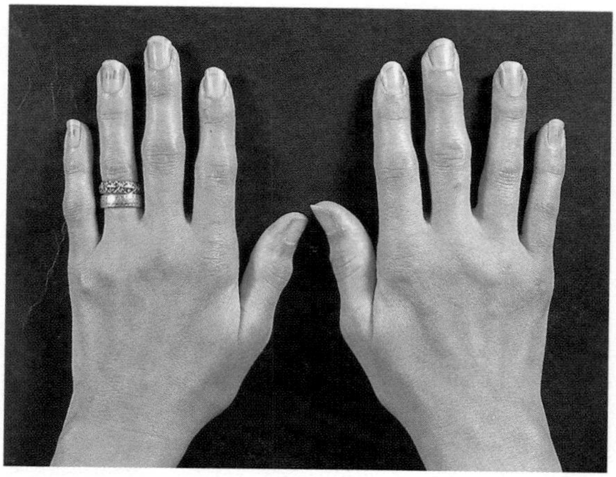

(a)

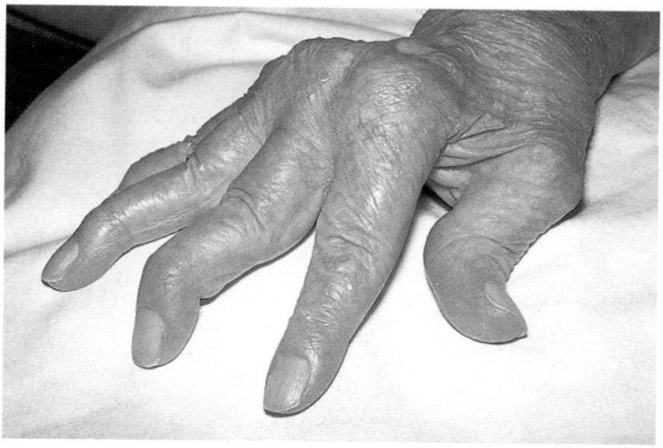

(b)

FIG. 20.7 (a) Early rheumatoid arthritis. Note the minimal spindling of the proximal interphalangeal joints of the index and the middle fingers. (b) Advanced arthritic changes. The middle and ring fingers show 'swan neck' deformity with hyperextension at the proximal interphalangeal joints and flexion at the distal interphalangeal joints. The thumb shows a Z deformity.

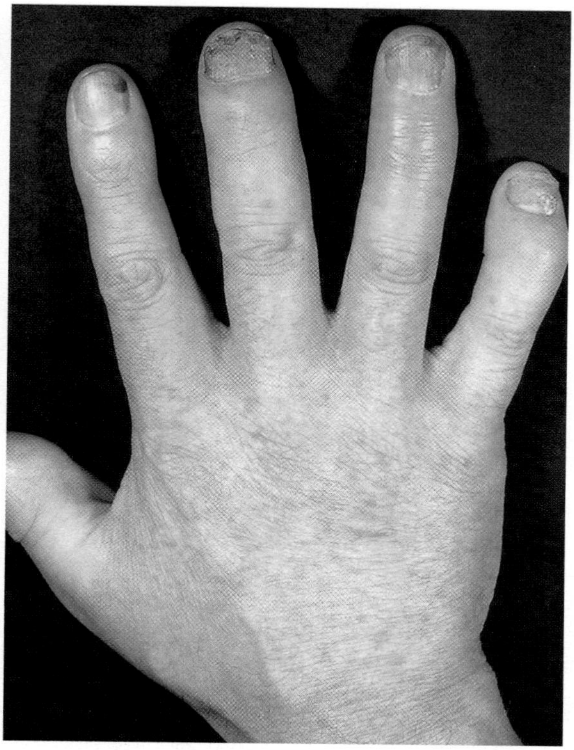

FIG. 20.8 Psoriatic arthritis. Here the distal interphalangeal joints are involved and there are typical psoriatic nail changes.

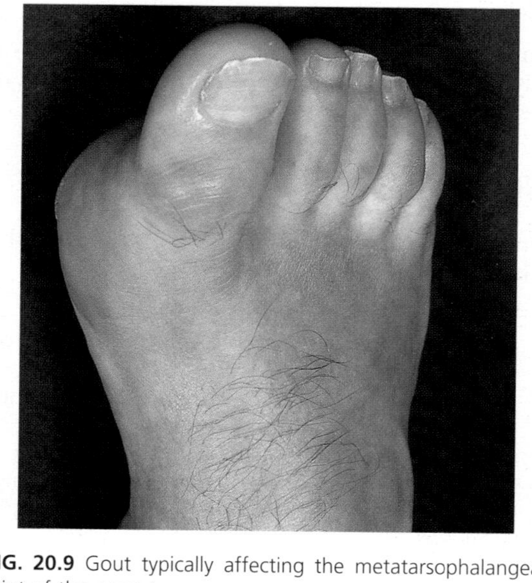

FIG. 20.9 Gout typically affecting the metatarsophalangeal joint of the great toe.

THE SPINE (See Revision Panel 20.2)

Each vertebra is joined to the next one by an intervertebral disc (a syndesmosis which is prone to mechanical disorders) and two posterior facet joints (synovial joints which are subject to osteoarthritis). Degenerative changes in the discs are known as *spondylosis*.

Symptoms

Pain

Disc lesions are commonest in the lower cervical and lower lumbar regions where they cause pain. If nerve roots are compressed there may be referred pain down the arm or leg – in the leg this is known as sciatica. Back pain may arise also from facet joints, disc sprain or prolapse or vertebral collapse.

Weakness and sensory changes

Collapse or disease of vertebrae may cause cord damage by direct pressure or ischaemia.

Deformity

Severe deformity such as scoliosis may interfere with cardiac or respiratory function.

Stiffness

This may be due to reflex muscle spasm or pathological changes in ligaments as in ankylosing spondylitis.

Signs

On looking at the patient with a spinal problem you may see:

- A pure lateral deformity termed *a tilt*.
- Spasm of the erector spinalis on the side of the pain.
- A permanently flexed curve of the spine: when this is over several vertebrae it is termed a *kyphosis* (Fig. 20.10), when there is a sharp angle at one point it is termed a *kyphos*.
- An abnormally extended position is called a *lordosis*.
- A lateral and rotational curve, often complex, is termed *scoliosis* (Fig. 20.11).

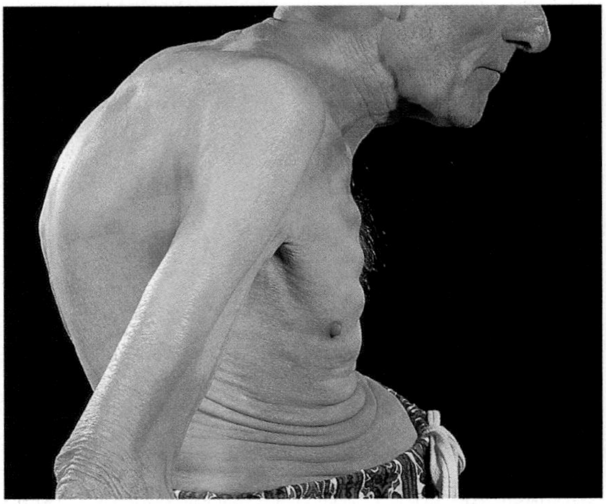

FIG. 20.10 Severe kyphosis as the result of collapse of multiple vertebrae due to myelomatosis. Note the anterior skin creases in the abdominal wall due to the trunk shortening.

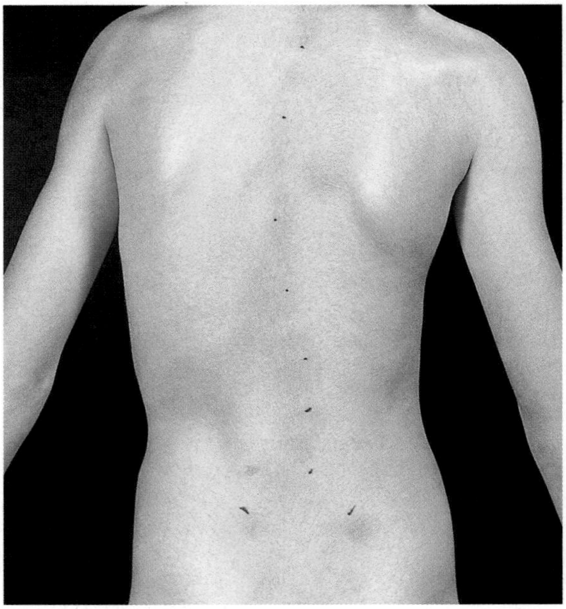

FIG. 20.11 Scoliosis.

Practical Point

If cord compression is not relieved within hours the damage will be permanent.

Revision Panel 20.2

Abnormalities of spine structure and function.

Physical signs	*Young patients*	*Middle-aged or elderly*
Stiffness and pain.	Ankylosing spondylitis. Disc lesions. Trauma.	As in the younger age groups. Spondylosis. Malignancy. Chronic infections e.g. tuberculosis.
Loss of height (shortening).	Extensive compression injuries.	Osteoporosis. Widespread malignant deposits in spine. Paget's disease.
Scoliosis.	Congenital. Acquired (idiopathic). Neurological (e.g. earlier polio).	Usually following problems in youth.
Kyphosis.	Congenital. Spinal tuberculosis. Ankylosing spondylosis. Scheuermann's disease.	As a result of disease whilst young. Osteoporosis. Tuberculosis. Widespread malignant deposits in spine.
Congenital and acquired change in shape of the skeleton.	Various forms of dwarfism in childhood such as achondroplasia (see Fig. 2.9) or rickets.	As a result of disease in childhood Paget's disease (see Fig. 2.5). Osteoporosis. Osteomalacia.

Where there is severe pain, and/or cord compression is suspected, full neurological examination is mandatory.

In particular check:

- Straight leg raising. If there is much pain and straight leg raising is limited to 20 or 30 degrees then a prolapsed disc is likely.
- Possible root level at which there might be damage.
- Any problems with micturition. Test sensation to pin prick round the anus; perianal anaesthesia indicates involvement of sacral roots, which also involves the bladder.

Practical Point

Back pain is unlikely to be of a serious nature when:

The patient gets on and off the examination couch without discomfort.

There is no associated spasm of the back muscles.

The spine moves fully in all directions.

21 Understanding AIDS

INTRODUCTION

AIDS, or acquired immune deficiency syndrome, is the end-stage of a chronic viral infection possibly caused by the human immunodeficiency virus (HIV) and is the result of a progressive impairment of cellular immune function. The disease may run through distinct stages, each causing different symptoms and signs.

Acute infection

Many individuals are completely asymptomatic but symptoms that do develop are usually suggestive of a viral illness. These include fever, myalgia, malaise, arthropathy, sore throat, headache, photophobia, nausea, vomiting and diarrhoea. You might find swollen glands and a rash and occasionally neurological problems such as facial palsy or weakness due to Guillain–Barré syndrome.

Asymptomatic chronic infection

Symptoms and signs are completely absent at this stage. Patients who know they have become infected may need help to deal with non-specific symptoms such as a mild temperature or nausea, vomiting and '24 hour diarrhoea'. Symptoms such as these are unlikely to be the first sign that the illness has progressed.

Persistent generalized lymphadenopathy

About one-third of patients will have easily palpable nodes in two sites other than the groin which persist for more than three months. These nodes will be mobile and symmetrical. Patients with AIDS are generally not aware of their swollen glands. If you do feel nodes in a patient in a high-risk group, ask if these are tender because lymph nodes enlarged due to most of the common illnesses are very tender.

Late chronic infection

Months or even years may pass before further problems arise. Constitutional symptoms and episodes of minor infection occur often:

- Fungal infections such as oral *Candida*.
- Bacterial skin infections such as impetigo.
- Viral infections such as re-activated herpes simplex or anogenital warts.

End-stage disease

By this stage, cellular immunodeficiency is well-advanced. Unusual tumours and neurological disease may become apparent and life-threatening opportunistic infections may affect particularly the lungs, skin and gut.

OPPORTUNISTIC INFECTIONS IN AIDS

Everyone is exposed to a wide range of potential pathogens but a competent immune system provides a high degree of protection. Immune suppression increases the risk of a life-threatening opportunistic infection with otherwise harmless bacterial, fungal, protozoan and viral organisms. Illness due to infection with common organisms such as *Streptococcus pneumoniae* or *Salmonella* species are usually more severe and may relapse unless a prolonged course of treatment is given.

In the lungs, *Pneumocystis carinii* is common. Often there are few signs in the chest despite marked dyspnoea and cyanosis. Atypical mycobacterium infections are almost diagnostic of AIDS but pulmonary tuberculosis is also seen.

In the gut, oral *Candida* is common, as is oral ulceration (Fig. 21.1) and hairy leukoplakia (Fig. 21.2). Acute oesophagitis follows infection with fungae or cytomegalovirus. Parasitic infection of the small bowel with *Cryptosporidium* may cause diarrhoea, malabsorption and weight loss.

A variety of non-malignant and malignant diseases affect the skin. The typical rash of herpes zoster may re-appear. Molluscum contagiosum, usually limited to the groin, is often generalized and labial or genital herpes simplex may be evident. Those who suffer from psoriasis may report a severe exacerbation.

Infection of the nervous system with herpes simplex virus, cytomegalovirus, herpes zoster and mycobacteria may cause encephalitis, cryptococcus a meningitis and toxoplasma multiple necrotic abscesses.

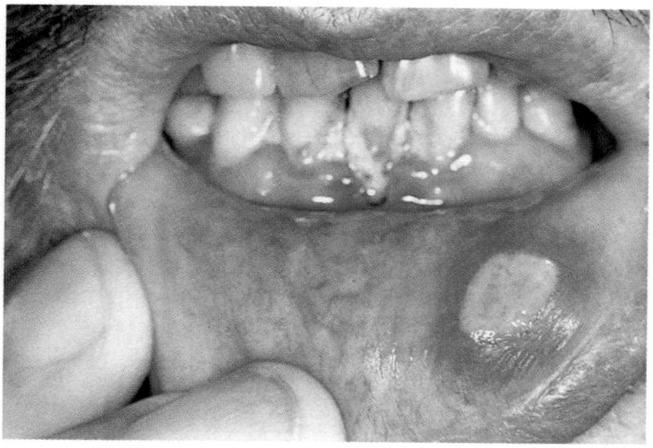

FIG. 21.1 Oral ulceration.

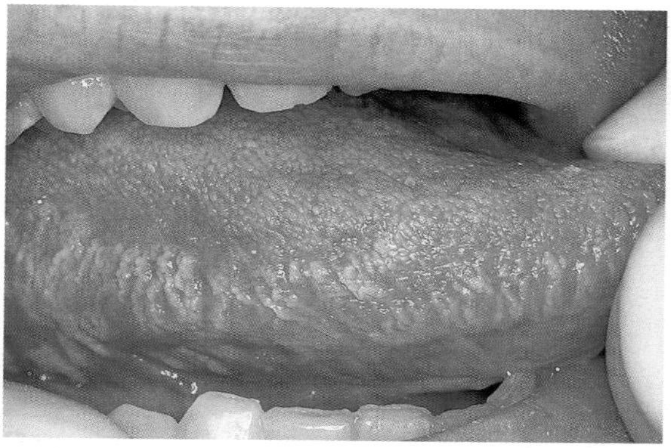

FIG. 21.2 Oral hairy leukoplakia.

MALIGNANCY AND AIDS

Although the distinctive subtle pink macules of Kaposi's sarcoma (Fig. 21.3) may appear on the skin and darken, this malignancy also can mimic an apparently innocent insect bite, or a fleshy mole, or a basal cell carcinoma. Similar lesions can occur in the lungs and gut. Lymphomas are usually extranodal and generally herald a quick decline. Symptoms of a systemic upset include weight loss, night sweats and malaise as well as features relating to the site of the tumour, such as obstruction or diarrhoea with gut involvement or headache and neurological signs with intracranial tumours.

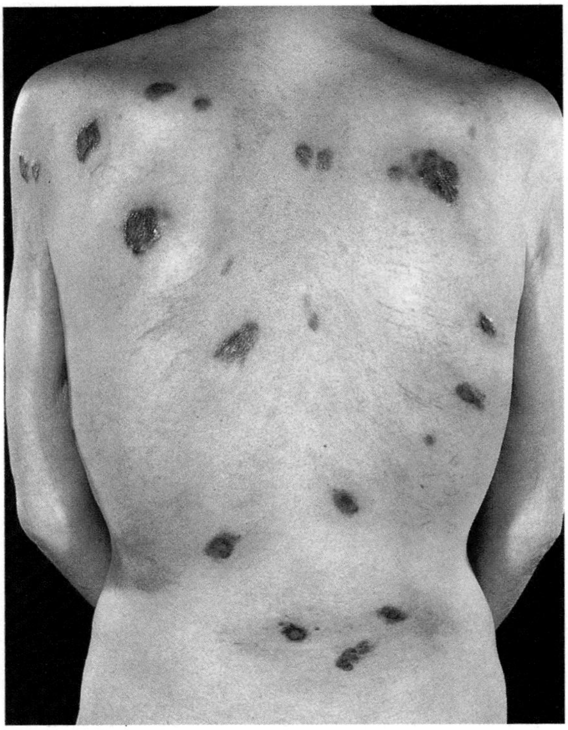

FIG. 21.3 Kaposi's sarcoma.

PSYCHOLOGICAL ASPECTS OF AIDS

News of a positive test for AIDS affects individuals in different ways. The typical stages of coming to terms psychologically with any diagnosis, such as shock, guilt, fear and anxiety, often do not apply to patients with AIDS because the social perception of the disease differs greatly from almost all other diseases. How patients handle the news depends on their own belief systems, personal resources and those of friends, family, colleagues and social support network, and previous experience with illness. Post-diagnosis counselling must be spread over several consultations so that important information can be reinforced.

You may be asked to discuss problems and uncertainties concerning:

- Day-to-day relationships with partners, friends, work colleagues and especially employers.
- Risk to daily contacts.
- Immediate and future and experimental treatment.
- Death and dying.

Despite media publicity, most patients newly diagnosed as HIV-positive remain well for some time. Although about half of all HIV-positive patients will develop AIDS within ten years, the number of patients who have not progressed to develop AIDS is increasing, so you can be fairly positive about the future. At least in the early days, not every non-specific symptom means that the disease has progressed. However, you will need to pass on these concerns to your seniors so that a more experienced member of the team can deal with the issues in a sensitive but truthful way.

Patients with AIDS are often triggered to seek help about their concerns and anxieties when:

- Specific 'negative' life events affecting the individual such as the death of a friend or the loss of a job raise concerns about general health.
- Events in society, such as 'positive' articles on advances in treatment which appear in newspapers or magazines may raise hopes of a 'cure' inappropriately.

Above all, you should remember that patients with AIDS are normal people trying to come to terms with a very abnormal situation – the fear that, at some stage, a symptom or sign may appear which indicates the finality of their illness. You should respond by allowing them to express their feelings and frustrations and inevitably strong emotions. Be prepared to offer psychological support and practical help where you can and seek the help of your seniors.

Learning to devise a differential diagnosis

22

Establishing the cause of a patient's symptoms generally requires:

- A well-taken and detailed history.
- A thorough systematic examination.
- Selected specific investigations.

Common diseases tend to present in characteristic ways and in most cases, as you gain experience, you will find you have a pretty good idea what is most likely to be wrong after simply taking the history. This will help direct your physical examination to look for specific clues which confirm your clinical suspicions (see Revision Panel 22.1 where examples are shown).

Revision Panel 22.1

Case 1

A 22-year-old student presents with a two-day history of headache, nausea, vomiting, a fever and is intolerant of bright lights. Her temperature is 38.5°C, there are no focal signs of infection but she has a stiff neck.

The most likely diagnosis is meningitis. A lumbar puncture will confirm the diagnosis.

Case 2

A 55-year-old man with a long history of angina presents two hours after the sudden onset of very severe pain spreading from the chest to the shoulder blades, much worse than his usual angina. He is cold, clammy and obviously in pain. Blood pressure is high and there is a 20 mmHg difference in pressure between the left and right arms. Electrocardiograph shows a sinus tachycardia only.

The differential diagnosis is a) aortic dissection; b) acute myocardial infarction; and c) unstable angina.

MAKING UP A DIFFERENTIAL DIAGNOSIS

In many cases, the history and examination point you towards a single diagnosis. In other cases, you may be less sure what is wrong, so you will need to consider a range of possibilities. You should now make a medical 'short list' of the two or three (or more) conditions that could explain the symptoms and signs. For example, an elderly patient may be confused due to a urinary or respiratory tract infection, an intracranial lesion or an accidental overdose.

This 'differental diagnosis' is important because:

- It allows others to see not only what diagnoses you have considered but also what you have (rightly or wrongly) omitted.
- It forms the basis for selecting appropriate investigations to confirm or refute each of your possible diagnoses.

The most likely diagnosis should go first and the rest should be ranked in descending order of importance.

WHAT TO DO IF YOU CAN'T MAKE UP A DIFFERENTIAL DIAGNOSIS

Sometimes things conspire against you. The patient may be confused, unable to remember anything or simply too ill to answer your questions; relatives may be unhelpful, or the symptoms just don't fit any pattern you can recognize.

If you really feel you have insufficient clues to make a diagnosis, it is good practice to go over the main points of the history again. Repeat parts of the examination you were unsure about. Try to get more information, from a friend or neighbour and contact the General Practitioner for some background details – patients sometimes 'forget' significant details of their medical history and treatment.

Having exhausted all avenues of information, you may still be no nearer a firm diagnosis. In these circumstances, it is essential to keep an open mind about the range of diseases that may explain the patient's symptoms. Make a list of all the common illnesses that you know that could conceivably account for your patient's problem.

You are most likely to have difficulty with a patient who presents with symptoms that do not fit into any classical pattern. Beware making a diagnosis of a rare disease until you have excluded common ones. Always remember that 'common diseases occur commonly' and most illnesses which prove difficult to diagnose turn out to be unusual presentations of common diseases. For example, a patient who presents with a fever that defies explanation despite extensive investigation in hospital *could* have Rocky Mountain Spotted Fever but a more likely diagnosis is a malignancy, connective tissue disorder or an infection due to a fastidious organism.

Practical Point

Remember:
Common diseases occasionally present with symptoms which are atypical.

The worst case scenario

At some stage, you may be forced to accept that the range of possibilities is very wide. For example, a headache is a very non-specific symptom of stress, cervical spondylosis, cerebral tumour, subarachnoid haemorrhage, meningitis, migraine, infection and many other illnesses.

Patients and relatives will be anxious to know what is wrong. A useful concept is to consider what is the most likely diagnosis and make this your *working diagnosis*. It is your best guess in the circumstances and forms the basis for your early management and initial investigations. You will almost certainly need to revise this:

- According to the response to treatment.
- When initial test results are available.
- If you acquire additional information.

What next?

A senior colleague will often check parts of the history and examination. An alternative differential diagnosis may emerge and further tests requested or some tests given higher priority.

DIAGNOSTIC POSSIBILITIES

To give you some idea of how to focus your thoughts on deriving a differential diagnosis breathlessness will be used as an example.

Breathlessness

Breathlessness is a common presenting symptom. It is often relatively easy to quickly eliminate many of the numerous causes so that just a handful remain. Speed may be important, but not at the expense of accuracy. As you gain experience, you will learn a useful short cut in emergency medicine of asking questions while you are examining the patient.

Adopt one of the following strategies:

The symptomatic approach – e.g. how quickly did the breathlessness develop? There are few causes of truly sudden onset of breathlessness. Have you had this before and what made it better?

The systematic approach – the commonest causes are due to cardiovascular and respiratory disease. Remember that haematological (anaemia), metabolic (diabetic ketoacidosis) and renal disease (uraemia) can cause breathlessness.

The probability approach – work out the likelihood of disease based on age, previously history and epidemiology. Pulmonary oedema is a common cause of acute breathlessness in an elderly man with a history of heart attack or valvular heart disease. Asthma is common in young children, pneumothorax in active thin people, emphysema and chronic bronchitis in middle-aged smokers and bronchopneumonia in the inactive elderly.

23 Ordering basic tests

The differential diagnosis simply ranks the most likely causes for a patient's symptoms based on the clinical impression. Sometimes you will be sufficiently confident in your diagnosis that you can start treatment. In emergencies, of course, you may be forced to do so. In most cases, however, it will be necessary to order a range of selected investigations to make sure that your clinical diagnosis is correct.

Carefully selected investigations can be very helpful because they may:

- Provide objective evidence that your clinical impression is correct.
- Define the extent of disease.
- Indicate the severity of disease.
- Provide a 'physiological' baseline prior to treatment.
- Monitor the impact of disease or the effect of treatment.
- Help avoid drug toxicity.

POINTS TO REMEMBER ABOUT TEST RESULTS

Biological variables generally have a Gaussian or normal 'bell-shaped' distribution, with 95% of the population falling within two standard deviations from the median. Blood test results are no different, so the expected 'normal' range provided with each result should apply to 95% of those tested. What about test results which fall outside the normal range?

THE ABNORMAL TEST RESULT

In statistical terms, results *just outside* this range may still be normal for the remaining 5% of the population. It is important to remember this because a *slightly* abnormal test does not necessarily indicate disease. A test result can be well outside the normal range for several reasons:

- The normal range may be inappropriate for the patient. Results may vary with age, sex, race and pregnancy.
- The test is truly abnormal and confirms the clinical diagnosis.
- The test has been affected by factors such as diet, drugs and serum proteins. Your local laboratory will advise.
- There may be evidence of a trend developing. Check previous and future results.
- Previously unsuspected pathology is discovered – this may warrant further investigation.
- A technical error has occurred. The laboratory will recommend repeating the test.

If there is any doubt about the relevance of a result, discuss alternative investigations with the appropriate department.

A WARNING ABOUT TESTS

The ideal test would reliably identify patients who genuinely have a specific disease. Few investigations come close to this because all tests are a compromise, balancing *sensitivity* (that is the test is good at identifying patients who really have a disease) against *specificity* (that is the test is good at proving patients are disease-free).

For example, a test with 95% sensitivity means 5% of tests would be 'false negatives' so those with disease would not be identified.

Similarly, a test with 95% specificity means 5% of tests would be 'false positives' and healthy individuals would be thought (wrongly) to be ill.

Altering a test to make it more sensitive reduces its specificity and vice versa.

Revision Panel 23.1

Example of investigation list in a patient complaining of breathless on exertion

Differential diagnosis	*Investigations*
Chronic airways disease.	Peak flow, chest X-ray, full lung function tests.
Ischaemic heart disease.	ECG, treadmill test.
Anaemia.	Full blood count.
Left ventricular dysfunction.	ECG, echocardiography.

WHICH TESTS SHOULD YOU REQUEST?

The purpose of investigation is to obtain conclusive objective evidence that there can be only one explanation for a patient's symptoms. Some tests are non-specific markers of disease. For example, raised C-reactive protein (CRP) and erythrocyte sedimentation rate (ESR) imply infection or inflammation, while other tests are positive only in the presence of a single disease.

Most of the common illnesses can be diagnosed with relatively simple tests (Revision Panel 23.1).

When considering which tests to request, start by reviewing the differential diagnosis list. Time spent thinking about what tests to organize (and the sequence in which you request them) is never wasted. It makes sense to aim first at the most likely cause of a patient's symptoms and consider what investigations are available to help confirm your clinical suspicions.

Invasive tests carry some risk of harming the patient, although training and expertise help minimize the risk; coronary angiography and liver biopsy are good examples. Wherever possible, consider whether non-invasive blood or urine tests and simple X-ray investigations (which generally cause the patient no harm or inconvenience) will provide you with the information you require.

Results which fall within the normal range may be described as 'negative'. They usually exclude or 'rule out' a putative diagnosis. Sometimes, however, a result may not become 'positive':

- For several hours after the onset of an illness e.g. creatine kinase takes up to 12 hours to appear in any great quantity in blood after a myocardial infarction.
- For several days after the onset of an illness e.g. viral titres are low for ten days or so after infection.
- For several months e.g. after infection with human immunodeficiency virus (HIV).

Results may be so far outside the normal range that the test can only be described as 'positive' and hence 'diagnostic' of disease. In most instances, this will be true, but occasionally, the result will be a 'false positive', implying that a disease is present when this is incorrect.

Negative results may be just as helpful as those that are positive; they may help to eliminate at least some of the causes in a long differential diagnosis list.

TESTS FOR DIAGNOSIS

As you gain experience and knowledge, you will find that your ability to develop a differential diagnosis improves, and with it, your ability to evaluate the most likely cause of a patient's illness. In addition, you will find it easier to work out which tests will give you a diagnosis quickly.

Most common diseases can be diagnosed quite simply:

- Suspected infections. Bacterial infection usually causes an abnormally high white cell count. For localized infection, specimens from throat, sputum, pleural fluid, stool, cerebrospinal fluid, urine and blood may be helpful; X-ray of chest; white cell scan to look for deep-seated infection.
- Chronic respiratory disease. Peak flow is reduced. Chest X-ray shows hyper-inflated lungs and 'flat' diaphragm.
- Heart attack. The electrocardiograph shows characteristic changes of ST segment elevation on the first day and Q waves develop later. Cardiac enzymes or troponin levels are raised.
- Joint diseases. Various immunological and antibody tests help distinguish one form of arthritis from another.

TESTS FOR MONITORING THE EFFECTS OF TREATMENT

Tests may be used to confirm that treatment is being effective, perhaps to ensure that serum levels of anticonvulsant drugs or digoxin are within a range considered to be optimum (the 'therapeutic window') or to make sure that treatment is not causing any important physiological changes. For example, diuretics and ACE inhibitors prescribed for heart failure may cause a deterioration in renal function, with a rise in serum creatinine and urea.

> **Practical Point**
>
> *Clinical problem*
>
> Patient admitted with severe central chest pain described as 'crushing' with radiation to the left arm.
>
> The diagnosis of acute myocardial infarction can be 'ruled out' with blood and electrocardiographic tests taken on consecutive days.
>
> Troponin and 'cardiac' enzymes such as creatine kinase are available in most hospitals.

POINTS TO REMEMBER WHEN ORDERING TESTS

There are dangers in thinking that tests are 'routine'. You should always be able to justify each test.

The most frequently requested blood tests such as the full blood count, erythrocyte sedimentation rate and C-reactive protein, urea and electrolytes, liver function tests, thyroid function tests and blood glucose, undergo automated analysis. You will usually find a chart in the treatment room or (in some hospitals) the junior doctors' handbook to indicate which sample bottle is required for each test.

Some tests require close attention to technique of collection or accurate timing of samples; these include blood cultures and cortisol measurement. Other tests demand individual analysis and requests must be discussed with the appropriate laboratory prior to collection of the sample.

If you request a test, make sure that you get the result and record it prominently in the notes before you permanently file it. This will help you when you are presenting on ward rounds. Try to get any outstanding results before a ward round. This will not only make you look very efficient but will allow your colleagues to consider whether further investigations are necessary.

TEST 'BATTERIES'

In some hospitals, a 'battery' of tests can be requested; one example is shown in Revision Panel 23.2

Revision Panel 23.2
A typical test battery

Sodium
Potassium
Urea
Creatinine
Albumin
γ-Glutamyltransferase (GGT)
Alkaline phosphatase
Alanine transaminase (ALT)
Bilirubin
Free T4
Thyroid-stimulating hormone (TSH)
Total cholesterol
Creatine phosphokinase (CPK)
Troponin I
Glucose

This approach produces more information than you need and inevitably will produce a few abnormal results which may generate even more unnecessary investigations. Stick to ordering only those investigations you feel are warranted by clinical circumstances.

It is probably more helpful to consider which tests will help prove that an infective cause is likely in a patient with a history of burning dysuria, a temperature of 38.5°C and a leucocytosis; or in an elderly patient arrange a range of tests which help differentiate acute confusion from mild but progressive dementia.

WHAT TO TELL THE PATIENT

Most patients will be reassured to be kept up-to-date with the way investigations are proceeding. It is important that you discuss any tests that are potentially unpleasant or carry recognized risks. Be prepared to spend time with your patient to explain why such tests are necessary and to answer any questions.*

Remember that:

- The benefits of any procedure (such as getting a diagnosis quickly) must outweigh any attendant risks.
- Unnecessary investigation will not be appreciated by your patient.
- Overinvestigation will not be appreciated by your boss or hospital.
- Potential complications of appropriate investigations must be discussed with the patient.
- Complications after inappropriate investigations are impossible to explain to patients and relatives.
- Patients have a right to know what risks accompany each investigation.
- Simple venepuncture can be traumatic for some patients.
- You must be able to justify the need for each test.
- Some tests are hazardous.
- Never arrange an invasive investigation if there is a reasonable non-invasive alternative.
- You may be causing unnecessary work for yourself.

Revision Panel 23.3
Summary

Tests should be carefully selected. This avoids subjecting your patient to unnecessary and potentially harmful investigations.

An abnormal value is not always a sign of disease.

Some tests demand close attention to detail. Check with your laboratory.

Request tests which are 'non-invasive' and low risk.

Always explain to your patient what each test involves, especially if investigations are 'invasive' and potentially harmful.

Discuss with your patient the results of tests as soon as you can.

*During your student years you should try to see as many investigations as possible. This will help you in later years to understand what patients go through when being investigated.

The problem, how it presents and what causes it

C

Breathlessness

Dyspnoea is the subjective awareness of being short of breath or the conscious awareness of the need for increased respiratory effort. Breathlessness related to strenuous physical exertion is universal but is abnormal when it occurs:

- At rest or with mild exertion.
- When lying flat necessitating having to sleep propped upright.
- When it causes the patient to wake from sleep.

It is mainly caused by diseases of the heart or lungs or by severe anaemia.

IS THE PATIENT ILL?

Many patients report breathlessness but are not seriously ill. Important clues to 'functional' dyspnoea (that is breathlessness which is not due to organic disease) are:

- A feeling of being unable to take a deep breath.
- Tingling in the lips and fingers; feeling faint; rapid breathing; a sensation of suffocation. These are often due to 'panic' and hyperventilation.
- Feeling out of breath all the time.
- Normal exercise tolerance.

Clues to genuine illness include:

- Adapting life to avoid all unnecessary exertion.
- Breathing through pursed lips, which helps to reduce the tendency for smaller airways to collapse.
- Using accessory muscles of respiration. Patients often sit leaning forward with shoulders hunched up and hands on hips.
- An audible wheeze – though some patients can generate this at will.
- A change in breathing pattern with short inspiration and prolonged expiration.
- Looking ill, fighting for breath or even looking 'shocked'.

Many patients report breathlessness following apparently trivial exertion. The cause is usually lack of fitness or weight gain over the years. A high proportion of the adult car-driving population in the UK is unused to taking exercise and is unfit.

In the acutely ill, you need to ask questions whilst you are examining. To develop your clinical skills to this standard means you need lots of practice. Try to see patients as soon as they arrive in hospital.

IS THE ILLNESS SERIOUS?

Some causes of breathlessness are life-threatening. As a general rule, acute onset of an illness in a previously well person or a sudden change in a patient known to have an underlying disease should always be considered to indicate a patient at high risk. Slowly progressive symptoms may indicate serious disease particularly if associated with weight loss, chronic cough or haemoptysis.

Clues to severity are:

- An associated tachycardia.
- An inability to complete a sentence.
- Low blood pressure, cold and clammy.
- Having to sit upright.
- Accompanying chest pain.
- Weight loss.

SOME COMMON CAUSES

A quick look at Revision Panel 24.1 shows the range of medical problems that may cause breathlessness. They cover all body systems and illnesses ranging from relatively harmless to life-threatening.

Revision Panel 24.1

Some causes of breathlessness

Cardiovascular	Pulmonary oedema. Congestive cardiac failure. Valvular heart disease. Cardiomyopathy. Coronary heart disease.
Respiratory	Asthma. Bronchiectasis. Bronchitis. Carcinoma. Emphysema. Fibrosing alveolitis. Pleural effusion. Pneumothorax. Pulmonary embolus.
Neuromuscular[a]	Guillain–Barré syndrome. Scoliosis. Ankylosing spondylitis. Myasthenia gravis. Hyperventilation. Brainstem infarction. Cheyne–Stokes respiration.
Drug-induced	Salicylate poisoning.
Haematological	Anaemia.
Renal[a]	Renal failure. Hypoalbuminaemia.
Trauma[a]	Chest wall injury.
Metabolic and endocrine[a]	Diabetic ketoacidosis. Obesity.
Other	Anxiety, hyperventilation and panic attack. Lack of fitness.

[a]In these disorders the breathlessness is usually a secondary feature of the basic problem.

SOME LESS COMMON BUT STILL IMPORTANT CAUSES

The list of possible causes of breathlessness embraces every body system. You need to bear in mind that:

- Pulmonary tuberculosis is still a very serious problem in many parts of the world such as the Indian subcontinent.
- In the developed world, pulmonary tuberculosis remains prevalent among those with AIDS (acquired immunodeficiency syndrome) and homeless people.
- Pulmonary fibrosis may develop insidiuosly.
- Multisystem disorders, such as rheumatoid arthritis, may be associated with lung disease.
- Symptoms may develop soon after initiating drug treatment with beta-blocking drugs used in the treatment of hypertension and angina, or much later after treatment with cytotoxic drugs such as methotrexate.

GROUPS AT RISK

Some patients are at increased risk of breathlessness. These include:

- 'Smokers'. Chronic lung disease including chronic bronchitis and emphysema and coronary heart disease are particularly common.
- Some occupational groups, such as miners, who are at risk of pneumoconiosis, or farmers who are at risk of an allergic alveolitis from mouldy hay.
- Some recreational groups such as those who keep caged birds may develop symptoms similar to farmer's lung.
- Anyone handling asbestos, used in fireproofing and insulation, may develop progressive pulmonary fibrosis years after exposure.
- Women who smoke and take the oral contraceptive pill are at increased risk of thromboembolic disease.

WHAT TO DO FIRST

Irrespective of the patient's presenting symptoms, three factors remain important:

- Knowledge of what illnesses are common in the young, middle-aged and elderly.
- A well-taken history and a careful examination paying particular attention to areas identified in your history as the potential cause of the present illness. This will allow you to construct a short differential diagnosis list.
- Carefully selected investigations – generally non-invasive before invasive.

Age, speed of onset and associated features will help towards diagnosis. Problems you will come across frequently in young people are:

- Asthma. Recurrent episodes of wheeze are often triggered by pollen, spores, exposure to pets or viral infection.
- Respiratory infection. Complaints of a productive cough, fever and haemoptysis with pain on inspiration suggest pneumonia.
- Pneumothorax. Sudden onset of breathlessness accompanied by unilateral chest pain is characteristic.
- Pulmonary embolus. Young women taking the oral contraceptive pill, especially smokers.

The spectrum of disease in middle-aged people is different:

- Severe chest pain with breathlessness is likely to be acute myocardial infarction.
- Acute breathlessness with a history of coronary heart disease is likely to be pulmonary oedema.

In the elderly, still other causes are common:

- Leg and abdominal swelling and liver tenderness suggests chronic heart failure.
- Chronic cough, haemoptysis and chest pain accompanying gradually progressive breathlessness is often due to carcinoma of the lung.

Revision Panel 24.2

Features associated with breathlessness which aid diagnosis

Wheeze	Usually a respiratory cause. Acute asthma. Chronic bronchitis and emphysema. Bronchiectasis. Acute pulmonary oedema.
Purulent sputum	Usually a respiratory cause. Chronic bronchitis. Bronchiectasis. Pneumonia.
Haemoptysis	Usually a respiratory cause. Pneumonia. Carcinoma. Pulmonary embolus.
Paroxysmal nocturnal dyspnoea	Usually a cardiac cause. Coronary heart disease. Valvular heart disease. Cardiomyopathy.
Chest pain	Usually a cardiac cause. Coronary heart disease.
Peripheral oedema	Usually a cardiac cause. Coronary heart disease. Cardiomyopathy. Cor pulmonale.
Clubbing	Usually a respiratory cause.
Raised jugular venous pressure/pulsation	Usually a cardiac cause.
Displaced apex beat	Usually a cardiac cause.
Palpitations	Usually a cardiac cause. Coronary heart disease. Valvular heart disease. Cardiomyopathy.

FINDING THE CAUSE

Remember to take a good history and examine thoroughly, after which you should be able to at least identify which physiological system is at fault.

It is often unnecessary (and potentially dangerous) to wait for confirmatory tests in desperately ill patients, for example the patient who is at death's door with left ventricular failure – a clinical trial of treatment is acceptable, as tests can be conducted once the situation is under control.

Fortunately dyspnoea is usually accompanied by other symptoms which help narrow the range of potential causes to a manageable few (see Revision Panel 24.2).

A logical sequence of questions will help establish the cause. Some clues are available in the history:

Speed of onset Pneumothorax and pulmonary oedema occur suddenly, while pneumonia and exacerbation of chronic bronchitis usually develop more slowly.

Age of patient Peanut inhalation occurs more frequently in the young, lack of fitness often becomes apparent in middle age and the elderly are more likely to have multiple causes including anaemia induced by non-steroidal drugs, chronic bronchitis and valvular heart disease.

Accompanying symptoms.

Previous medical problems Coronary heart disease predisposes to acute pulmonary oedema and immunosuppressive therapy after transplant increases the risk of infection.

WHAT TO DO NEXT

Your differential diagnosis will dictate which simple investigations you need to request to provide supporting evidence for one diagnosis and to eliminate all others. Typical investigations are shown in Revision Panel 24.3. Not every test will be necessary in every patient. You will soon gain sufficient experience to help you select which are the most appropriate.

Revision Panel 24.3

System under suspicion	Test
Cardiovascular	ECG, 'cardiac enzymes' and troponin, echocardiography, 24-hour tape recording and chest X-ray.
Respiratory	Chest X-ray, sputum and blood cultures, spirometry and blood gas analysis. Invasive procedures include pleural aspiration, bronchoscopy and node biopsy.[a]
Haematological	Full blood count; bone marrow.[a]
Metabolic	Cortisol, urea, thyroid function tests, glucose, blood gases.

[a]The decision to request one of these tests will usually be made by a more senior doctor.

Chest pain

Chest pain is a common cause of admission to hospital and a frequent symptom reported in the Outpatient Department. It often causes great anxiety through either its severity or frequency or its impact on employment prospects and on lifestyle.

Almost any structure within the thorax and chest wall can cause chest pain. Some pains are temporarily inconvenient and self-limiting (most musculoskeletal causes), some are immediately life-threatening (like myocardial infarction or a dissecting aneurysm).

IS THE PATIENT ILL?

Many patients who complain of chest pain may not necessarily look particularly unwell. Even so, chest pain can be a very debilitating symptom, leading many patients to suspect that they are seriously ill. The patient is unlikely to be ill if chest pain is:

- Constant and niggling having lasted for days or weeks without any disturbance to normal activities.
- Ill-defined or associated with tingling in the fingers or lips.
- Relieved by change of posture, heat or manipulation.
- Described by pointing at a localized area on the chest wall, particularly the left submammary region.

IS THE ILLNESS SERIOUS?

Symptoms which suggest a potentially serious cause include:

- Pain which is severe, probably the worst a man has ever experienced or the second worst (to chilbirth) that a woman has experienced.
- Pain which is of very sudden onset.
- Pain which radiates to either arm, throat, neck or back.
- Pain which is associated with other symptoms especially syncope or progressive breathlessness.
- Pain which is worse on exertion.

Chest pain which is potentially life-threatening arises predominantly from the cardiovascular and respiratory systems.

Important signs to look for are those due to 'shock' and a low cardiac output, such as:

- Pale and clammy skin.
- Low blood pressure.
- Tachycardia.
- Pulmonary oedema.
- Poor urine output.
- Clouded consciousness.

SOME COMMON CAUSES

The most frequent causes are musculoskeletal problems, gastro-oesophageal reflux (Fig. 25.1), myocardial ischaemia or infarction and pulmonary thromboembolism. Acute chest pain suggestive of a heart attack is a common cause of admission to hospital.

SOME LESS COMMON BUT STILL IMPORTANT CAUSES

Dissecting aneurysm of the aorta is life-threatening. Although the pain may be like that of a

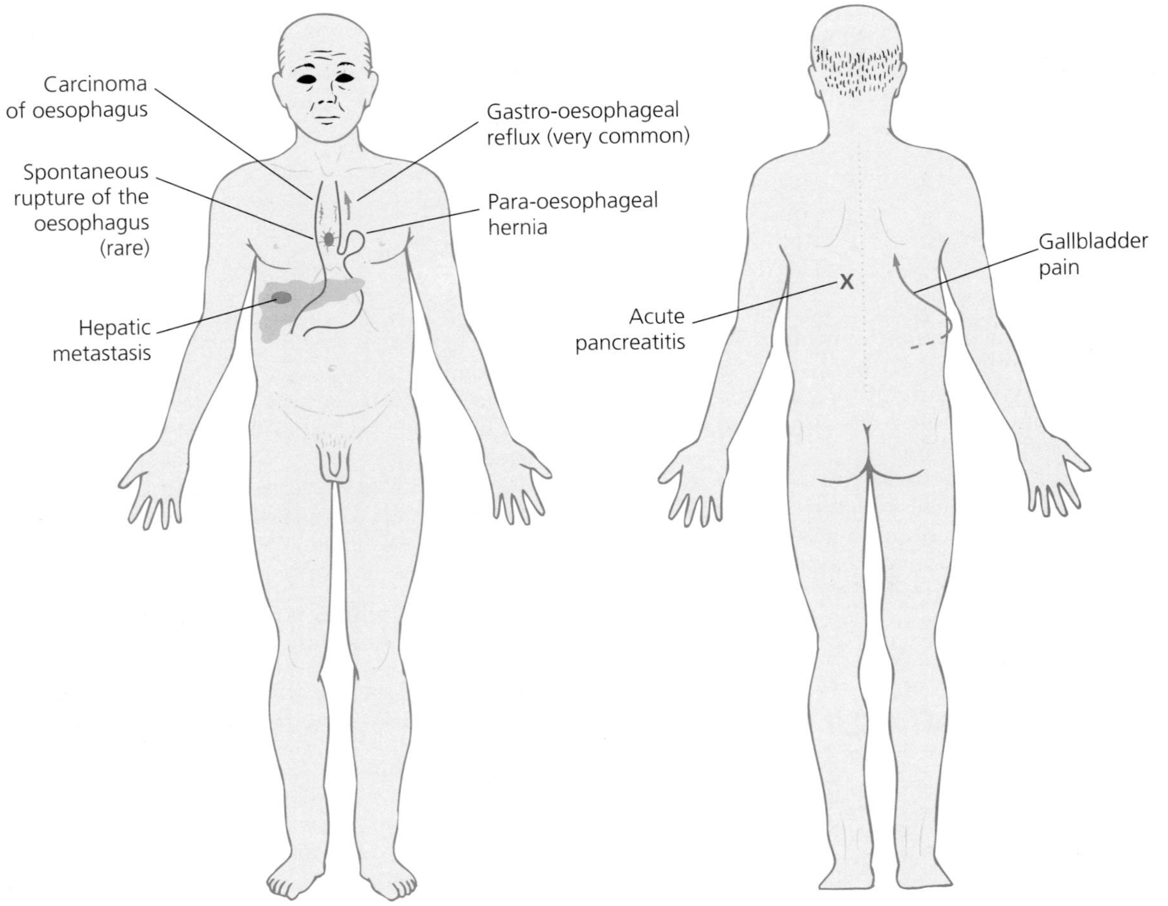

FIG. 25.1 Do not forget the possibility of gastrointestinal conditions causing chest pain.

myocardial infarction (sudden onset and severe), features which should raise your suspicions include pain which radiates through to the back, absent limb pulses and very different pulse and blood pressure in each arm in the absence of typical changes on the electrocardiograph.

Herpes zoster may present with pain, followed a few days later by the typical rash in dermatomal distribution.

Carcinoma of the bronchus can cause a variety of symptoms, most frequently cough and haemoptysis. A late symptom may be persistent ache in the chest. Pleurisy may occur as a result of direct invasion of the chest wall or secondary to pneumonia.

GROUPS AT RISK

Those most at risk of a cardiovascular cause will usually have one or more risk factors such as:

- Smoking habit.
- High cholesterol.
- History of hypertension, diabetes mellitus, cerebrovascular or peripheral vascular disease.
- Family history of coronary disease in young or middle age.

Smokers are also at greater risk of carcinoma of the bronchus and vascular disease generally.

Chest pain during unusual exertion such as digging the garden or moving snow from the drive may well be due to angina; when it occurs afterwards it is likely to be due to muscle stiffness. However it must be remembered that unusually strenuous exercise can also precipitate a bout of angina or even a heart attack. Pleurisy from pulmonary embolism may be the first indication of a deep vein thrombosis after prolonged bed rest, surgery or severe illness.

You should enquire about use of the contraceptive pill in young women (and hormone replacement therapy in older women). Both are associated with a slightly higher risk of thromboembolic disease, particularly in those who also smoke.

FINDING THE CAUSE

Remember that, in every case, the process of establishing a diagnosis follows a standard pattern:

- Experience of, and background information on, disease prevalence will limit the possible causes to just a few.
- A well-taken history will help you formulate a reasonable differential diagnosis.
- This will guide your clinical examination and allow you to pay special attention to specific areas.
- Your differential diagnosis will determine which investigations you will need to consider.

Age, speed of onset and associated features will help towards diagnosis (see Revision Panel 25.1).

A logical sequence of questions will help establish the cause. First decide if the pain is life-threatening. This is usually:

- Of sudden onset.
- Severe and associated with a feeling of impending doom.
- Accompanied by features of shock – the patient is cold, clammy, breathless and hypotensive.

Always enquire about:

- A family history of a similar problem.
- Predisposing risk factors for cardiovascular or thromboembolic disease.
- Previous medical history.

Next, establish where the pain might be coming from. Generally:

- Cardiac pain is persistent, feels like a heavy weight or constricting band around the chest, radiates to the jaw, shoulders and/or arms, is associated with breathlessness, nausea and vomiting and is brought on by exertion and relieved by (but can occur on) rest. Pericardial pain is relieved by sitting forward.
- Respiratory pain causes a sharp, stabbing pain made worse with deep inspiration particularly when the pleura is involved and is often accompanied by a cough and breathlessness. Pulmonary embolus may be accompanied by haemoptysis and signs of circulatory shock.

Revision Panel 25.1

Features associated with chest pain which aid diagnosis

Character of pain
If 'constricting', tight' or 'crushing', consider myocardial infarction or ischaemia; a 'tearing' pain through to the back may be due to a dissection of the aorta.

Location
If very localized, suspect muscle pain; if in the distribution of intercostal nerves, remember that the pain of herpes zoster may precede the rash by several days.

Radiation
Around the chest suggests cardiac disease, epigastrium to throat gastrointestinal disease, right scapula pain gallbladder disease.

Severity
Life-threatening pain is usually severe.

Persistence
Pain which does not go away is generally due to chest wall pain; occasionally carcinoma of the bronchus may present with a boring persistent pain.

- Gastrointestinal problems (Fig. 25.1 and Revision Panel 25.2) may cause 'burning' retrosternal pain with radiation to the jaw in reflux oesophagitis and pain referred to the right scapula in gallbladder disease. The latter is often preceded by months or years of attacks related to meals.
- Musculoskeletal pain is often associated with very localized chest wall tenderness and can be reproduced on movement.

Practical Point

As a general rule, diseases which are of sudden dramatic onset are the result of 'tubes which block or tubes which burst'.

WHAT TO DO NEXT

Having considered life-threatening disease and the most likely system involved, arrange appropriate tests and ensure that analgesia is prescribed and administered frequently enough to be effective.

Revision Panel 25.2
Some causes of chest pain

Cardiovascular
Coronary heart disease, chronic stable angina, unstable angina and myocardial infarction. Pericarditis. Aortic aneurysm.

Respiratory
Acute tracheitis. Carcinoma of the bronchus. Pneumothorax. Pulmonary embolus. Pneumonia and associated pleurisy.

Haematological
Anaemia. Leukaemia.

Gastrointestinal
Subphrenic abscess. Hepatic enlargement from metastases, hepatitis, congestive cardiac failure. Carcinoma of the oesophagus. Reflux oesophagitis. Hiatus hernia. Gallstones.

Neuromuscular
Herpes zoster. Scoliosis.Chest wall injury. Muscle strain. Costochondritis. Ankylosing spondylitis. Osteoporosis and osteomalacia. Paget's disease.

Other
Anxiety, hyperventilation and panic attack.

Headache

26

SOME COMMON CAUSES

Headache is an almost universal symptom. Whilst there are innumerable causes of headaches, most are perfectly innocent. Tension headaches, migraine and extracranial causes account for the majority (Revision Panel 26.1).

Revision Panel 26.1
Some important causes of headache

Migraine[a].	Tension headaches[a].
Extracranial causes[a] (e.g. cervical spondylosis).	Hypertension.
Meningitis/encephalitis.	Cranial arteritis.
Other febrile illnesses[a].	Raised intracranial pressure.

[a]Common causes

FIRST THINGS FIRST

The diagnosis depends on the speed of onset, periodicity and any accompanying symptoms and signs. Your first priority is to establish whether a headache might be due to a serious condition. You should ask:

- Did the headache come on suddenly?
- Did it develop over an hour or two?
- Did you feel hot and sweaty with it?

SUDDEN VERY SEVERE HEADACHES WHICH ARE SERIOUS

The character of the pain and its speed of onset are characteristic. The patient may complain of a sudden excruciating headache ('just like being hit on the back of the head with a hammer'). The important cause to consider is an intracranial catastrophe, almost always an intracranial haemorrhage. Bleeding may occur:

- In young and older patients from a congenital berry aneurysm or from an arteriovenous malformation into the subarachnoid space.
- In older patients mainly secondary to hypertensive cerebrovascular disease.

Consciousness may be disturbed; some patients will be mentally alert while others will be deeply unconscious. The Glasgow Coma Scale (shown on page 211) is a useful way of monitoring conscious level. You should examine the nervous system carefully as focal neurological signs are not uncommon.

Rarely, acute pyogenic meningitis, particularly meningococcal, may be associated with a very rapid onset of headache over a few minutes. More typically, however, it emerges slowly, accompanied by fever, nausea, vomiting and neck stiffness (Fig. 26.1).

PERIODIC HEADACHES

Headaches that are periodic or recurrent gradually escalate over an hour or two. The

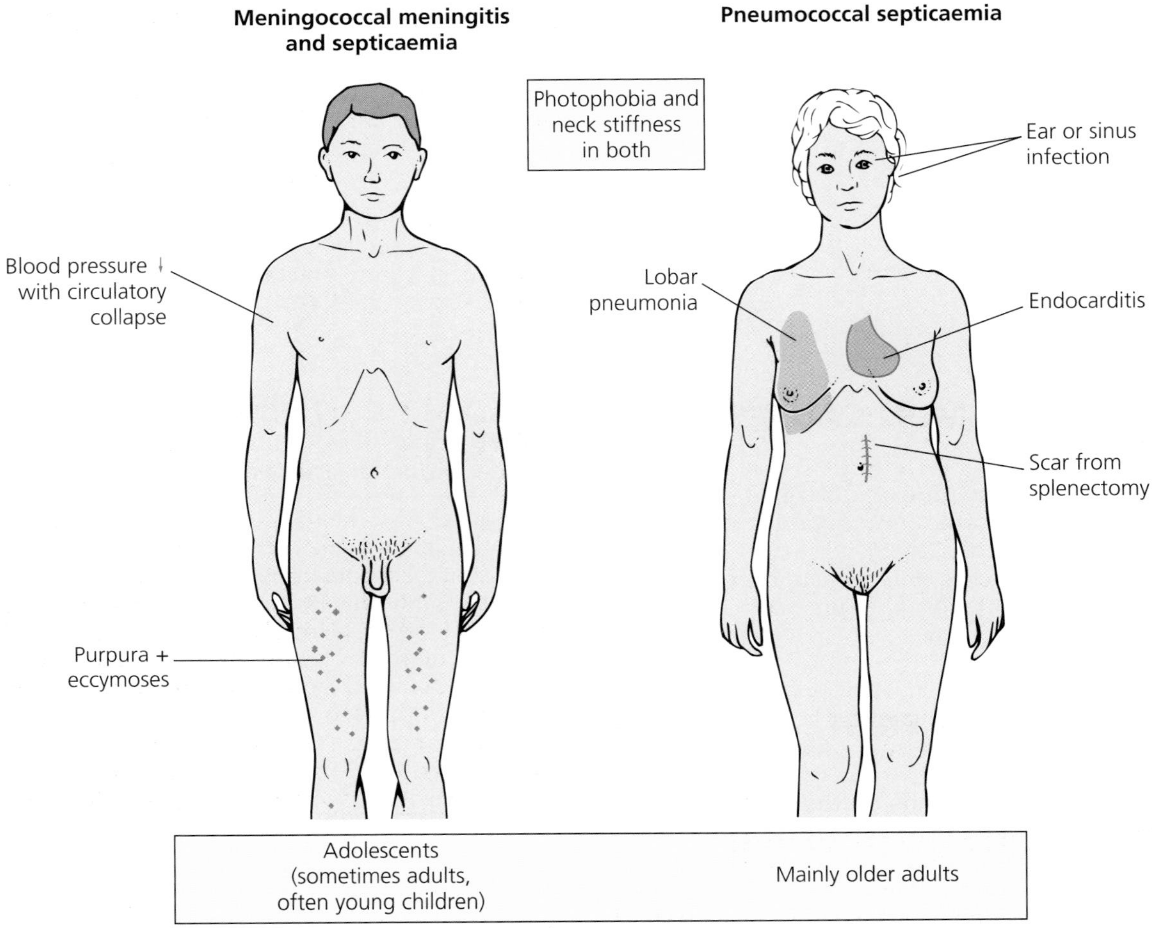

FIG. 26.1 Clinical pointers in acute pyogenic meningitis.

differential diagnosis comprises migraine, cluster headaches and tension headaches.

The main points that will help you identify migraine are:

- A history of headache going back to childhood or adolescence.
- Symptoms which precede the headache, particularly visual disturbance ('prodromal' symptoms).
- Headaches occurring at any time of the day or night.
- Attacks that are quite disabling, forcing the patient to lie down in a quiet, dark room for a few hours or even days.

Migrainous neuralgia, or cluster headache, is a less common form of migraine, which affects males more frequently than females. Clues to ask about include:

- Sudden onset, often awakening the patient from sleep.
- Intense hemicranial pain around the eye, which may be red and watery (Fig. 26.2).
- Headaches occurring in clusters, say every day or night for several days or even weeks, then disappearing for months or years at a time.

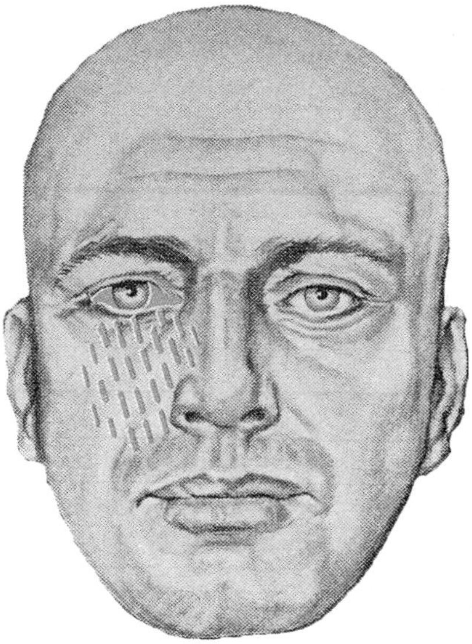

FIG. 26.2 Migranous neuralgia. Intense cranial pain around the eye, which may be red and watery.

Tension headaches are very common and are felt all over the head. Ask if the headache tends to occur during periods of stress.

HEADACHES WITH FEVER

Patients presenting with headaches as part of a febrile illness form an important diagnostic group. Acute meningeal infections, particularly by meningococcus, pneumococcus and *Haemophilus influenzae*, may cause singularly abrupt onset headache. The onset may extend over days with encephalitis and chronic forms of meningitis, such as tuberculous or cryptococcal meningitis. In all these patients, be sure to enquire about and look for:

- History of nausea and vomiting.
- Neck stiffness when trying to put chin to chest.
- Light sensitivity or 'photophobia'.

Many febrile infective states, particularly influenza, tonsillitis and glandular fever, can cause a headache. Neck stiffness, photophobia and disturbed conciousness are not dominant features of these illnesses.

HEADACHE IN HYPERTENSION

Despite the general belief that high blood pressure causes headache, hypertension does not usually cause symptoms. Symptoms which suggest hypertension as the cause are:

- A headache worse on wakening.
- Occipital in site.
- Pounding in character.
- Worsened by physical exertion.

HEADACHE IN ELDERLY PATIENTS

Whilst all the headaches described above occur in patients of all ages, one condition, cranial or temporal arteritis, is particularly hazardous for the elderly. Early diagnosis is absolutely critical. Involvement of the retinal vessels can lead to blindness, a catastrophe which can usually be averted by prompt therapy with high dose steroids.

Cranial arteritis (Fig. 26.3) (temporal arteritis or giant cell arteritis) almost invariably occurs in patients over the age of 65 years.

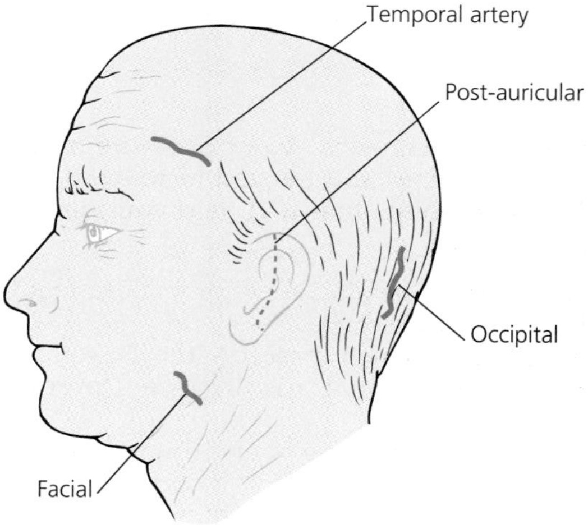

FIG. 26.3 Vessels affected in cranial arteritis.

Revision Panel 26.2

Common causes of a headache

Speed of onset	*Cause of headache*	*Common diseases*	*Associated physical signs*
Seconds to minutes.	Intracranial bleeding.	Subarachnoid haemorrhage. Cerebral haemorrhage.	Neck stiffness with subarachnoid bleeding, disturbed consciousness, abnormal neurological signs at onset.
Minutes to an hour.	Migraine.	Classical migraine. Cluster headaches. Migrainous variants.	None except in cluster headaches where there may be ocular signs (see text).
Hours (occasionally minutes).	Infections of the meninges or of the central nervous system.	Encephalitis. Pyogenic meningitis. Viral meningitis.	Fever, photophobia and neck stiffness.
Hours.	Other infections with fever.	Influenza, malaria, typhoid, glandular fever.	Signs of primary disease, no neck stiffness.
Days to months to years.	Raised intracranial pressure.	Cerebral tumour, subdural haematoma.	Papilloedema, other neurological signs according to site of primary lesion.
	Cranial arteritis.		Tenderness over cranial arteries in elderly patients.
	Hypertension.		Blood pressure considerably elevated.

Practical Point

The first symptom of cranial arteritis may be unilateral blindness.

Characteristically:

- Pain is localized over the scalp.
- The temporal, facial and occipital arteries may be tender, nodular, and non-pulsatile.

HEADACHE DUE TO RAISED INTRACRANIAL PRESSURE

In routine clinical work these are relatively uncommon and their characteristics are dominated by the underlying cause. In general these headaches are:

- Worsened by coughing and straining.
- Progressive in nature.
- In the later stages associated with vomiting and papilloedema.

Abdominal pain

When confronted with a patient with abdominal pain, you need to ask three basic questions:

How long have you had it?
- Acute (minutes or hours).
- Subacute (days).
- Chronic (weeks).

Where is it?
- Upper, central or lower.
- Right or left-sided.
- Does it radiate elsewhere?

What is it like?
- Colicky.
- Variable.
- Constant.

With clear answers to these questions, and taking into account the age, sex and race of your patient, you are well on the way to making a clinical diagnosis.

ACUTE COLICKY ABDOMINAL PAIN

Colicky pain arises from any tube containing smooth muscle. It rises to a crescendo over a period of seconds to minutes, fades away and may disappear only for the cycle to repeat itself minutes later. Features to look for are shown in Revision Panel 27.1.

Revision Panel 27.1
What to look for in a patient with severe acute colicky abdominal pain

Location of pain	*Physical signs*	*Distinguishing symptoms*	*Common problem*
Central.	Generalized tenderness. Possible fever.	Associated anorexia, nausea, vomiting and diarrhoea.	Gastroenteritis.
Central.	Depends on underlying cause (herniae, masses, distention etc).	Vomiting or constipation depending on site of obstruction (see text).	Acute intestinal obstruction.
Central, may radiate to angle of right scapula.	Mild obstructive jaundice after 24–48 h.	Possible previous gallbladder disease. Dyspepsia.	Gallstone and biliary colic.
Unilateral, loin to genitalia.	Tenderness in loin.	Unilateral pain, strangury.	Ureteric colic.

Acute gut colic due to intestinal obstruction

The important causes of intestinal obstruction at various times of adolescence and adult life are shown in Revision Panel 27.2.

Gut colic is unusual with obstructions above the pylorus. Small bowel colic is felt centrally and large gut colic below the umbilicus. It is important to realize that intestinal obstruction commonly results from the presence of adjacent abdominal masses.

Associated symptoms with the gut colic of intestinal obstruction, dependent of course on the site of the obstruction, are vomiting, distension and constipation.

The vomiting of upper (small gut) intestinal obstruction is profuse, watery and bile-stained. With lower (large gut) intestinal obstruction the vomit is thicker, brown and foul smelling. Higher small gut obstruction is not associated with very much distension because of the vomiting but obstruction to the left side of the colon causes considerable distension. When obstruction is complete there is absolute constipation with an empty gut below the obstruction.

Revision Panel 27.2
Causes of intestinal obstruction

Teenagers and adolescents
Inflammatory masses (appendicitis).
Intussusception of Meckel's diverticulum or a polyp.
Hernia.
Adhesions.

Adults
As in teenagers.
Crohn's disease.
Local inflammation due to appendicitis or diverticulitis.
Carcinoma of colon.

Elderly
As in adults.
Sigmoid volvulus.
Gut ischaemia.

Gallstone colic

This occurs when the gallbladder contracts to force a stone down the cystic duct. The pain is very severe, epigastric and usually accompanied by vomiting. If the stone gets into the common bile duct it is then more correctly termed biliary colic. If the stone obstructs the duct it will cause jaundice.

Ureteric colic

Ureteric colic is an intensely severe pain due to the passage of a stone or blood clot down the ureter. Typically:

- It starts in the renal angle.
- It radiates round the flank into the groin and penis and scrotum in the men and labia majora in women
- The patient may roll on the floor prostrated by the severity of the pain.
- Sweating and vomiting occur.
- The patient may experience strangury, an intense desire to pass urine which results in the passage of no more than a few drops.
- Once the stone or clot enters the bladder the pain stops immediately.

SUDDEN ONSET OF SEVERE PERSISTENT ABDOMINAL PAIN

As a general rule in medicine, this type of pain is caused by 'things that burst and things that get blocked'. In the abdomen, there are three conditions which give rise to excruciatingly severe persistent abdominal pain of sudden onset (see Fig. 27.1).

- Perforated peptic ulcer.
- Acute pancreatitis.
- Rupture of an abdominal aneurysm.

Perforated peptic ulcer

This abdominal emergency occurs usually between the ages of 40 and 60 years. Suspect a perforation in an older patient, particularly

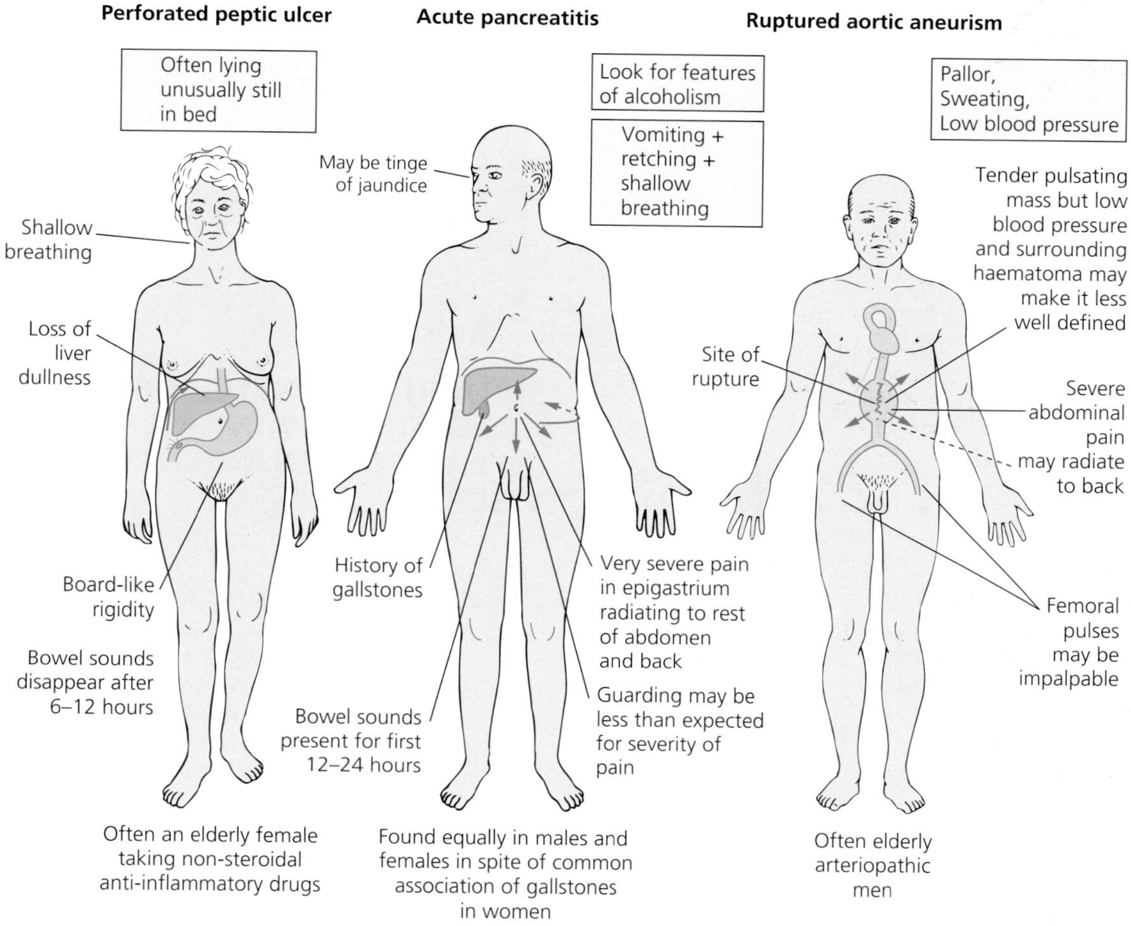

FIG. 27.1 Signs to look for in the adult patient with sudden onset severe abdominal pain.

if non-steroidal anti-inflammatory drugs are being used. There may not always be a preceding history of peptic ulceration.

The pain is sited initially in the epigastrium but may spread later all over the abdomen. There may be referred pain to the left shoulder tip.

On examination the patient is clearly seriously ill (Fig. 27.1) with tachycardia, shallow respiration but not fever. Characteristically, the abdomen is rigid like a board, is extremely tender, initially in the epigastrium but later all over the abdomen. Bowel sounds are absent. If much gas has escaped through the perforation into the peritoneal cavity, the area of liver dullness will be obscured and an erect chest X-ray will show a dense black shadow of air under the diaphragm.

Be concerned if your patient's pain eases and he or she begins to feel better after a few hours. Peritonitis is almost certainly developing. Clues to look for are a softening of a previously rigid abdomen and a progressive tachycardia.

Practical Point

As a general rule continuing abdominal pain which is severe and of sudden onset is caused by 'things that burst' and 'things that get blocked' For example:

Gut perforation.
Acute pancreatitis.
Ruptured aneurysm.

Acute pancreatitis

This too is a life-threatening condition. Suspect this in middle-aged and elderly patients where the history suggests:

- Heavy alcohol intake.
- Biliary tract disease.
- Pancreatic duct obstruction.
- Viruses (i.e. mumps).
- Abdominal trauma.

About 30% of UK patients will have no history of any of these.

Clues to diagnosis include:

- Severe epigastric pain radiating to the back.
- Nausea and extreme vomiting.
- Prostration, tachycardia, shallow rapid respiration and shock.

On examination the initial signs may be difficult to differentiate from those of a perforated peptic ulcer but there is no gas within the peritoneal cavity. Mild jaundice may develop after 2–3 days and in severe cases there is discolouration in the flank (Grey Turner's sign) or at the umbilicus (Cullen's sign (see Fig. 6.12)).

Rupture of an abdominal aneurysm

An aneurysm may lurk for years, causing few symptoms before rupturing unexpectedly. Suspect a ruptured aneurysm in anyone over 60 years of age who:

- Has a history of persistent abdominal and aching back pain.
- Presents with abdominal pain and low blood pressure.
- Presents with a combination of severe abdominal pain and blood loss.

Practical Point

Severe pain and guarding may prevent you feeling an abdominal aneurysm when it ruptures.

SUBACUTE ONSET SEVERE ABDOMINAL PAIN DUE TO INFLAMED ORGANS OR VISCERA

The features of these illnesses are summarized in Revision Panel 27.3. Pain may develop over a variable period lasting from a few hours to a few days. Local signs of inflammation or peritoneal irritation appear and complications may occur. In practical terms the site of pain will direct you towards the diagnosis.

RIGHT UPPER QUADRANT PAIN

Pain in this quadrant is generally due to disease affecting:

- Gallbladder.
- Right kidney.
- Liver.

Differentiating between these is usually straightforward. Gallbladder pain is generally referred to the back and the tip of the right scapula and may be made worse by moving or deep breathing. Kidney pain is referred down the abdomen to the groin and liver pain is fairly localized.

The most common cause of right upper quadrant pain in women is acute cholecystitis. Here a small stone becomes stuck in the cystic duct, the organ becomes inflamed and subsequently infected. Recurrent attacks may become progressively worse and nausea and vomiting are common.

Revision Panel 27.3

The features of subacute severe abdominal pain involving inflamed organs.

Site of pain	*Patients*	*Disease*	*Sequelae and complications*
Right upper quadrant			
■ Gall bladder	Women > Men.	Acute cholecystitis.	Inflammatory mass, peritonitis.
■ Right kidney	Women > Men.	Acute pyelonephritis.	Chronic pyelonephritis or pyonephrosis.
■ Liver	Both sexes, older age groups.	Metastases.	–
■ Intrathoracic cause	All ages, both sexes.	See text.	–
Central abdominal shifting after a variable time to right iliac fossa.	All ages and both sexes.	Acute appendicitis.	If untreated perforation with peritonitis or appendix abscess.
Unilateral or bilateral loin pain with also anterior pain over kidneys.	Mainly women in reproductive period of life.	Acute pyelonephritis.	May develop chronic pyelonephritis or pyonephrosis.
Left iliac fossa.	Men and women from age 50 onwards.	Acute diverticulitis.	Peritonitis, pericolic abscess, fistulae.
Mainly suprapubic but also in both iliac fossae.	Sexually active women.	Acute salpingitis.	Pyosalpinx or tubovarian mass.

Accompanying signs you should look for include:

- Fever.
- Abdominal distension.
- Tenderness and guarding in the right upper quadrant.
- Sharp pain during inspiration as the acutely inflamed gallbladder moves into contact with the examining hand – a 'positive Murphy's sign'.

Practical Point

Murphy's sign

This sign is elicited by asking the patient to breathe in whilst you palpate the tender area. As the gallbladder moves down with inspiration, there is a sharp pain when the inflamed organ nudges the examining fingers. When the gallbladder is significantly distended and inflamed, you may be able to feel a diffuse tender mass.

A right pyelonephritis may also give right upper quadrant pain but there will also be much loin tenderness with dysuria and frequency.

LESS COMMON CAUSES TO LOOK OUT FOR

Common diseases occur commonly but there are several conditions that may produce similar symptoms – painful necrotic secondaries in the liver, subphrenic abscess and other liver abscesses or hydatid cysts.

Remember too that the pathology may be above the diaphragm. Pleurisy due to underlying pneumonia or pulmonary embolism or

Practical Point

Chest pathology such as pleurisy or herpes zoster may cause upper abdominal pain.

infection with herpes zoster may cause tenderness and guarding in the right upper quadrant and even a false positive Murphy's sign.

LEFT UPPER QUADRANT PAIN

You will come across acute left upper quadrant pain with features of local inflammation much less frequently. As with right-sided pain, the cause may not always be below the diaphragm.

If the past history includes a blood or lymphopoetic disorder causing splenic enlargement, suspect a splenic infarction. Guarding may obscure the splenomegaly so listen for a splenic friction rub.

The elderly may present with acute ischaemic lesions of the large gut in the region of the splenic flexure. Local colicky pain with tenderness and local guarding are easy to detect.

RIGHT LOWER QUADRANT PAIN

Of all abdominal conditions, pain in the right lower quadrant can be a diagnostic nightmare for physicians, surgeons and gynaecologists. You will soon encounter the common three: appendicitis, Crohn's disease and salpingitis.

Although many illnesses present in a characteristic way, you cannot rely on this in appendicitis. Most patients lose their appetite early and feel nauseated but reports of diarrhoea should make you question, but not exclude, the diagnosis. Also in the history, ask if initial central pain has worsened and moved to the right iliac fossa. This may occur over hours or even days. Sometimes the pain may start in the right iliac fossa or may remain centralized and sometimes there is abdominal colic and distension.

Practical Point

It is unusual for acute appendicitis to be associated with diarrhoea.

On physical examination check for:

- Low-grade fever and dirty tongue.
- Tenderness with guarding in the right iliac fossa.
- Release pain (see page 92).
- Tenderness well out in the loin suggesting a retrocaecal appendicitis.
- Rupture of the appendix producing generalized signs of peritonitis over the lower abdomen.
- An appendix mass or abscess due to appendicitis being untreated for days or even weeks.

Acute Crohn's disease affecting the terminal ileum may be indistinguishable from acute appendicitis but if the local guarding is not severe you may be able to palpate a thickened terminal ileum.

Of the gynaecological causes of acute right iliac fossa pain with inflammation, salpingitis is the most common. Some simple clues that differentiate this from appendicitis are:

- Bilateral pain and tenderness.
- A mucopurulent vaginal discharge.
- Urinary frequency and dysuria.

LEFT LOWER QUADRANT PAIN

This mostly occurs in the second half of life due to acute diverticulitis, usually affecting the sigmoid colon.

The acute attack typically causes pain in the left lower abdomen made worse by movement. On examination there is tenderness, guarding and abdominal distension. With increasing inflammation the patient becomes toxic with fever and not infrequently rigors.

Tiredness

28

Very few textbooks have sections devoted to tiredness. This is mainly because it is such a vague term that is used by patients to convey all manner of sensations and symptoms, and partly because doctors know that, in the main, no organic cause will be found for it. Indeed there are few doctors who do not experience 'heart sink' when they hear their patient's primary complaint is tiredness. Nevertheless, tiredness is a symptom that occurs in a wide variety of unrelated diseases and a logical and systematic approach will ensure that any underlying disease process will not be missed.

SIMPLE PHYSIOLOGICAL TIREDNESS

For healthy people tiredness is the body's way of indicating that physical rest or sleep is required. Sleep is a normal physiological response to activities as diverse as a prolonged period of duty on the wards, caring for a new baby, or a gruelling marathon. All undertaking such activities are entitled to feel tired.

Rather different is the tiredness that really equates with boredom. The reluctant schoolboy isn't 'tired' of going to school. So it is important that you take the history carefully and assess your patient's lifestyle in detail if necessary!

The isolated symptom of tiredness may mean very little. If, however, you elicit from the history any of the following points, consider investigations carefully as these associated symptoms often herald potentially serious disease:

- Weight loss.
- Anorexia.
- Fever.
- Night sweats.
- Progressive breathlessness.
- Enlarged lymphatic glands.
- Pallor.

> **Practical Point**
>
> *Tiredness may simply be due to:*
> Boredom.
> Lack of sleep.
> Excessive physical activity.
> Long hours of work.

Some patients may complain of tiredness when what they actually mean is weakness of the muscles. Revision Panel 28.1 gives some indication of the wide range of serious symptoms that may cause the patient to complain of tiredness. It is not meant to be comprehensive.

TIREDNESS IN ASSOCIATION WITH PSYCHIATRIC SYMPTOMS

Tiredness and fatigue are extremely common symptoms in association with psychiatric ill-

Revision Panel 28.1

Warning symptoms that may accompany tiredness

System	*'Red flag' warning*	*Possible disease*[a]	*Physical signs*
Cardiovascular	Increasing breathlessness.	Cardiomyopathy. Heart failure.	Cardiomegaly. Heart failure.
Respiratory	Increasing breathlessness. Haemoptysis. Night sweats. Cough.	Carcinoma of bronchus. Pulmonary tuberculosis. Fibrosing alveolitis.	Clubbing. Abnormal signs in the lungs.
Gastrointestinal	Loss of weight. Anorexia. Change in bowel habit.	Gut carcinomas. Malabsorption. Inflammatory bowel disease.	Anaemia. Hepatomegaly. Abdominal masses.
Central nervous system	Muscle weakness.	Motor neuron disease. Myopathies. Myasthenia.	Muscle weakness. Muscle wasting.
Endocrine	Change in weight.	Hyperthyroidism. Hypothyroidism.	Features of: thyrotoxicosis. myxoedema.
Blood	Complaint by patient of pallor.	Iron deficiency anaemia. Pernicious anaemia. Leukaemia.	Pallor. Tongue and other mucosal changes.
Lymphatic system	Enlarged glands. Night sweats.	Lymphoma.	Generalized lymphadenopathy. Splenomegaly.

[a]This is not an exhaustive list of possible causes.

nesses, particularly depression. Here, symptoms may well include:

- Apathy.
- Feelings of guilt.
- Difficulty in concentration.
- Early morning wakening.
- Retardation.
- Diurnal mood changes.

These complaints may be associated with somatic symptoms including poor appetite, anorexia and headache. The range of associated symptoms is so vast that there is usually little difficulty in confusing these with 'red flag' warning symptoms. Depression and anxiety states are the most common psychiatric disorders in which tiredness is the presenting complaint.

CHRONIC FATIGUE SYNDROME

Achieving prominence in the Western world in recent years, chronic fatigue syndrome affects primarily adolescents and young adults. It pursues a protracted course over months or years before remitting spontaneously. No organic cause has been demonstrated for this curious complaint but overwhelming and incapacitating tiredness and weakness are dominant features.

A SIMPLE SERIES OF QUESTIONS

Working your way through a simple series of questions should help you decide whether the patient has a specific illness.

Ask about the following:

- Is the patient doing too much at work or socially?
- Is the patient simply bored?
- Are there any accompanying symptoms that suggest underlying organic disease?
- Is the patient clinically depressed?
- Are there any features to suggest chronic fatigue syndrome?

29 Loss of weight

The recognition of loss of weight has been dealt with in Chapter 2. Between 5 and 10 kg must be lost before there is any significant change in physical appearance. Its causes in the young, middle-aged and the elderly are listed in Revision Panel 29.1. As has already been emphasized, these causes are dominated by geographical, cultural and ecological factors. As an example, one of the most common causes of weight loss in adolescent girls in the Western world is anorexia nervosa whereas in Central Africa this disease is virtually unknown in the indigenous population where malnutrition has, in places, reached epidemic proportions. Revision Panel 29.1 indicates, in broad terms, some of the differences which might be expected.

WEIGHT LOSS IN BABIES

In the underdeveloped world this is common and almost invariably due to malnutrition and infections such as gastroenteritis. In the

Revision Panel 29.1

Loss of weight in the young, middle-aged and elderly in the developed and underdeveloped world

Age group	*Cause of loss of weight*	*Developed world*	*Underdeveloped countries*
Young	Malnutrition	Rare	+++
	Infections	+	+++
	Diabetes	+	+
	Malabsorption including inflammatory bowel disease	+	+
	Tuberculosis	Rare	++
	Anorexia nervosa	++	Rare
	AIDS (acquired immunodeficiency syndrome)	+	+++
Middle age	Malignancy	++	++
	Diabetes	++	+
	Thyrotoxicosis	+	+
	Malabsorption	+	+
	Cardiac cachexia	+	+
	Chronic hypoxia	++	+
	Malnutrition and neglect	Rare	++
Old age	As in middle age		
	Senile cachexia	++	++
	Malnutrition and neglect	++	++

Western world malnutrition, though still occurring, is most unusual.

WEIGHT LOSS IN THE YOUNG

Malnutrition and infections are the prime causes of weight loss, and indeed death, in children and adolescents as well as babies in underdeveloped countries.

> **Practical Point**
>
> The cause of loss of weight at various ages is dominated by geographical, cultural and ecological factors.

Patterns of disease alter but infections are now a relatively uncommon cause of weight loss in the Western world. The widespread menace of HIV (human immunodeficiency virus) infection in Central Africa and the Far East brings it to the fore as a frequent cause of weight loss in children and young adults but in parts of North America it is also a serious problem. Of all the chronic infections tuberculosis remains common in Africa, the Indian subcontinent and in China. In the Western world it is now rare.

The syndrome of anorexia nervosa is a common cause of severe weight loss in adolescent females in developed countries. As distinct from the other causes of weight loss the young girl with gross wasting is little distressed by her cachectic appearance and indeed often denies it entirely. Instead of looking ill the anorexic is bright and alert. As with

Revision Panel 29.2

Interacting factors

Disease	*Inadequate or unavailable nutrition*	*Difficulties with food intake*	*Anorexia*	*Mal-absorption*	*Hyper-metabolism*
Malnutrition, food fads, slimming diets, elder abuse.	+++	–	–	–	–
Mechanical problems with swallowing e.g. bulbar palsy.	–	+++	–	–	–
Malignant obstruction to swallowing e.g. carcinoma of oesophagus or stomach.	–	+++	++	–	–
Coeliac disease, Crohn's disease.	–	–	+	+++	–
Malignancy.	–	*a*	+++	*b*	+
Diabetes, thyrotoxicosis.	–	–	–	–	+++
Chronic infections.	–	–	+++	–	–
Cardiac cachexia, chronic hypoxia.		–	++	+++	+
Metabolic states e.g. uraemia, hypercalcaemia.	–	–	+++	–	–

[a]Except with malignant disease of upper gastrointestinal tract. [b]Except with small gut malignancies

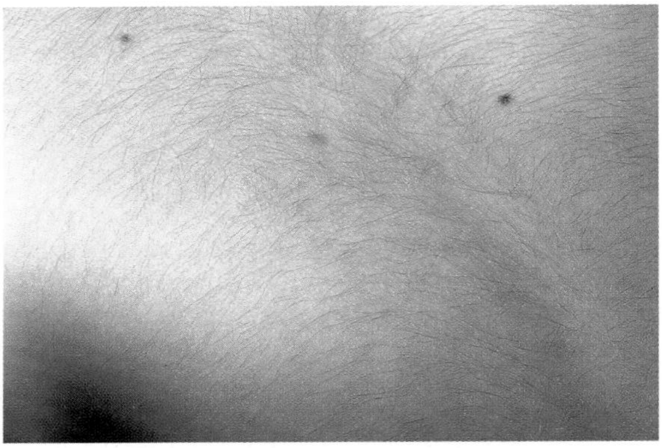

FIG. 29.1 Profuse growth of soft, downy, lanugo hair over back and shoulders.

some other wasting diseases there may be a profuse growth of soft, downy, lanugo hair over the back and shoulders (Fig. 29.1).

WEIGHT LOSS IN ADULTS

Since weight loss is a cardinal feature of so many systemic illnesses the cause is best sought by attempting first to define the mechanism of the weight loss and then to focus on the specific diseases that might be responsible.

Excluding dehydration, weight loss is due to one or more of the following:

- Inadequate or unavailable nutrition.
- Poor nutrition due to anorexia.
- Mechanical difficulties with swallowing or pain after food.
- Malabsorption.
- Malignancy.
- Hypermetabolism.
- Severe heart failure.
- Chronic anoxic states.

With many diseases several factors may interact together (see Revision Panel 29.2).

Swollen legs

30

Swelling of the legs, or peripheral oedema, tends to occur when excess tissue fluid is redistributed under the influence of gravity. Oedema can be temporarily dispersed by fingertip pressure ('pitting') but longstanding oedema feels hard due to accompanying fibrosis. Swelling may be generalized, so that rings become tight, clothes feel too small and constricting and the face looks puffy.

IS THE PATIENT ILL?

Severe oedema is usually pathological, causing at first gross engorgement of the ankles, then both legs, followed by abdominal distension or ascites, sacral, genital and arm swelling and even pleural or pericardial effusions. Such gross oedema is a sign of severe but not immediately life-threatening disease.

Even 'mild' ankle swelling may add over 4 kg to body weight.

IS IT SERIOUS?

Bilateral swollen ankles when unaccompanied by any other abnormality are not usually serious and do not necessarily indicate 'disease'. For example, almost anyone can develop swelling involving just the dorsum of the foot and ankle after sitting on a long-haul flight for many hours. Under similar circumstances, swelling of *one* calf may suggest deep venous thrombosis and a risk of potentially life-threatening thromboembolic disease.

SOME COMMON CAUSES

Generalized swelling always indicates severe sodium and water overload. Heart failure, kidney failure and liver failure are likely culprits.

SOME LESS COMMON BUT STILL IMPORTANT CAUSES

(Fig. 30.1)

Some middle aged and elderly women may have a variable degree of oedema, aggravated by standing, for which there is no serious cause (idiopathic oedema).

Practical Point

Fluid balance is difficult to assess clinically and regular weighing is the best simple way in the short term. A dry tongue does not always mean dehydration – mouth breathing is common. Sacral and leg oedema do not necessarily indicate fluid overload.

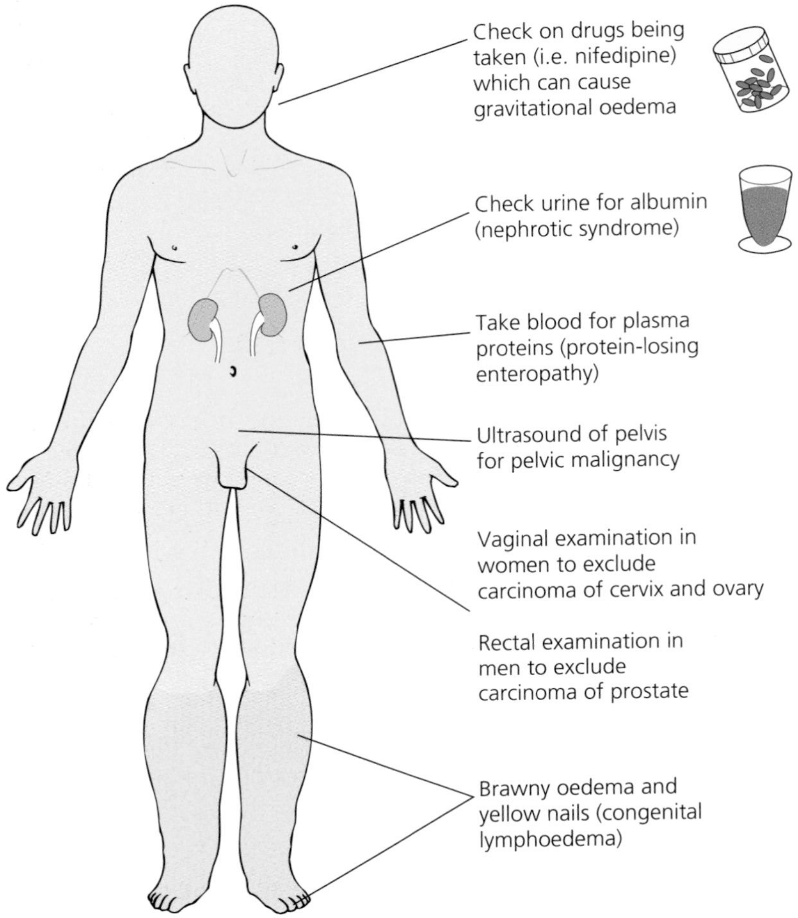
Check on drugs being taken (i.e. nifedipine) which can cause gravitational oedema
Check urine for albumin (nephrotic syndrome)
Take blood for plasma proteins (protein-losing enteropathy)
Ultrasound of pelvis for pelvic malignancy
Vaginal examination in women to exclude carcinoma of cervix and ovary
Rectal examination in men to exclude carcinoma of prostate
Brawny oedema and yellow nails (congenital lymphoedema)

FIG. 30.1 Further steps to take for the patient who, on routine clinical examination, has swollen legs without any obvious cause.

Longstanding non-pitting oedema accompanied by pigmentation suggests chronic (but benign) venous insufficiency. Bilateral gross swelling is the norm in congenital lymphoedema. Gastrointestinal disease may produce hypoproteinaemic oedema by malabsorption and/or protein-losing enteropathy.

Weight change associated with the menstrual cycle can produce abdominal swelling and irritability.

Lymphatic obstruction from malignant disease causes a brawny oedema which does not readily 'pit' due to its high protein content.

GROUPS AT RISK

Mild transient swelling may occur:

- After a period of relative immobility such as during a long car or plane journey, giving a feeling of 'tight shoes'.
- In otherwise healthy elderly people, with oedema developing during the day and disappearing overnight.
- In pregnancy.
- After removal of a plaster cast following a lower limb fracture.
- After a period of prolonged bed rest.

FINDING THE CAUSE

It is usually fairly straightforward to establish the cause of oedema. You should always assume that oedema is pathological until you are confident that you have excluded the major general and local causes.

Symptoms and accompanying signs to look out for are:

- In middle-aged and elderly patients, exertional and nocturnal dyspnoea and raised jugular venous pressure, tachycardia and pleural effusion suggestive of heart failure.
- Jaundice due to liver disease, with oedema due to a low albumin.
- Fatigue and pallor of renal failure.
- Varicose veins and pigmentation leading to chronic venous insufficiency.
- Unilateral ankle swelling and tenderness due to deep vein thrombosis.
- Palpable lymph nodes and/or abdominal mass which may indicate lymphoma or carcinoma.

Practical Point

There are no consistent signs that reliably diagnose deep vein thrombosis. Clinical suspicion based on the history is the most helpful indicator but formal investigation is usually necessary.

WHAT TO DO NEXT

How best to confirm the cause depends on what investigations are readily available to you. Urea, electrolytes and albumin will identify renal and liver failure and are universally available, as is echocardiography to determine ventricular function. Venography or ultrasound are useful in diagnosing deep vein thrombosis. The investigation of suspected malignancy is more complex and should be discussed with seniors.

31 Hot joint

Many rheumatological conditions can cause inflammation in a group of joints such as rheumatoid disease or systemic lupus. When a *single* joint is affected, the most important diagnosis to consider is an infected or septic joint. Although emergencies due to joint disease are not common, when they do occur, prompt diagnosis and treatment is essential. Failure to act can lead to avoidable morbidity and mortality (see Revision Panel 20.1).

IS THE PATIENT ILL?

The patient with acute pain and swelling affecting the small joints in a symmetrical peripheral polyarthritis may be clearly disabled but is not usually ill. Signs of systemic upset are fever, nausea, vomiting and rigors.

IS THE ILLNESS SERIOUS?

Signs of inflammation, exquisite tenderness and extreme pain on the smallest movement in any direction indicate significant joint disease. Always suspect serious disease when:

- A single joint is affected.
- One joint seems much worse than others in a patient with known joint disease.
- There is a history of an infected lesion such as an ingrowing toe nail, a boil or ulcerating lesion.
- Signs of systemic upset are present.

SOME COMMON CAUSES

Acute swelling of a single joint often follows trauma, particularly in joints which are degenerative. Gout can be exquisitely tender and generally affects weightbearing joints; attacks may be mild and self-limiting or severe and recurrent. An acute arthritis can develop in haemophiliac patients. Patients with existing rheumatoid disease may experience a flare up in which some joints are more affected than others. Septic arthritis is the most important diagnosis to be considered as without prompt recognition and treatment, severe destruction and deformity of the joint may result and death from septicaemia has been reported.

GROUPS AT RISK

Gout accompanies many illnesses and can be triggered by various drugs such as diuretics and salicylates.

Those susceptible to septic arthritis include those who:

- Have existing joint disease especially rheumatoid disease.
- Are elderly.
- Are chronically debilitated.
- Are immunocompromised e.g. after a course of steroids.

Infection may also be introduced during an intra-articular injection.

FINDING THE CAUSE

A good history is essential because there are numerous arthropathies that may present with pain and swelling – symptoms associated with the underlying problem such as bowel or lung disease will aid diagnosis. Look for evidence of trauma and previous similar attacks in the same or other joints, or of existing joint disease. Blood should be taken for urate, erythrocyte sedimentation rate, C-reactive protein and for blood cultures. Joint aspiration is the most important diagnostic procedure but someone experienced should perform this. You should contact your laboratory and advise them that samples are on the way for microscopy and culture.

WHAT TO DO NEXT

Once you suspect a septic arthritis, you must get help from one of your seniors. Drainage of the joint and appropriate antibiotic treatment are essential. An infected joint requires urgent treatment. Delay may mean irreparable damage, destruction and deformity of the joint surface and, at worst, overwhelming infection and death.

32 Palpitations

Patients, particularly the elderly, often report that they suffer from 'palpitations'. This is a rather vague term so it is important that you try to establish what the patient means. Palpitations seem to cover a wide range of symptoms, including:

- Awareness of the normal heart beat.
- Feeling lightheaded.
- Dizziness.
- A skipping or racing heart beat.
- Thumping in the chest.
- Pounding in the ears.
- Irregular heart beat.
- Sensation of missed beats.
- Forceful beats.

IS THE PATIENT ILL?

Most patients with palpitations are not ill. Most of the symptoms listed above are benign and are simply due to a sudden, unexpected, unpleasant (but transient) awareness of the heart beat during times of stress.

Palpitations which are due to an unusually fast or unusually slow heart rate are fairly easy to recognize if they are present when you see the patient, but they can be notoriously difficult to define when they are intermittent, infrequent or last for a few minutes only.

A patient may be quite ill if a change in heart rate is accompanied by a fall in blood pressure or pulmonary oedema. The elderly or those with valvular heart disease or pre-existing coronary heart disease are particularly prone. Chronic heart block or atrial fibrillation with a controlled ventricular rate may be remarkably well-tolerated.

IS THE ILLNESS SERIOUS?

Palpitations that are pathological are generally due to heart rates that are inappropriately fast or slow, sometimes accompanied by a fall in blood pressure. Clues that indicate a serious abnormality include:

- A history of falls.
- A sensation of dizziness.
- Unexplained syncope or near collapse.
- Associated symptoms of breathlessness or chest pain.

SOME COMMON CAUSES

Fibrosis of the myocardial conducting tissue can lead to heart block while myocardial ischaemia can trigger atrial fibrillation or a malignant ventricular arrhythmia. An abnormally fast heart beat or *tachyarrhythmia* usually gives a barely palpable pulse, while an abnormally slow heart beat may feel heavy or forceful.

Ventricular extrasystoles become more common with advancing age. The pause which follows an extrasystole allows greater left ventricular filling time and so a more forceful beat.

An overactive thyroid can cause a rapid pulse, as can left ventricular failure, stress, anxiety, fever, or excessive nicotine or caffeine consumption. Bradycardia can be caused by digoxin toxicity, hypothyroidism and hypothermia.

SOME LESS COMMON BUT STILL IMPORTANT CAUSES

Raised intracranial pressure, myocarditis and electrolyte disturbances (particularly low potassium and magnesium) sometimes cause a noticeable change in cardiac rate.

GROUPS AT RISK

The elderly or those with valvular heart disease or pre-existing coronary heart disease are particularly prone to episodes of 'palpitations'. Those who feel under stress either socially or at work also report palpitations more frequently than most. Some people become aware of their heart beat when sitting quietly or when going to bed.

FINDING THE CAUSE

You will need to get as clear a description as you can of what the patient means by palpitations. Is the heart going fast or slow? Teaching how to take the pulse during an event is useful.

If the patient has noticed an odd heart rhythm, suggest tapping it out on the desk. A chaotic rhythm is likely to be atrial fibrillation, a slow beat heart block.

Ask how any pulse change starts. Sinus tachycardia builds up and declines gradually, while pathological ventricular or supraventricular tachycardia start abruptly, like flicking a switch.

Ask what seems to start off an event. Anxiety, nervousness, emotion and excitement are powerful triggers.

Rates greater than 150 per minute usually indicate a rhythm other than sinus tachycardia, especially when accompanied by symptoms of light-headedness or near-syncope.

WHAT TO DO NEXT

It is important to try and correlate the patient's symptoms with some abnormality on the electrocardiograph or 24-hour tape recording. You may need to request several recordings. If symptoms are infrequent, an electronic memo device is available which the patient can activate the moment an episode of palpitations occurs.

Once an abnormal rhythm has been identified, you can consider other tests to find the underlying cause or where appropriate commence treatment. This may mean a pacemaker, suppression of potentially lethal arrhythmias or treatment for a thyroid problem.

Most patients who become aware of a normal heart beat respond to simple reassurance.

Revision Panel 32.1

Summary: Some causes of 'palpitations'

Cardiac disease: ischaemia, dilated cardiomyopathy, valve disease, heart failure.

Excess caffeine: tea, coffee and many carbonated drinks contain significant quantities of caffeine. Cutting down or changing to decaffeinated drinks can be very effective strategies.

Anaemia causes a 'high output' state. High altitude has a similar effect.

Lack of fitness: unusual or unaccustomed exercise can draw attention to a prominent rise in heart rate.

Anxiety: look for associated features (tingling in lips and fingers, hyperventilation, lump in throat).

Drugs: especially cardioactive drugs like beta-blockers and calcium channel blockers. Don't forget eye drops may be absorbed systemically and can cause a severe bradycardia. Vasoactive drugs like nifedipine (used to treat angina or hypertension) can cause a reflex tachycardia when not prescribed concomitantly with a beta-blocker.

Thyroid disease, both over- and underactive can cause marked change in pulse rate. Hyperthyroidism is one cause of atrial fibrillation.

33 Dizziness

It is important to find out what your patient means by this vague symptom. The various sensations described as dizziness include:

- Feeling unsteady when walking or standing up.
- Patients feeling as if they or their surroundings are moving.
- Light-headedness on exertion, including walking, standing or bending, straining, coughing or micturating.
- Anxiety about passing out.
- A racing heart beat.
- Faintness triggered by some unpleasant sight or smell.

You will need to distinguish between:

- Vertigo. Your patient senses that the world is spinning or that he is spinning within the world; there may be associated nausea and vomiting.
- Light-headed or giddiness.
- Impending loss of consciousness.

IS THE PATIENT ILL? IS THE ILLNESS SERIOUS?

Dizziness is not usually a life-threatening problem, though it can severely affect quality of life and day-to-day activities. Warnings of potentially serious disease are:

- Evidence of vascular disease, coronary heart disease or arrhythmia.
- Evidence of brainstem disease – double vision, muscle weakness and difficulty with the muscles used for speech (dysarthria).
- Evidence of disease affecting the cochlear apparatus – hearing loss and tinnitus.

SOME COMMON CAUSES

Almost everyone will be familiar with the most common cause – prolonged standing in hot surroundings or standing up quickly after sitting or lying. Many suffer sensations of unsteadiness with travel or motion sickness.

With advancing age, wear and tear in the neck or *cervical spondylosis* causes bony encroachment on to the blood supply to the brain. Vessels may be 'pinched' when turning the head or looking upwards.

Autonomic dysfunction from diabetes and Parkinson's disease or from anti-hypertensive drugs prevent the normal rise in blood pressure on standing up, causing *postural hypotension* (see Chapter 14).

Viral infections can cause a *vestibular neuronitis.*

Dizziness can be precipitated by changes in head position (benign positional vertigo).

A single attack of dizziness with sensory deafness may be due to acute labyrinthitis, with symptoms of nausea, vomiting and prostration and obvious nystagmus.

SOME LESS COMMON BUT STILL IMPORTANT CAUSES

Neurological damage as in brainstem infarction, multiple sclerosis, posterior fossa lesions, acoustic neuroma or cerebellar disease may be associated with dizziness. Whilst they are very disabling, they are relatively uncommon. Dizziness, which is made worse on closing the eyes, is usually due to posterior column disease.

Recurrent attacks of intense vertigo with increasing nerve deafness suggest Meniere's disease, which can be very disabling.

GROUPS AT RISK

Because a range of diseases can precipitate dizziness, only a few people can be considered to be at special risk – those with vascular disease, the elderly, or those taking anti-hypertensive medication.

FINDING THE CAUSE

True vertigo may arise from two sorts of lesions:

- Central lesions may be due to cerebellar and brainstem disease. You may be able to elicit signs e.g. difficulties with speech articulation (dysarthria), swallowing (dysphagia), blurred or double vision (diplopia) and cranial nerve palsies.
- Peripheral lesions of the VIIIth cranial nerve or the labyrinth itself. Often associated are buzzing or ringing in the ears (tinnitus), nystagmus and hearing loss.

If you suspect that symptoms are suggestive of impending loss of consciousness, look for abnormalities of pulse and cardiac rhythm and check for postural hypotension with sitting then standing blood pressure. Collapse of cardiac origin is usually brief. Prolonged unconsciousness from asystole or a ventricular arrhythmia will be fatal if the rhythm does not terminate quickly. Collapse on exertion may be due to valvular heart disease or a rhythm abnormality. Syncope after exertion is more likely to be due to venous pooling.

WHAT TO DO NEXT

Up to half of all patients complaining of dizziness do not have a diagnosis despite extensive tests. Fortunately, although morbidity is high, mortality is generally low. It is useful to know that repeating previously normal investigations rarely helps establish a diagnosis.

Revision Panel 33.1

Some causes of dizziness

Neurological disease.	Cerebellar ataxia, multiple sclerosis, posterior column disease, brainstem infarction, posterior fossa lesion, acoustic neuroma.
Associated with presumed viral infection.	Vestibular neuronitis.
Motion sickness.	
Degenerative disease.	Cervical spondylosis.
True rotational vertigo.	*Peripheral:* tinnitus, nystagmus, hearing loss due to VIIIth nerve damage. *Central:* difficulties with speech, swallowing and vision.
Associated with change in position of the head.	Benign positional vertigo.
Cardiovascular disease.	Syncope or near syncope from abnormal rate, rhythm, low blood pressure or poor left ventricular output.

34 Collapse

Collapse is a common cause of acute medical admission. There are many causes, spanning nearly every major body system (See also Chapter 15).

IS THE PATIENT ILL?

Almost every instance of collapse is abnormal and most patients will have an underlying problem. A few exceptions include:

- Fainting in the heat.
- Fainting when observing something unpleasant.
- Venous pooling after exertion.
- Fainting after passing urine (micturition syncope) or coughing (cough syncope).
- Carotid hypersensitivity.

IS THE ILLNESS SERIOUS?

Almost all causes of collapse that produce unconsciousness are potentially life-threatening. Particularly hazardous are:

- Most heart rhythm abnormalities (especially during a myocardial infarction).
- Structural cardiac abnormalities such as aortic stenosis or hypertrophic cardiomyopathy.
- Hypoglycaemia and hyperglycaemia.
- Intracranial catastrophes.
- Massive blood loss.

SOME COMMON CAUSES

The most common causes of unconsciousness requiring admission to hospital are overdose (including alcohol), intracranial lesions (stroke, head injury and subarachnoid haemorrhage), epilepsy and hypotension due to cardiac disease.

SOME LESS COMMON BUT STILL IMPORTANT CAUSES

Meningitis and encephalitis, septicaemia, massive blood loss, anaphylaxis, hypothermia, hypo- and hyperglycaemia, and myxoedema can all be fatal. Abnormalities of electrolytes, often due to drug treatment, may cause extreme confusion and unconsciousness. In patients who have recently returned from abroad, malaria may present as prostration or collapse.

GROUPS AT RISK

At particular risk are those known to have epilepsy, cardiovascular or cerebrovascular disease. Patients with multiple medical problems may suffer from polypharmacy and the ever-present potential for previously unknown drug interactions or drug overdose from simple confusion. Recent trauma or travel also increase the risk of unexplained collapse.

FINDING THE CAUSE

While it is important to establish a cause, the priority is always to control airway, breathing and circulation, to apply resuscitation if necessary, to treat any urgent problems and to accumulate information from any and every available source to help establish the underlying cause. Enquire about:

- Previous illnesses (especially epilepsy, cardio- or cerebrovascular disease or drug overdose) and operations.
- Available medication.
- Drugs of abuse.
- Recent trauma or travel.

Check clothing and wallet for outpatient appointment cards or Medi-Alert cards.

Completely undress the patient and check for signs of head or neck trauma and examine the pupils. If pinpoint, give naloxone to reverse any narcotic overdose. Assess vital signs, check for neck stiffness and record conscious level using Glasgow Coma Scale. Check for needle marks.

Attach and record an electrocardiograph (ECG) and treat any arrhythmia.

Take blood for urgent full blood count, electrolytes, glucose, liver function, amylase and toxicology. Cross-match blood and give intravenous fluids if you suspect blood loss.

WHAT TO DO NEXT

Many patients will have no external evidence of injury. Once you have treated any immediately life-threatening problems and provided life support where appropriate, you will need to focus on the underlying problem and reassess at intervals to ensure that your diagnosis is correct, your management is effective and your patient is improving.

Revision Panel 34.1

Some causes of collapse leading to unconsciousness

Common	*Less common*
Overdose (including alcohol).	Meningitis and encephalitis.
Hypoglycaemia.	Liver or renal failure.
Intracranial lesion: stroke, subarachnoid haemorrhage, head injury.	Septicaemia.
Post-ictal epilepsy.	Hyperglycaemia.
Cardiogenic cause: arrhythmia or infarction.	Hypothermia.
Respiratory failure.	Subdural haematoma.
	Massive blood loss.
	Malaria in tropics.

35 Rectal bleeding

The cause of rectal bleeding in adults can usually be determined by a careful consideration of the history and full physical examination which includes rectal examination and proctosigmoidoscopy.

IS THE BLEEDING LIKELY TO BE SERIOUS?

Common things occur commonly and by far the most likely cause of rectal bleeding is haemorrhoids, usually referred to as piles. Nevertheless, one of the greatest errors you can commit is to attribute all rectal bleeding to haemorrhoids without first conducting a full examination and investigation.

Haemorrhoids may bleed at any stage in life but are more likely to do so in patients:

- In late pregnancy.
- With portal hypertension.
- With large pelvic masses.

The bleeding is associated with defaecation, especially when the patient is constipated. The blood is fresh, venous in colour (dark red) and is not mixed with the faeces. Other useful diagnostic pointers include:

- Blood is splattered around the pan after defaecation.
- Blood is also noted on the toilet paper after wiping.
- The patient may notice a lump at the anus when haemorrhoids are more severe (see Revision Panel 6.13).

Rectal carcinomas

These frequently present with rectal bleeding. Early diagnosis is essential as they can be cured surgically. The disease occurs predominantly in middle and old age. There are some important features which differentiate rectal carcinomas from piles. The 'red flag' warning symptoms that should alert you to the fact that you are *not* dealing with simple haemorrhoids are:

- Bleeding is not usually profuse but the blood is mixed with the stools.
- Stools contain mucus.
- The patient may complain of apparent incomplete emptying of the bowel after defaecation.
- Perineal pain or tenesmus is common.
- Diarrhoea may occur (also in carcinomas of the descending and sigmoid colon).

Rectal and colonic polyps

These are common causes of rectal bleeding without associated bowel upset. Always ask if other members of the family have had bowel polyps as there is a (rare) syndrome of familial polyposis.

Diverticulitis

This common condition, a poorly recognized cause of rectal bleeding, usually presents with left iliac fossa pain, constipation, or as an acute abdominal emergency. When rectal bleeding occurs it is often profuse, fresh and unheralded. Bleeding may be massive and associated with shock.

Ischaemic colitis and angiodysplasia

Ischaemic colitis is found usually at the splenic flexure and angiodysplasia is found usually at the caecum. These are relatively rare causes of rectal bleeding.

Infective diarrhoeas

In medical practice, acute and chronic diarrhoeas are often associated with rectal bleeding though the diarrhoea dominates the clinical picture. *Salmonella*, *Shigella* or *Entamoeba histolytica*, are likely to be associated with fever, abdominal pain, anorexia, vomiting and malaise. If you suspect an infective diarrhoea clinically you must ask about family, friends or colleagues who might also have been affected and about travel abroad. Antibiotics can induce pseudomembranous colitis.

Chronic inflammatory bowel disease

Bleeding is commonly associated with diarrhoea in chronic inflammatory bowel disease, more so in ulcerative colitis than in Crohn's disease (see also Chapter 36).

COULD THE BLEEDING BE FROM HIGHER UP IN THE GASTROINTESTINAL TRACT?

Blood from lesions higher in the gastrointestinal tract such as the oesophagus, stomach and duodenum is black and sticky with the consistency of tar (melaena). This is the result of the denaturing effect of gastric acid and gut enzymes on blood. Iron tablets and bismuth salts (used to treat ulcers) also turn the stools black. Making sure that you take a good drug history will save you from embarrassment.

WHAT TO LOOK FOR IN THE PATIENT WHO COMPLAINS OF RECTAL BLEEDING

In your general examination:

- Ensure your patient is not anaemic by checking the haemoglobin level.

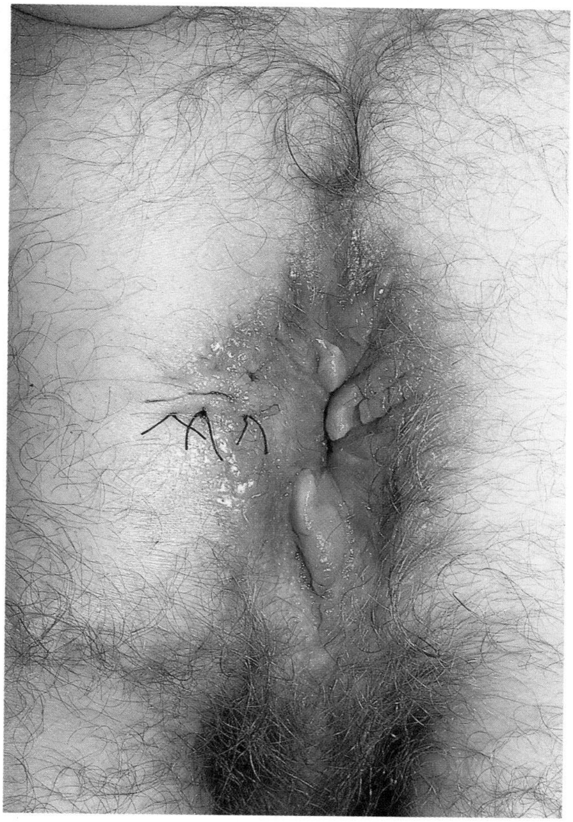

FIG. 35.1 Fistulae suggestive of anal Crohn's disease. Note the recent biopsies.

- Look for signs of loss of weight and dehydration in patients with a long history of heavy blood loss and associated symptoms which might suggest a serious cause.

In your examination of the abdomen, check carefully for signs of:

- Hepatomegaly.
- Abdominal masses.
- Inguinal lymphadenopathy. A tumour of the rectum may spread down to the lymphatics of the anal canal or the ischiorectal fossae.
- Second and third degree piles.
- Anal fissure.
- Anal carcinoma.
- Fistulae suggestive of anal Crohn's disease (Fig. 35.1).

You should routinely perform a rectal examination looking for:

- Rectal carcinoma – 90% of rectal cancers are palpable on rectal examination.
- Rectal polyps.
- Strictures suggestive of rectal Crohn's disease.

Finally, you should perform proctoscopy to:

- Assess first-degree haemorrhoids. They cannot be diagnosed with the finger.
- View rectal polyps or carcinomas.
- Visualize and biopsy the rectal mucosa in cases of chronic inflammatory bowel disease.

Sigmoidoscopy is a useful skill which you should learn at the first opportunity and which is essential as a further investigation.

Revision Panel 35.1
Causes of rectal bleeding

Disease	*Features of the rectal bleeding*
Haemorrhoids.	Fresh blood with defaecation, not mixed with faeces, often splatters pan.
Rectal carcinoma.	Blood and mucus streaking stools, sense of incomplete emptying of rectum, change in bowel habit.
Diverticulitis.	Bleeding often profuse and unexpected.
Rectal polyps.	Intermittent bleeding without other symptoms.
Chronic inflammatory bowel disease.	Usually associated with diarrhoea.

Change in bowel habit

36

DIARRHOEA

This term is used to imply an increase in:

- Stool frequency.
- Stool volume with a change to sloppy or liquid consistency.

There is a wide differential diagnosis but questioning, particularly about the onset of the diarrhoea, usually narrows the field quickly (see Revision Panel 36.1). This is a rough classification but it does act as a useful start to your questioning which can then be directed in detail to the more likely possibilities.

ABRUPT ONSET DIARRHOEA

Sudden onset diarrhoea is nearly always due to infection or toxin ingestion, so it is essential that you ask carefully about family, friends or workmates who have taken similar food who might also be affected. Notifications of cases of food poisoning in the UK are currently increasing at an alarming rate. Common foods that are often responsible include:

- Cooked meats.
- Dairy products.
- Inadequately cooked 'fast foods'.
- Re-heated meals.

Recent travel abroad, particularly in the tropics, is important and a significant proportion of bacteriologically proven gut infections in the UK are imported from abroad either by holidaymakers or business travellers.

Commonly associated symptoms include anorexia, vomiting, crampy abdominal pain, headache, aches and pains in the limbs and faintness on standing. Much can be learned from stool gazing so make sure that you inspect the stools yourself. The characteristic appearances of the stools in small intestinal and colorectal diarrhoea are listed in Revision Panel 36.2.

Revision Panel 36.1

Causes of diarrhoea in relation to onset

Abrupt onset.	Infections or toxins
After taking drugs or unusual medication (days).	Antibiotics, oral iron.
With changes in lifestyle (days to months).	High fibre diet, stress, anxiety.
After surgery (days).	Post-gastrectomy, gut resection.
Subacute or chronic onset often with weight loss, abdominal pain or mucus per rectum (weeks to months).	Chronic inflammatory bowel disease, colon or rectal carcinoma, malabsorption syndromes, pancreatic disease.
In frail bedfast patients.	Spurious diarrhoea.

Revision Panel 36.2

Characteristic appearance of stools in small intestinal and colorectal diarrhoea

Stool appearance	*Faecal microscopy*	*Infecting organism*
Large volume watery stools (secretory) (small intestine)	(*Vibrio cholerae*).	*Vibrio cholerae*.[a] *Escherichia coli* (enterotoxogenic). *Campylobacter jejuni*. Salmonellae. *Clostridium perfringens*. *Staphylococcus aureus*.
Large pale and bulky (malabsorption) (small intestine)	Fat globules.	*Giardia lamblia*. *Strongyloides stercoralis*.[a] Tropical sprue.[a]
With blood and mucus (invasive) (colorectal)	Pus and blood.	*Entamoeba histolytica*.[a] *Yersinia enterocolitica*.[a] *Campylobacter jejuni*. *Clostridium difficile*. Shigellae.[a] Enteroinvasive *E. coli*.

[a]These are mainly of tropical origin.

DIARRHOEA DUE TO DRUGS AND DIETARY CHANGES

Many patients develop diarrhoea whilst taking medication, particularly antibiotics. With some antibiotics, such as clindamycin, there may be an associated pseudomembranous colitis. Laxatives are freely available so don't forget the possibility of secret purgative abuse. Changes in diet, particularly the high fibre diets, may induce 'windy' diarrhoea with abdominal bloating.

MORE SERIOUS DIARRHOEA OF SUBACUTE OR CHRONIC ONSET

This sort of diarrhoea is likely to present diagnostic difficulties. In practical terms you can make the diagnosis from associated symptoms.

Diarrhoea with blood and mucus

Diagnoses to consider include:

- Chronic inflammatory bowel disease. The stools in ulcerative colitis are usually more bloody than Crohn's. Anal changes are only seen in Crohn's – think of this diagnosis if the patient has particularly fleshy looking and succulent piles.
- Carcinoma of rectum and colon. A sensation of incomplete emptying of the bowel after defecation is virtually diagnostic of rectal carcinoma.
- Amoebic colitis. This may be difficult to distinguish from ulcerative colitis when seen in temperate regions. It may persist for many years after leaving the tropics.
- Non-specific procto-colitis. The alternative name is 'gay bowel' syndrome as it results from anal intercourse.

Bulky, pale offensive diarrhoea (steatorrhoea)

You should consider the following:

- Pancreatic carcinoma. The stools are often grossly fatty, as with chronic pancreatitis. Increasingly severe back and abdominal pains are frequently reported. With

tumours in the head of the pancreas there is obstructive jaundice with a distended, palpable gallbladder.
- Chronic pancreatitis. This may be difficult to distinguish from pancreatic cancer but the course is often relapsing.
- Coeliac disease. Diarrhoea may not be a prominent symptom. All age groups are affected. Syndromes such as iron and/or folate deficiency anaemia may dominate the clinical syndrome in adults.
- Crohn's disease or tuberculosis. There is usually extensive small gut involvement with both of these.

Frequent stools without blood or mucus

This is a common presenting problem which may be due to:

- Nervous diarrhoea or irritable bowel syndrome (IBS). It is often characterized by a flurry of bowel actions in the early morning but nothing later in the day. There may be bloating and colicky pain with IBS. The diarrhoea never occurs at night.
- Thyrotoxicosis. Suspect this if the patient is very nervous and is losing weight. Rare endocrinological syndromes causing diarrhoea include the Zollinger–Ellison syndrome, medullary carcinoma of the thyroid and the carcinoid syndrome.

Faecal soiling with mucus (spurious diarrhoea)

The impaction of a mass of faeces in the rectum which causes liquid stool to seep round it is a common symptom in the bedridden, confused, frail elderly.

FAECAL INCONTINENCE

Sometimes faecal incontinence is misinterpreted by patients, but usually more by their carers, as diarrhoea. Its causes are:

- Faecal impaction.
- Sphincter muscle weakness or nerve damage.
- Dementing illnesses and confusion.

Practical Point

In the absence of local neuromuscular problems, faecal incontinence is likely to be due to impaction or organic brain disease.

CONSTIPATION

Many claim they are constipated simply because they do not conform to the single, morning bowel action expected by many living in the Western world. What constitutes 'normal' is variable. For some, one bowel action every three or four days is usual. Constipation might be described more accurately as straining with the passage of hard small stools.

CHRONIC CONSTIPATION

Constipation which has been going on for years is likely to be due to lifestyle and habits more than anything else. You should enquire about:

- Degree of (in)activity.
- Amount of dietary roughage (fibre).
- Fluid intake.
- Inconvenient or inappropriate toilet facilities.
- General debility.

RECENT ONSET CONSTIPATION

This must be taken much more seriously as there may well be an organic cause. There may well be other symptoms to point the way to the definitive cause (see Revision Panel 36.3).

Revision Panel 36.3
Conditions responsible for recent onset constipation

Disease	*Some associated symptoms*
Strictures of descending colon, sigmoid and rectum, malignant and benign.	Progressive and colicky abdominal pain, distension, perhaps bleeding with mucus.
Myxoedema.	Tiredness, weight gain, cold intolerance.
Drug ingestion.	Codeine for pain, oral iron.
Depression.	Apathy, poor concentration, insomnia.
Pain on defaecation.	Anal fissure.

ALTERNATING CONSTIPATION AND DIARRHOEA

Although much prominence is given in many textbooks to this symptom as a feature of carcinoma of the colon, it is, in clinical practice, very rare.

Haematemesis

37

Vomiting blood indicates bleeding from the oesophagus, stomach or duodenum. Revision Panel 37.1 shows the sites from which gastrointestinal bleeding occurs in UK residents.

LIKELY CAUSES

The causes of upper gastrointestinal bleeding outside the UK are very different, mainly due to the high prevalence of alcoholic liver disease in France, Germany, Italy and North America. Here up to 50% of haematemeses are related to cirrhosis or alcoholic gastropathy. Elsewhere there may be other local influences on the figures, such as the high incidence of gastric ulceration in parts of India.

You will often get clear leads from the history as to the cause of the haematemesis (see Revision Panel 37.1). In addition, questioning about the vomiting itself (Revision Panel 37.2) may also yield critical information:

- Effortless, very profuse vomiting of relatively fresh blood is common with bleeding varices (Figs 37.1, 37.2).
- Torrential vomiting of bright red blood occurs with rupture of an aneurysm into the oesophagus.
- Streaks of blood appearing after an episode of retching or vomiting is characteristic of Mallory–Weiss syndrome.
- Vomiting of fresh blood suggests recent (and possibly continuing) bleeding.
- Vomiting of altered, stale blood suggests slower bleeding which may have already stopped.
- Vomiting of fresh blood with melaena suggests continuing substantial bleeding.

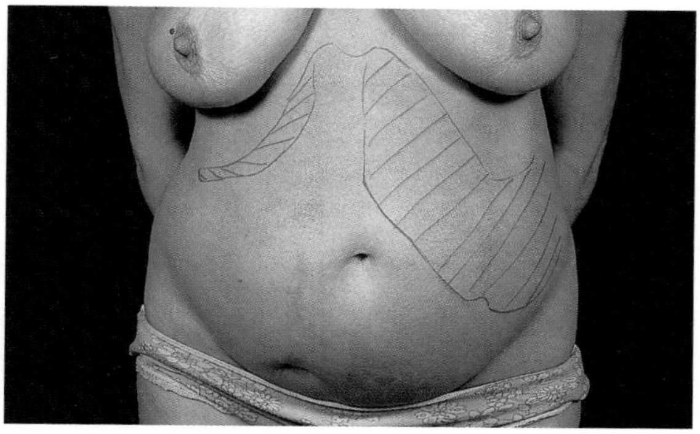

FIG. 37.1 The spleen is likely to be palpable in patients with portal hypertension though not usually as large as in this case. Signs suggestive of chronic liver disease may be apparent.

- Small amounts of stale blood with recurrent vomiting in an anorexic patient may indicate carcinoma of the stomach – frank haematemesis is unusual with this disease.

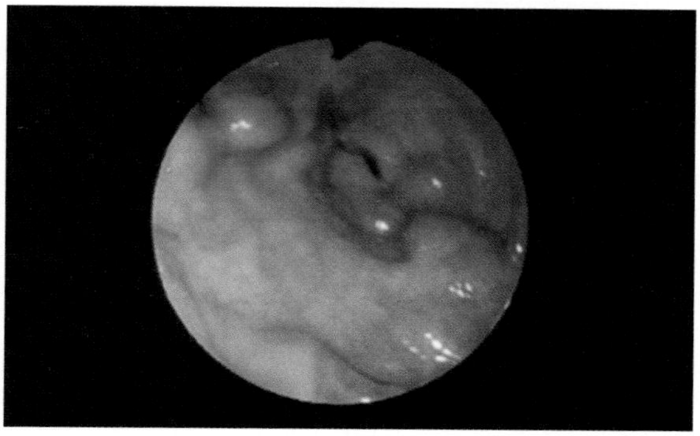

FIG. 37.2 Profuse vomiting is very common with bleeding varices (endoscopic view).

Revision Panel 37.1

Causes of gastrointestinal bleeding in the UK

Cause	*Frequency %*	*Features in the history (see also Chapter 6)*
Oesophagitis/hiatus hernia	8	History of acid reflux, heartburn or discomfort on swallowing.
Mallory–Weiss bleeding	2	Recurrent forceful vomiting, as after an alcoholic binge, preceding an episode of frank haematemesis.
Oesophageal varices	5–10	Long history of heavy alcohol intake, known cirrhotic.
Gastric erosions	10	Often no obvious cause, may be associated with ulcerogenic drugs such as aspirin, non-steroidal, anti-inflammatory agents, steroids.
Chronic gastric ulcers	30	Relapsing history of dyspepsia and upper abdominal pain.
Chronic duodenal ulcers	20	Relapsing history of dyspepsia and abdominal pain.
Duodenitis	5	Often no significant history.
Carcinoma of stomach	5	Loss of weight, anorexia, dyspepsia, abdominal pain.
Blood dyscrasias and others	20	

Practical Point

Central venous cannulation may be needed to assess central venous pressure or to give fluids and blood quickly

THE EXAMINATION

Haematemesis is an acute medical emergency requiring admission to hospital.

You must first assess the extent and rate of the bleeding by checking for:

- Pulse.
- Blood pressure lying and sitting if possible. A fall in blood pressure with change of posture is suggestive of a large loss of circulating volume.
- Clinical evidence of anaemia.

Look at the vomit (and melaena if present) and try to assess how much blood has been lost. Remember that vomiting of blood is a highly dramatic and frightening event to both patient and observers; those around may overestimate the volume of blood lost.

Next, look for:

- Evidence of wasting in keeping with carcinoma of the stomach.
- Stigmata of chronic liver disease such as jaundice, spider naevi, clubbing, leuconychia and liver palms.
- Tell-tale lesions on the lips and tongue of hereditary haemorrhagic telangiectasia (Osler–Weber–Rendau disease) which may extend down the gullet and bleed into the gut.

Do not expect to gain too much information from examination of the abdomen in patients with haematemesis:

- In many cases it will be normal.
- An epigastric mass of a carcinoma of the stomach may be palpable.
- The spleen is likely to be palpable in patients with portal hypertension (Fig. 37.1).

It is important to perform a rectal examination to check for melaena.

WHAT TO DO NEXT

A definitive diagnosis must be made by directly visualizing the upper gastrointestinal tract with endoscopy.

Revision Panel 37.2

Questions for patients presenting with haematemesis

Has this happened before?
Any abdominal pain?
Any history of dyspepsia?
Any history of liver disease?
Any painkillers or other tablets taken recently?

38 Haemoptysis

Haemoptysis is an alarming symptom for a patient because it raises the spectre of malignancy, especially in smokers. After thorough investigation many patients turn out to have a relatively benign problem.

The first thing to establish is whether the haemoptysis is serious. Some simple pointers as to whether haemoptyses are likely to be serious are shown in Revision Panel 38.1 but do remember that they are only pointers and not strict guidelines.

WHEN TO ARRANGE URGENT INVESTIGATION

While patients with haemetemesis and melaena generally require urgent admission to hospital, this is not necessarily true with haemoptysis.

Of the patients who develop haemoptysis there are four situations which require urgent investigation, management and appropriate treatment. These 'Red Flag' situations are:

- Coughing up of large amounts of blood. There is no 'cut-off point' but more than 200 ml in 24 hours carries a high mortality.
- Haemoptysis in middle-aged or elderly smokers which is due to carcinoma of the bronchus until proved otherwise.
- Haemoptysis in the postoperative period or after prolonged immobility, particularly if associated with pleurisy, which is very likely to be due to pulmonary embolism and requires urgent investigation.
- Haemoptysis associated with systemic symptoms.

Revision Panel 38.1

Indicators of serious and benign causes of haemoptysis

Usually serious	*Usually not serious*
Large volume of blood.[a]	Trace or single episode.
Long-term smoker.[a]	Non-smoker.
Recent surgery and/or prolonged immobility.[a]	Active.
Spontaneous and recurrent.	Recent upper or lower respiratory tract infection.
Middle-aged or elderly.	Young.
With other symptoms such as weight loss.[a]	

[a]These warrant urgent investigation and treatment

OTHER CAUSES OF HAEMOPTYSIS

Having assessed whether a patient with a haemoptysis is likely to have a serious condition or need urgent investigation, your next task is to make a specific diagnosis, bearing in mind that no specific cause is found in many patients with haemoptysis (see Revision Panel 38.2).

Revision Panel 38.2

Causes of haemoptysis

Frequency	*Disease*	*Clinical presentation*
Common.	Respiratory infections, particularly pneumonia.	Signs of chest infection. Haemoptysis rarely profuse, sputum streaked with blood.
	Bronchiectasis.	Recurrent with the profuse sputum.
	Pulmonary embolism.	Postoperative or bed-ridden patients. Often associated with pleurisy with infarction of a segment of lung.
	Pulmonary tuberculosis.[a]	Both in active and passive disease.
	Carcinoma of bronchus.	Often first sign of the disease.
	Chest trauma.	Particularly in association with fractured ribs.
Less common.	Mitral stenosis.[a]	Rare in developed world, still common in India, Africa and Far East. Recurrent small haemoptyses.
Rare.	Benign tumours such as bronchial adenomas.	Often the only symptom.
	Arteriovenous malformations.	Often the only symptom.
	Blood dyscrasias.	Evidence of abnormal bleeding elsewhere.
	Aspergilloma.	Features often those of primary disease.
	Pulmonary vasculitis.	
	Foreign body.	Particularly in children.

[a]Common in underdeveloped world.

WHAT TO DO NEXT

Bronchoscopy is indicated in those cases where the diagnosis is uncertain, where clinical and radiological examinations are negative, and a serious cause remains possible.

39 Jaundice

Jaundice can be complicated. Generally, the main problem clinically is to decide whether jaundice is due to:

- Disease of the liver itself as a result of hepatitis or cirrhosis.
- Defective drainage of bile or obstructive jaundice.

Other causes, such as acute haemolysis, rarely pose a diagnostic problem as it is the anaemia rather than the jaundice that dominates the clinical picture. If you notice a lemon coloured tinge to the skin, this is characteristic of an unconjugated hyperbilirubinaemia, the result of massive destruction of red cells. The presence of leg ulcers and splenomegaly are much more likely in the haemolytic anaemias, particularly the haemoglobinopathies.

With these in mind, the best advice for medical students (and junior doctors) is to keep things simple.

TAKE A VERY DETAILED HISTORY

In the majority of patients with jaundice you can surprisingly reach an accurate diagnosis from the history alone.

For many patients the cause of their jaundice depends on their age and their lifestyle, as Revision Panel 39.1 shows.

INFECTIOUS HEPATITIS (Fig. 39.1)

Here, prodromal illness gives a clue towards diagnosis. Ask about:

- Anorexia.
- Fever.
- Malaise.
- Backache.
- Upper abdominal pain lasting for a few days.
- Dark urine and pale stools, signs of a 'cholestatic' type jaundice.
- Duration of jaundice – typically this is two to three weeks.

Not infrequently the illness may drag on for several weeks. Return of appetite heralds recovery which may be dogged by several weeks of tiredness and poor health.

Hepatitis A

Hepatitis A is spread by ingesting contaminated food or drink: the *faecal–oral* route. Outbreaks do occur in the UK but most cases are sporadic, particularly in children and young adults. Ask your patient about:

- Travel in areas with poor hygiene, especially subtropical or tropical regions, in the last two to six weeks.
- Prodromal illness lasting a few days.

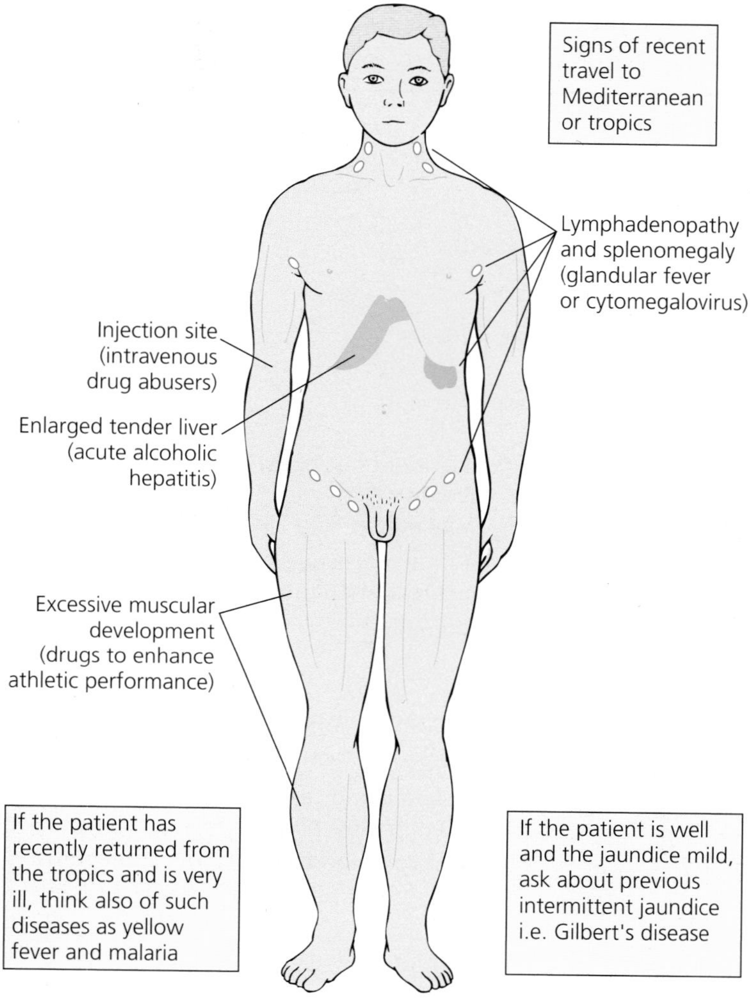
Signs of recent travel to Mediterranean or tropics
Lymphadenopathy and splenomegaly (glandular fever or cytomegalovirus)
Injection site (intravenous drug abusers)
Enlarged tender liver (acute alcoholic hepatitis)
Excessive muscular development (drugs to enhance athletic performance)
If the patient has recently returned from the tropics and is very ill, think also of such diseases as yellow fever and malaria
If the patient is well and the jaundice mild, ask about previous intermittent jaundice i.e. Gilbert's disease

FIG. 39.1 What to look for in a young adult with acute jaundice.

Most patients recover satisfactorily. You can reassure your patient that:

- The prognosis is good.
- There is no chronic carrier state.
- Chronic hepatitis A does not occur.
- Fulminant hepatitis rarely follows hepatitis A.

Hepatitis B

Hepatitis B is spread by contaminated blood and body fluids. You should suspect hepatitis B in a patient who presents with an infectious type hepatitis if they belong to one of the high-risk groups listed in Revision Panel 39.1. You can usually distinguish hepatitis B from hepatitis A by:

- A longer incubation period of six weeks to six months (and sometimes longer).
- A history of arthralgia and a rash.

The clinical course of the illness is much more variable, from a trivial illness to fulminant disease with an appreciable death rate.

Revision Panel 39.1

Who is at risk of jaundice

Groups or populations at risk	*Disease*
Children/young adults; travellers; adventurous eaters; holiday makers from Mediterranean or tropics; close contacts.	Hepatitis A.
Intravenous drug abusers; sexually promiscuous; homosexuals; those with needle stick injuries; health professionals.	Hepatitis B.
Anyone having had blood transfusions and those involved in intravenous abuse.	Hepatitis C.
Those at risk of water borne infection in Indian subcontinent.	Hepatitis E.
Children and young adults.	Infective mononucleosis. Cytomegalovirus.
Barmen; hoteliers; those in entertainment world.	Alcoholic hepatitis or cirrhosis.
Middle-aged and elderly women.	Primary biliary cirrhosis. Active chronic hepatitis.
Patients undergoing psychotrophic therapy, those taking illicit drugs to enhance athletic performance, tablets for another primary illness.	Drug jaundice.
Those involved in industrial accidents.	Jaundice due to toxins.
Recurrent jaundice in late pregnancy.	Cholestatic jaundice of pregnancy.
Middle-aged or elderly.	Obstructive jaundice due to pancreatic or common bile duct carcinoma.
Middle-aged and elderly (women>men).	Stones in common bile duct +/ – cholangitis.

Hepatitis C

The acute illness is now rarely seen after blood transfusion because of screening of blood products but it occurs in intravenous drug abusers on a worldwide basis.

Hepatitis E

This illness is spread by the faecal–oral route and, in many repects is difficult to differentiate clinically from hepatitis A on other than serological grounds. However, it is currently restricted to the Indian subcontinent.

JAUNDICE AS PART OF ANOTHER ILLNESS

Jaundice may develop as part of the clinical spectrum of other infectious diseases such as infectious mononucleosis (glandular fever). Be suspicious if you find:

- A nasty sore throat.
- Generalized lymphadenopathy.
- Rash.
- Splenomegaly.

Enquire about the health of your patient's partner – kissing is a recognized route of transmission in teenagers.

Practical Point

Gilbert's syndrome may cause mild intermittent jaundice in many healthy people. The jaundice often worsens with intercurrent illnesses such as influenza.

Toxoplasmosis and cytomegalovirus infection may present similarly. If you are faced with anyone participating in leisure activities on canals, lakes or river water who is ill, has haematuria and renal failure, think of infection from rat urine causing leptospirosis icterohaemorrhagicia (Weil's disease).

DRUG JAUNDICE

Many drugs are toxic to hepatocytes. This can be dose-related, as invariably happens after an overdose of paracetamol; or unpredictable, in which a single tablet taken weeks previously may trigger jaundice. These idiosyncratic reactions give rise to diagnostic difficulties. Some drugs which can cause jaundice unpredictably are listed in Revision Panel 39.2.

Suspect drug-induced jaundice when:

- An older patient develops a hepatitic-type illness.
- There is a clear relationship between administration of the drug and the onset of jaundice (usually one to six weeks).
- When the type of jaundice corresponds to that known to occur with the drug.
- There is associated urticaria.

Practical Point

Jaundice may be due to the liver congestion of heart failure.

Revision Panel 39.2

Some drugs which cause liver damage unpredictably

Halothane	Methyldopa
Chlorpromazine	Rifampicin
Co-trimoxazole	Co-amoxiclav
Phenelzine	Flucloxacillin

CHRONIC LIVER DISEASE

Jaundice is a relatively late sign of chronic liver disease, appearing with the many stigmata of chronic liver disease such as:

- Spider naevi.
- Liver palms.
- Clubbing (see Chapter 2).

The aetiology of chronic liver disease varies from one part of the world to the other and Revision Panel 39.3 indicates how a reasonable clinical diagnosis can be reached before serological tests and liver biopsy are performed to establish a precise diagnosis.

It is generally believed that cirrhosis is the only effect of alcohol abuse. This is not true. Acute alcoholic hepatitis (included in Revision Panel 39.3 for convenience) and fatty liver are other important complications.

OBSTRUCTIVE JAUNDICE

The diagnosis of extrahepatic biliary obstruction is usually straightforward. This mainly affects those in middle and old age.

Pain is an important symptom:

- Painless jaundice which becomes progressively deeper (even a greenish-olive hue), accompanied by dark urine (which contains bile) and pale stools (which are bile-free) is usually due to a carcinoma of the head of the pancreas or a cholangiocarcinoma.

Revision Panel 39.3
Clinical features of chronic liver disease (CLD)

Disease	*Geographical distribution*	*Clinical features pointing to the aetiology*
Alcoholic cirrhosis.	North America; Europe; wide distribution throughout world.	Features of alcohol abuse such as facial plethora, Cushingoid facies, tremor, sweating. Signs of cirrhosis: liver may be shrunken, normal size or enlarged; spleen+, stigmata of CLD, may be ascites and oedema.
Alcoholic hepatitis.[a]	As above.	May be as the result of 'binge drinking'. Liver enlarged and tender. Spleen not enlarged. Not necessarily signs of CLD unless associated cirrhosis.
Alcoholic fatty liver.	As above.	Jaundice unusual. Liver very enlarged. Spleen not enlarged. No signs of CLD unless associated cirrhosis.
Chronic hepatitis B infection.	Throughout world but common in tropics.	Non-specific apart from signs of CLD.
Chronic hepatitis C infection.	Worldwide.	Non-specific apart from signs of CLD.
Primary biliary cirrhosis.	Western Europe.	Almost exclusively middle-aged and elderly women. Marked pruritus. Scratch marks. Pigmentation. Signs of CLD.
Active chronic hepatitis.	Europe and North America.	Signs of CLD. Other autoimmune phenomena.

[a]Not strictly chronic liver disease.

- Gallstones occur frequently in young women. A gallstone stuck in the bile duct triggers biliary colic which is very painful.

Courvoisier's law fairly reliably suggests that when the gallbladder is palpable, the jaundice is likely to be due to a carcinoma (Fig. 39.2). The converse of the law, i.e. that obstructive jaundice without a palpable (non-distended) gallbladder is likely to be due to stones is not reliable.

Obstructive jaundice usually produces dilated bile ducts, seen easily on abdominal ultrasound. If the bile ducts are not dilated, the possibilities are:

- The ducts have not yet had time to dilate.
- The patient is in the cholestatic phase of infectious hepatitis.
- It is a cholestatic drug reaction.

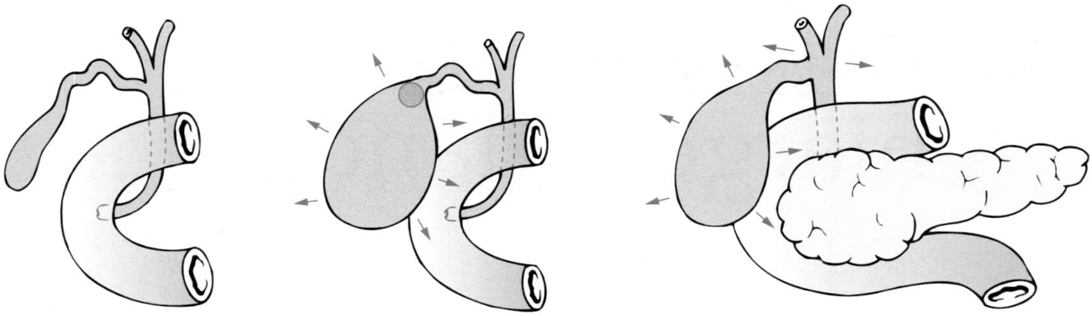

Normal gallbladder
Not palpable

Mucocele of gallbladder
Stone in neck
Non-dilated ducts
Palpable distended gallbladder

Carcinoma of head of pancreas
Dilated ducts
Dilated gallbladder
Liver diffusely distended

FIG. 39.2 When a gallbladder is palpable, the jaundice is likely to be due to a carcinoma.

40 Anaemia and enlarged glands

These are disorders in which the definitive diagnosis requires a full blood count and other haematological investigations. Nevertheless, the doctor seeing the clinically anaemic patient for the first time should be able to arrive at a realistic diagnosis on clinical examination.

SYMPTOMS COMMON TO ALL ANAEMIC PATIENTS

Those due simply to a low haemoglobin level are:

Tiredness This non-specific symptom is mainly related to the rate of fall in the haemoglobin level. For example, a slow fall over several months to 7 g/dl may be unassociated with symptoms, whereas a swift fall over a day or two with bleeding would cause severe tiredness and weakness. A slightly low haemoglobin of 10 g/dl rarely causes symptoms.

Pallor Some patients and their relatives may notice increasing pallor.

Breathlessness (in the absence of cardiological or respiratory disease) Note that severe anaemia may cause high output heart failure.

Excessive bruising and bleeding This may be present with the leukaemias or with coagulation defects.

SYMPTOMS RELATED TO THE CAUSE OF THE ANAEMIA

Swollen glands In the lymphomas this may be the primary symptom.

Fever and sweating, particularly at night This is a feature of generalized lymphoma.

Skin itching Without a rash this may herald serious underlying disease such as lymphoma.

Vulnerability to infections.

Pains Bone pains may characterize infiltrative disease of the bone marrow such as myeloma.

PHYSICAL SIGNS TO BE LOOKED FOR IN THE ANAEMIC PATIENT

Anaemia

The diagnosis of anaemia on clinical grounds is fraught with difficulties. The conjunctiva in the healthy elderly is often pale whereas in the anaemias it may be reddened unduly by

Revision Panel 40.1
Signs associated with anaemia

Site	*Iron deficiency*	*B12 or folate deficiency*	*Haemolytic anaemia*
Sclerae	White.	May be icteric.	Icteric.
Nails	Koilonychia if anaemia is severe and longstanding (Fig. 40.1).	Normal but may be clubbed with . malabsorption.	Normal.
Tongue	Smooth.[a]	Smooth and sore.[a]	Normal.
Lips	Cheilosis.	Cheilosis.	Normal.
Fundi	Normal.	Retinal haemorrhages if anaemia is severe.	Normal.
Leg ulcers	Do not occur.	Do not occur.	Common in haemoglobinopathies.
Splenomegaly	Rare.	Rare.	Common except with sickle cell disease.

[a]See Fig. 6.6.

rubbing or conjunctivitis. In assessing anaemia you should also take into consideration the colour of the nail beds, the fingers and the tongue. It is only when the haemoglobin falls below 7 or 8 g/dl that a confident diagnosis of anaemia can be made on clinical grounds. You may get some clues as to the type of the anaemia from associated signs, which are listed in Revision Panel 40.1.

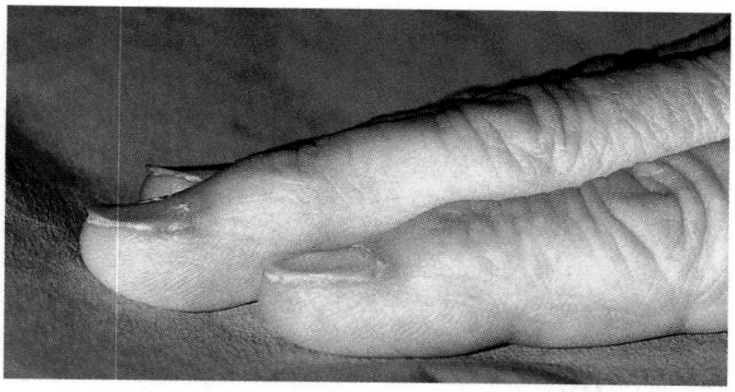

FIG. 40.1 Koilonychia. This is a feature of longstanding iron-deficiency anaemia with depleted iron stores. It is a relatively rare physical sign in the Western world but is frequently seen in underdeveloped countries. In addition to the spoon shape, the nails are longitudinally ridged and unduly brittle.

Excessive bleeding

This may occur as:

- Purpura – spontaneous bleeding from small vessels into the skin (Fig. 40.2) and mucous membranes; the lesions are a few mm in diameter, do not blanch with pressure and fade to a brownish colour over a few days.
- Ecchymoses – larger bruises into the skin (Fig. 40.3).
- Overt bleeding from the nose, mouth, kidneys and gastrointestinal tract.
- Internal bleeding into joints or retroperitoneal spaces.

Practical Point

Purpura usually indicate serious disease and an urgent blood count is warranted.

The bleeding in various haemorrhagic disorders tends to follow characteristic patterns which are summarized in Revision Panel 40.2. The list is not intended to be comprehensive.

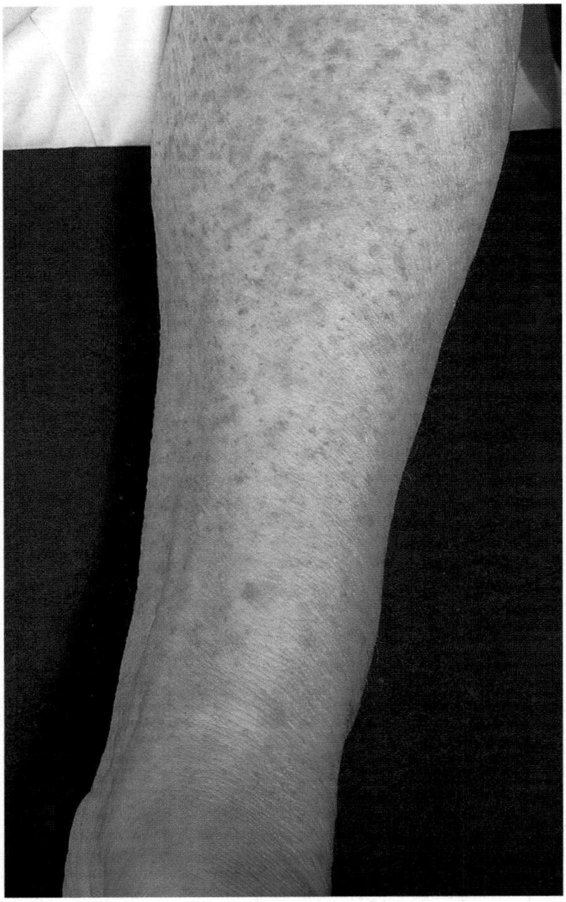

FIG. 40.2 Purpura in Henoch–Schönlein purpura. Purpura are extravasations into the skin which are usually a few mm in diameter, do not blanch on pressure and fade to a brownish colour after a few days. They are usually due to thrombocytopenia or to defects of the blood vessels as in anaphylactoid or Henoch–Schönlein purpura.

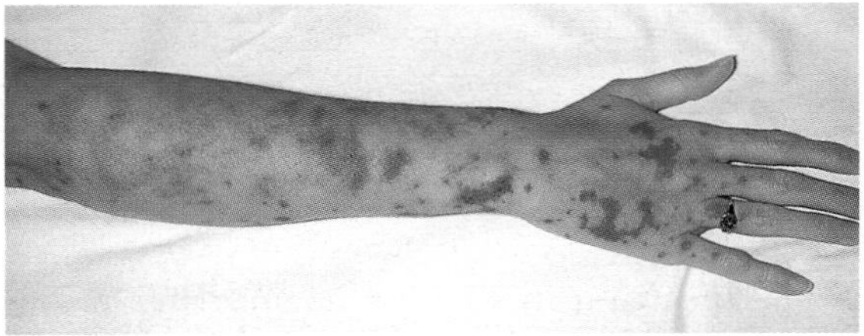

FIG. 40.3 Ecchymoses in a patient with severe coagulation problems due to acute hepatic necrosis.

Splenomegaly

The significance and assessment of spleen size is critical in patients with haematological disorders and has already been discussed in Chapter 6 (see Figs 6.21–6.23). Its size should be measured in cm as the maximum distance below and medial to the left costal margin.

Lymph node enlargement

Several points have to be borne in mind when assessing lymph node size:

- Many normal people have palpable nodes in the neck, axillae and groins but nodes of more than 1.5 cm diameter should always be regarded with suspicion.
- Lymphoid tissue tends to atrophy with age; therefore the young tend to have larger nodes than the old.
- Recurrent trauma to hands and arms as with farmers and gardeners may cause some mild enlargement of the axillary nodes.
- Epitrochlear nodes are virtually never palpable in health.
- Tonsillar nodes may be recurrently infected in childhood and may remain palpable throughout life.

Palpate nodes in the neck from behind, working in a systemic manner through the submental region, then the anterior triangle and finally to the posterior triangle. Pay particular attention to the region behind the lower end of the sternocleidomastoid muscle where enlarged glands are easily missed. Palpate axillary nodes sitting facing the patient. Slide the left hand into the patient's right axilla and vice versa for the other side. Hook your fingers when palpating high in the axillae so as not to miss glands high on the medial wall.

Practical Point

Learn to palpate epitrochlear glands. If they are enlarged without a local cause, then the patient is likely to have a significant generalized lymphadenopathy.

Revision Panel 40.2
Sites of bleeding with various haemorrhagic disorders

Basis for bleeding	*Causes*	*Common sites of bleeding*
Thrombocytopenia	Infiltration of marrow. Drugs (including chemotherapy). Idiopathic thrombocytopenia purpura.	Skin, nose, central nervous system, fundi.
Vascular defects	Vasculitis.	Skin (purpura), gut, kidneys.
	Infections e.g. Meningococcal septicaemia.	Skin (purpura).
	Henoch–Schönlein purpura.	Skin (purpura), kidneys, gut.
	Drugs.	Skin (purpura).
	Scurvy.	Skin and mucous membranes.
Coagulation defects	Hereditary defects of clotting i.e. Haemophilia.	Soft tissues and joints.
	Liver disease.	Various sites.
	Excessive anticoagulation.	Gut, skin, retroperitoneal spaces and other various sites.
Hyperviscosity	Macroglobulinaemia.	Fundi, nose and skin.

The main causes of lymphadenopathy are shown in Revision Panel 40.3.

Revision Panel 40.3
Causes of generalized lymphadenopathy

Group	*Disease*	*Relative frequency as a cause of generalized lymphadenopathy in young adults*	*Relative frequency as a cause of generalized lymphadenopathy in older patients*
Infections	Glandular fever.	Common.	All becoming less common with increasing age
	Cytomegalovirus.	Occasional.	
	Rubella.	Common.	
	Toxoplasmosis.	Occasional.	
	Brucellosis.	Occasional.	
	Secondary syphilis.	Occasional.	
	Persistent generalized lymphodenopathy.	Occasional.	
	Non-specific response to viral infections.	Common.	
Leukaemia	Acute.	Occasional.	Occasional.
	Chronic lymphatic.	Does not occur.	Fairly common (Fig. 40.4).
Lymphoma	Hodgkin's disease.	Generalized lymphadenopathy in late disease.	In late disease only.
	Non-Hodgkin's lymphoma.	Occasional.	Fairly common.
Carcinomatosis		Occasional	Occasional.
Tuberculosis		Localized lymphadenopathy common but generalized lymphadenopathy unusual.	Localized lymphadenopathy common but generalized lymphadenopathy unusual.
Sarcoidosis		Occasional.	Occasional.

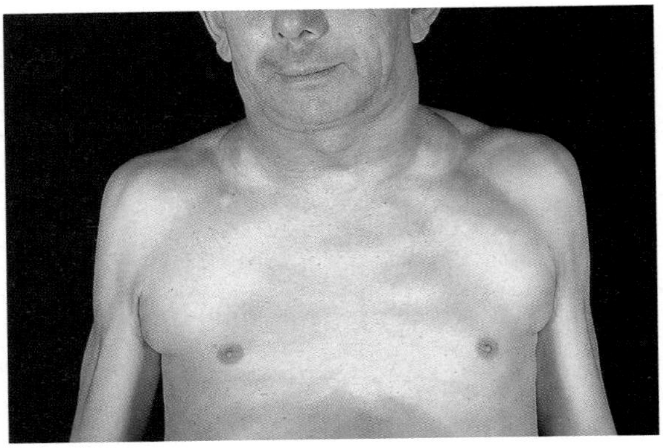

FIG. 40.4 Gross axillary lymphadenopathy in an elderly patient with chronic lymphatic leukaemia.

Infections

These commonly complicate the anaemias and haematological malignancies. In broad terms they are the result of:

Neutropenia As in the leukaemias, patients with bone marrow infiltration, or during chemotherapy. Various infections and/or septicaemia.

Immunosuppression With human immunodeficiency virus (HIV) infection, myeloma or malignancy. Moniliasis and other opportunistic infection common.

Hypersplenism As in Felty's syndrome.

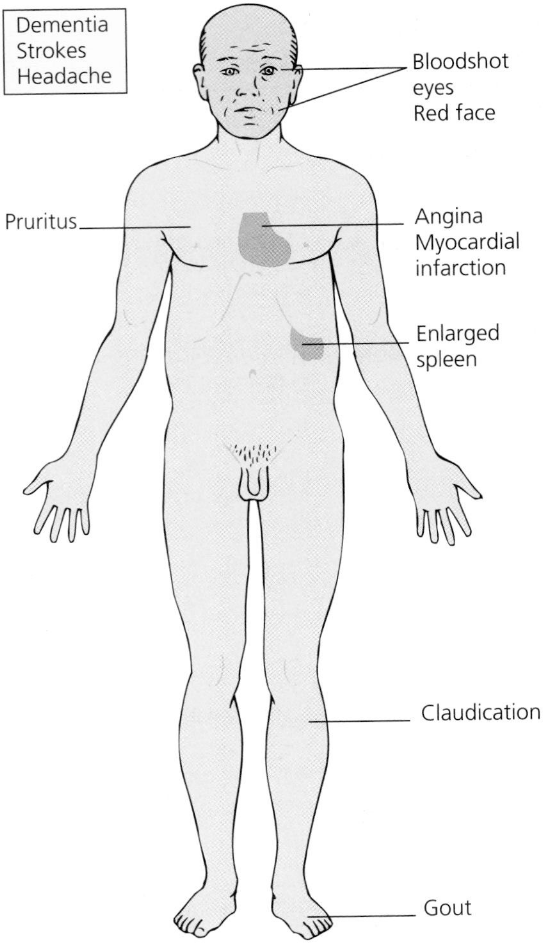

FIG. 40.5 The clinical features of polcythaemia rubra vera.

THE MYELOPROLIFERATIVE SYNDROMES

Practical Point

Massive splenomegaly in the Western world is likely to be due to myelosclerosis or chronic myeloid or lymphatic leukaemia.

This group of diseases is characterized by proliferation of one or more of the components of the bone marrow. They are closely related. Transitional forms occur and evolution from one to the other may take place in the course of the disease. The commonest diseases in the group area:

- Polycythaemia rubra vera (PRV) (Fig. 40.5).
- Chronic myeloid leukaemia.
- Essential thrombocythaemia.
- Myelosclerosis.

A common feature of these diseases is splenomegaly which may be gross in chronic myeloid leukaemia and myelosclerosis. The physical signs of polycythaemia rubra vera are summarized in Fig. 40.5. Remember that

Revision Panel 40.4
Causes of polycythaemia

Primary	Polycythaemia rubra vera.
Secondary (anoxic)	Due to residence at high altitudes. Cardiac or pulmonary disease. Heavy smoking.
Secondary (inappropriate erythropoietin secretion)	Renal disease such as carcinoma, hydronephrosis. Cerebellar haemangioblastoma. Uterine fibroids.
Relative	Stress polycythaemia. Dehydration. Plasma loss e.g. burns.

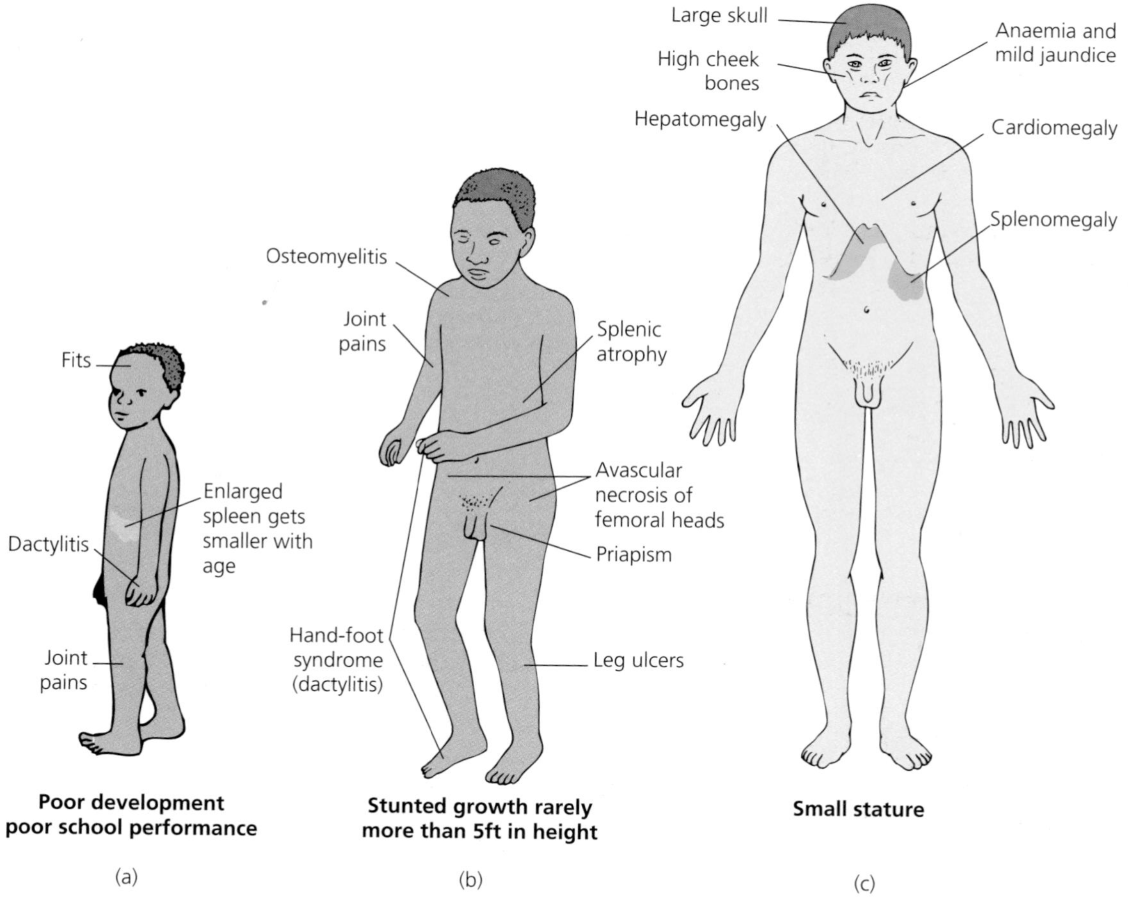

FIG. 40.6 Physical signs in the haemoglobinopathies. (a) A young child with sickle-cell disease Hb-SS. (b) A young adult with sickle-cell Hb-SS. In this disease growth is stunted and mental development is impaired. In early life the spleen is enlarged but as the years pass it becomes smaller with recurrent episodes of splenic infarction. Dactylitis occurs mainly in childhood. (c) The physical signs in a non-Black adolescent with thalassaemia major.

there are several pathophysiological causes of polycythaemia (See Revision Panel 40.4).

CONSIDER THE POSSIBILITY OF A HAEMOGLOBINOPATHY

These are relatively common diseases in many parts of the world characterized by the production of an atypical haemoglobin or by the suppression of normal haemoglobin formation. The two most important are sickle cell disease and thalassaemia (Fig. 40.6).

Sickle cell disease

Sickle cell disease is common in Black people in the Americas, Africa and in West Indian migrants in the UK. In the homozygous state it carries significant morbidity and mortality. The principal physical signs in the child and in the adult are shown in the diagrams. Those with sickle cell trait (10–20% of Black people) have few problems except in anoxic states.

Thalassaemia

Thalassaemia is found in many parts of the world in a broad band extending through the Mediterranean region, the Middle East, the Indian subcontinent and south-east Asia. Children with homozygous B chain disease are stunted with chipmunk type faces due to expansion of the bone marrow cavity in the facial and skull bones. The have gross splenomegaly and hepatomegaly and have limited survival into adult life.

Revision Panel 40.5

Summary

Anaemia is a secondary feature of a range of diseases.

Look for associated symptoms and signs that may act as pointers to the basic diagnosis.

Do not attempt to diagnose mild degrees of anaemia on clinical grounds.

Make the definitive diagnosis on a blood count and other appropriate investigations.

Consider haemoglobinopathy as a cause of apparently unexplained anaemia in a patient with appropriate ethnic background.

Limb weakness

41

BASIC STEPS

The possible causes of progressive limb weakness depend very much on the age and general condition of your patient but in all cases you will need to ask about:

- The time course – has the weakness been remorselessly progressive or has it been fluctuant?
- The pattern of the muscle weakness – is it generalized, or localized to specific muscle groups?
- Wasting – are the muscles getting thinner?
- Associated diseases – is the patient diabetic?
- Any associated symptoms – is there any evidence of sensory disturbance?
- Family history – are any other family members affected?

If you are dealing with a child or young adult with progressive weakness, suspect muscular dystrophy or myotonia. You should:

- Enquire carefully for a possible family history.
- Establish which muscle groups are affected. Duchenne, facio-scapulo-humeral and limb girdle syndromes have characteristic patterns of muscle weakness.
- Examine for myotonia dystrophia. Facial appearance is characteristic and if you shake hands with your patient he may have difficulty letting go.

If you are dealing with a seriously ill elderly patient, always consider non-neurological causes:

- General frailty. Check for evidence of weight loss, general debility and malignancy.
- Disuse atrophy. This usually occurs in patients who have been immobile and bedfast?
- Arthritis. Wasting is localized to specific muscle groups operating appropriate joints.

Having excluded these causes, you will now need to consider lesions of the corticospinal tract, lesions of anterior horn cells, neuropathy, defects in neuromuscular transmission and acquired muscle disorders.

Lesions of the corticospinal tract

Weakness is most obvious in the shoulder abductor and extensor muscles, the wrist dorsiflexors, hip flexors and foot dorsiflexors. Slowness, clumsiness and stiffness may be more troublesome than muscle weakness. Examine for signs of a spastic paraparesis and consider possible causes – cord compression, multiple sclerosis, cerebrovascular disease and cervical myelopathy.

Motor neuron disease

There is selective loss of *lower motor neurons* from pons, medulla and spinal cord with loss of *upper motor neurons* from the pre-central gyrus. Limb weakness may result from two clinical syndromes. In progressive muscular atrophy (PMA), weakness, wasting and fasciculation of the muscles, especially of the small muscles of the hand due to loss of lower motor neurons will be fairly obvious. In amyotrophic lateral sclerosis (ALS), the loss of upper motor neurons is associated with weakness, spasticity, clonus and brisk tendon reflexes with extensor plantar responses.

Revision Panel 41.1

Causes of peripheral neuropathy

Western World
Undetermined causes.[a]
Diabetes.[a]
Alcohol.[a]
B12 deficiency.
Drugs (such as isoniazid, vincristine).
Paraneoplastic arthritis.
Amyloidosis.
Hereditary (peroneal muscular atrophy).
Postinfective (Guillaine–Barré).

Tropics as above
Leprosy.[a]
Pellagra.
Thiamine deficiency.

[a]Common

Peripheral neuropathy

This is a common syndrome due to a wide variety of diseases (see Revision Panel 41.1). You should look for:

- Symmetrical distal sensory loss in the legs more than the hands.
- Symmetrical distal weakness and wasting.
- Loss of deep tendon reflexes, particularly the ankle jerks.

Defects in neuromuscular transmission

Myasthenia gravis is rare. The most characteristic feature that distinguishes this from other causes of muscle weakness is fatigability. Myasthenia often affects the external ocular muscles but can also affect the muscles of swallowing and speech, neck, proximal limbs and trunk. Distal muscle groups are rarely affected.

Acquired muscle disorders

This rare group of diseases characterized by weakness and wasting of limb muscles may be due to acquired immunologically mediated inflammatory diseases such as polymositis and dermatomyositis or secondary to a variety of causes such as thyrotoxicosis and steroid therapy.

PUTTING IT ALL TOGETHER

A summary of the site and frequency of the pathological lesions and the clinical conditions involved is shown in Revision Panel 41.2.

Revision Panel 41.2

Generalized wasting due to starvation or malignant disease[a]	*Lesions of corticospinal tract as in multiple sclerosis, cervical myelopathy*[a]	*Lesions of upper and lower motor neurons as in motor neuron disease*[b]
Disuse atrophy. All muscles weak and wasted. No fasciculation. No sensory loss. Reflexes normal.	Often stiffness and clumsiness rather than weakness. No fasciculation. Spasticity. Brisk reflexes. Extensor plantar responses.	Generalized wasting, weakness and fasciculation of muscle groups. No sensory loss. Steadily progressive and fatal.
Peripheral neuropathy[a]	*Defective neuromuscular transmission as in myasthenia gravis*[b]	*Muscle disease e.g. muscular dystrophy but associated with wide spectrum of diseases*[b]
Distal wasting and weakness of muscles. Legs more involved than arms. Distal sensory symptoms and signs. Many causes (see Revision Panel 41.1)	Muscle weakness without wasting. Weakness fluctuating throughout day with fatigability. Ocular and bulbar muscles commonly involved.	Weakness and wasting with particular muscle groups affected according to basic disease. Some inherited, some metabolic, some inflammatory.

[a]Common. [b]Rare.

Index

Page numbers in **bold** refer to Revision Panels, those in *italics* refer to figures.